Evidence-Based Management of Pancreatic Malignancy

Guest Editor

RICHARD K. ORR, MD, MPH

SURGICAL CLINICS
OF NORTH AMERICA

www.surgical.theclinics.com

Consulting Editor
RONALD F. MARTIN, MD

April 2010 • Volume 90 • Number 2

SAUNDERS an imprint of ELSEVIER, Inc.

W.B. SAUNDERS COMPANY

A Division of Elsevier Inc.

1600 John F. Kennedy Blvd., Suite 1800, Philadelphia, PA 19103-2899

http://www.theclinics.com

SURGICAL CLINICS OF NORTH AMERICA Volume 90, Number 2

April 2010 ISSN 0039–6109, ISBN-13: 978-1-4377-1876-8

Editor: Catherine Bewick

Developmental Editor: Donald Mumford

Surgical Clinics of North America (ISSN 0039–6109) is published bimonthly by Elsevier Inc., 360 Park Avenue South, New York, NY 10010-1710. Months of publication are February, April, June, August, October, and December. Business and Editorial Offices: 1600 John F. Kennedy Blvd., Suite 1800, Philadelphia, PA 19103-2899. Periodicals postage paid at New York, NY and additional mailing offices. Subscription prices are $291.00 per year for US individuals, $475.00 per year for US institutions, $145.00 per year for US students and residents, $356.00 per year for Canadian individuals, $590.00 per year for Canadian institutions, $401.00 for international individuals, $590.00 per year for international institutions and $200.00 per year for Canadian and foreign students/residents. To receive student/resident rate, orders must be accompanied by name of affiliated institution, date of term, and the *signature* of program/residency coordinator on institution letterhead. Orders will be billed at individual rate until proof of status is received. Foreign air speed delivery is included in all *Clinics* subscription prices. All prices are subject to change without notice. POSTMASTER: Send address changes to *Surgical Clinics*, Elsevier Health Sciences Division, Subscription Customer Service, 3251 Riverport Lane, Maryland Heights, MO 63043. **Customer Service (orders, claims, online, change of address): Telephone: 1-800-654-2452 (U.S. and Canada); 314-447-8871 (outside U.S. and Canada). Fax: 314-447-8029. E-mail: journalscustomerservice-usa@elsevier.com (for print support); journalsonlinesupport-usa@elsevier.com (for online support).**

Reprints. For copies of 100 or more, of articles in this publication, please contact the Commercial Reprints Department, Elsevier Inc., 360 Park Avenue South, New York, New York 10010-1710. Tel. (212) 633-3812, Fax: (212) 462-1935, e-mail: reprints@elsevier.com.

The *Surgical Clinics of North America* is also published in Spanish by McGraw-Hill Interamericana Editores S.A., P.O. Box 5-237 06500 Mexico D.F. Mexico; and in Portuguese by Interlivros Edicoes Ltda., Rua Comandante Coelho 1085, CEP 21250, Rio de Janeiro, Brazil; and in Greek by Paschalidis Medical Publications, Athens Greece.

The *Surgical Clinics of North America* is covered in *MEDLINE/PubMed (Index Medicus), EMBASE/Excerpta Medica, Current Contents/Clinical Medicine, Current Contents/Life Sciences, Science Citation Index,* and *ISI/BIOMED.*

Printed and bound in the United Kingdom

Transferred to Digital Print 2011

Contributors

CONSULTING EDITOR

RONALD F. MARTIN, MD
Staff Surgeon, Department of Surgery, Marshfield Clinic, Marshfield, Wisconsin; Clinical Associate Professor, University of Wisconsin School of Medicine and Public Health, Madison, Wisconsin; Colonel, Medical Corps, United States Army Reserve

GUEST EDITOR

RICHARD K. ORR, MD, MPH
Director of Surgical Oncology, Marsha and Jimmy Gibbs Regional Cancer Center, Spartanburg Regional Medical Center, Spartanburg, South Carolina; Associate Professor of Clinical Surgery, Medical University of South Carolina, Charleston, South Carolina

AUTHORS

DAVID B. ADAMS, MD, FACS
Professor and Head, Section of Gastrointestinal and Laparoscopic Surgery, Medical University of South Carolina, Charleston, South Carolina

TOMS AUGUSTIN, MD, MPH
Resident in General Surgery, Department of Surgery, Guthrie-Robert Packer Hospital, One Guthrie Square, Sayre, Pennsylvania

KATHLEEN K. CHRISTIANS, MD
Associate Professor, Department of Surgery, Medical College of Wisconsin, Milwaukee, Wisconsin

CARRIE K. CHU, MD
General Surgery Resident, Department of Surgery, Emory University School of Medicine, Atlanta, Georgia

ELLEN W. COOKE, MD
Radiation Oncology Resident, Department of Radiation Oncology, University of Utah, Huntsman Cancer Hospital, Salt Lake City

PETER V. DRAGANOV, MD
Division of Gastroenterology, Hepatology and Nutrition, University of Florida, Gainesville, Florida

MOHAMAD A. ELOUBEIDI, MD, MHS
Department of Gastroenterology and Hepatology and the Pancreatico-biliary Center, the University of Alabama at Birmingham, Birmingham, Alabama

DOUGLAS B. EVANS, MD
Professor and Chairman, Department of Surgery, Medical College of Wisconsin, Milwaukee, Wisconsin

LISA HAZARD, MD
Assistant Professor of Radiation Oncology, Department of Radiation Oncology, University of Utah, Huntsman Cancer Hospital, Salt Lake City

GRANT HUTCHINS, MD
Nebraska Medical Center, University of Nebraska, Omaha, Nebraska

TIMOTHY KINNEY, MD
Director of Endoscopy, Assistant Professor of Medicine, Department of Medicine, Division of Gastroenterology, Hennepin County Medical Center, University of Minnesota, Minneapolis, Minnesota

DAVID A. KOOBY, MD
Associate Professor of Surgery, Division of Surgical Oncology, Department of Surgery, Emory University School of Medicine and the Winship Cancer Institute, Atlanta, Georgia

E. JAMES KRUSE, DO
Assistant Professor, Department of Surgery, Surgical Oncology Section, Medical College of Georgia, Augusta, Georgia

ALYSANDRA LAL, MD
Assistant Professor, Department of Surgery, Medical College of Wisconsin, Milwaukee, Wisconsin

RONALD F. MARTIN, MD
Director of Surgical Education and Residency Program Director, Department of Surgery, Marshfield Clinic and Saint Joseph's Hospital, Marshfield, Wisconsin; Clinical Associate Professor of Surgery, University of Wisconsin School of Medicine and Public Health, Madison, Wisconsin

SHARMILA P. MEHTA, MD
Physician, Palmetto Hematology/Oncology Internal Medicine, Marsha and Jimmy Gibbs Regional Cancer Center, Spartanburg Regional Health Systems, Spartanburg, South Carolina

KATHERINE A. MORGAN, MD, FACS
Associate Professor, Section of Gastrointestinal and Laparoscopic Surgery, Medical University of South Carolina, Charleston, South Carolina

J. LAWRENCE MUNSON, MD
Assistant Clinical Professor of Surgery/Hepatobiliary Surgeon, Department of General Surgery, Lahey Clinic Medical Center, Burlington, Massachusetts

F.W. NUGENT, MD
Associate Professor of Medicine and Vice Chair, Department of Hematology/Oncology, Lahey Clinic Medical Center, Burlington, Massachusetts

RICHARD K. ORR, MD, MPH
Director of Surgical Oncology, Marsha and Jimmy Gibbs Regional Cancer Center, Spartanburg Regional Medical Center, Spartanburg, South Carolina; Associate Professor of Clinical Surgery, Medical University of South Carolina, Charleston, South Carolina

SAM PAPPAS, MD
Assistant Professor, Department of Surgery, Medical College of Wisconsin, Milwaukee, Wisconsin

EDWARD QUEBBEMAN, PhD, MD
Professor, Department of Surgery, Medical College of Wisconsin, Milwaukee, Wisconsin

KEITH STUART, MD
Professor of Medicine and Chair, Department of Hematology/Oncology, Lahey Clinic Medical Center, Burlington, Massachusetts

THOMAS J. VANDERMEER, MD, FACS
Chief, Section of General Surgery, Director, General Surgery Residency Program, Guthrie Health, Sayre; Assistant Professor of Surgery, SUNY Upstate Medical University, Sayre, Pennsylvania

SHYAM VARADARAJULU, MD
Department of Gastroenterology and Hepatology and the Pancreatico-Biliary Center, the University of Alabama at Birmingham, Birmingham, Alabama

JENNIFER E. VERBESEY, MD
Transplantation Fellow, Department of Transplantation, Lahey Clinic Medical Center, Burlington, Massachusetts

KASHIF A. ZUBERI, MD
Resident in General Surgery, Department of Surgery, Marshfield Clinic and Saint Joseph's Hospital, Marshfield, Wisconsin

Contents

> The increase in surgery for pancreatic cancer during the last 3 decades can be correlated with a gradual decline in operative mortality and postoperative complications. Although not all surgeons (nor all hospitals) can have equal outcomes, the definition and tabulation of these outcomes have been difficult. This article asks several pertinent questions: (1) what is the scientific rationale for pancreatic resection? (2) what are the best available results at this time? (3) who should be performing pancreatic resections? The article analyzes results of resection for adenocarcinoma of the exocrine pancreas, and excludes duodenal and ampullary cancers, pancreatic endocrine tumors, and tumors of less malignant potential.

> A high-quality pancreatic protocol computed tomography (CT) is the primary imaging modality for diagnosing and staging pancreatic malignancy. The main limitation of CT is the lack of sensitivity for early pancreatic lesions. Endoscopic ultrasound (EUS) provides an excellent complement to CT for both diagnosis and staging of pancreatic cancer, and allows easy access for needle aspiration and tissue diagnosis. Magnetic resonance (MR) can be helpful for evaluating small hepatic nodules or cystic lesions of the pancreas, but in general, the role of MR and positron emission tomography remains limited to special situations when the results of CT and EUS are equivocal.

> Accurate staging of pancreatico-biliary cancer is essential for surgical planning and for identification of locally advanced and metastatic disease that is incurable by surgery. The complex regional anatomy of the pancreatico-biliary system makes histologic diagnosis of malignancy at this region difficult. The ability to position the endoscopic ultrasound transducer at endoscopy in direct proximity to the pancreas and the bile duct, combined with the use of fine-needle aspiration, enables accurate preoperative staging of cancer, especially cancer too small to be characterized by CT or

MRI. Endoscopic ultrasonography (EUS) identifies patients unlikely to be cured by surgery due to vascular invasion or regional nodal metastasis, thereby limiting procedure-related morbidity and mortality. This article focuses on the utility and recent advances of EUS in the evaluation of pancreatico-biliary cancer.

The surgeon who wishes to perform successful resections for malignant processes involving the pancreas has to be conversant with a broad range of topics. There are extensive collections of data that usually give excellent guidance, but sometimes also provide conflicting advice. No matter what the data suggest might work best, the surgeon and local collaborators must be able to deliver the quality care cited in some of these reports; usually it is the best results that are published. There is a difference between results that are statistically significant, clinically significant, and important to the patient, and these concepts should never be confused.

Solid lesions of the body and tail of the pancreas challenge all the diagnostic and technical skills of the modern gastrointestinal surgeon. The information available from modern computed tomography (CT), magnetic resonance (MR), and endoscopic ultrasound (EUS) imaging provide diagnostic and anatomic data that give the surgeon precise information with which to plan an operation and to discuss with the patient during the preoperative visit. A preoperative evaluation includes a thorough history and a pancreas protocol CT scan, supplemented by MR imaging and EUS when needed, to differentiate between the various potential diagnoses. These same modalities can be essential in proper staging in the case of malignant lesions, thus aiding in management decisions. Most lesions ultimately require operative resection, barring metastatic disease, with the notable exception of autoimmune pancreatitis.

The American Hepato-Pancreatico-Biliary Association and Society of Surgical Oncology published a consensus statement in 2009 on the subject of vein resection and reconstruction during pancreaticoduodenectomy (PD), and concluded that PD with vein resection and reconstruction is a viable option for treatment of some pancreatic adenocarcinomas. This article describes the current approaches and recent advances in the management, staging, and surgical techniques regarding portal vein resection. With proper patient selection, a detailed understanding of the anatomy of the root of mesentery, and adequate surgeon experience, vascular resection and reconstruction can be performed safely and does not impact survival duration. Isolated venous involvement is not a contraindication to PD when performed by experienced surgeons at high-volume centers as part of a multidisciplinary and multimodal approach to localized pancreatic cancer.

Pancreatic cancer is the tenth most common cancer in the United States and the fourth leading cause of cancer death. Afflicting approximately 37,000 Americans yearly, more than 80% of patients are unresectable and, therefore, incurable at the time of their diagnosis. Although surgical resection offers the only opportunity for cure, it remains largely unsuccessful; most patients who are candidates for surgical resection relapse and die in fewer than 5 years. This mortality leaves a 5-year overall survival of about 4% for patients diagnosed with pancreatic cancer. Perhaps the most daunting realization for physicians involved in the management of this disease is the understanding that these numbers have not changed in more than 30 years. As surgery remains the foundation of curative therapy for pancreatic cancer, this article reviews the data on adjuvant chemotherapy and adjuvant chemotherapy with radiotherapy as efforts to boost cure rates.

Surgery is generally considered as the only curative therapy for pancreatic cancer; however, even with optimal surgery, long-term cure is achieved in very few patients, thus highlighting the need for adjuvant therapies. Radiation therapy, usually in combination with chemotherapy, plays a role in the setting of unresectable, nonmetastatic pancreatic cancer. Its role in the adjuvant setting remains controversial and as yet undefined. This article reviews the role of radiation therapy in the adjuvant and definitive settings, and describes recent improvements in the delivery of radiotherapy that allow for improved dose delivery with decreased toxicity.

Pancreatic cancer is rarely curable, and because of its location causes significant symptoms for patients in need of palliation. The common problems of incurable pancreatic cancer are biliary obstruction, duodenal obstruction, and pain. Approaches include surgical, endoscopic and radiologic interventions. This article discusses the palliative options and controversies related to these symptoms.

Metastatic pancreatic cancer is often one of the most challenging malignancies a medical oncologist faces. Although the primary endpoint of many studies remains overall survival, palliation and quality of life are now more commonly being addressed. The author discusses the most common chemotherapeutic modalities for the treatment of metastatic pancreatic cancer, such as single agent chemotherapy, combination therapy, targeted therapy, and second line treatment.

Intraductal papillary mucinous neoplasm (IPMN) is an intraductal mucin-producing epithelial neoplasm that arises from the main pancreatic duct (MD-IPMN), secondary branch ducts (BD-IPMN), or both (mixed type; Mix-IPMN). Neoplastic progression from benign adenoma to invasive adenocarcinoma has not been proven but is generally thought to occur. With increasing recognition of IPMN, our understanding of the diagnosis and management of the tumors is evolving. At present, treatment options for patients with IPMN range from observation to pancreatic resection depending on the natural history of the lesion. This review focuses on currently available data that guide management decisions for patients with IPMN.

Cystic neoplasms of the pancreas are increasingly recognized because of expanding use and improved sensitivity of cross-sectional imaging studies. Major advances in the last decade have led to an improved understanding of the various types of cystic lesions and their biologic behavior. Despite significant improvement in imaging technology and the advent of endoscopic ultrasound-guided fine-needle aspiration (EUS-FNA) the diagnosis and management of pancreatic cystic lesions remains a significant clinical challenge. Previous "operate in all cases of pancreatic cyst" strategies have been refined and largely replaced using EUS and cyst fluid analysis as the crux for a more practical management approach. The first diagnostic step remains the differentiation between pancreatic pseudocyst and cystic neoplasm. If a pseudocyst has been effectively excluded, the cornerstone issue becomes to determine the malignant potential of the pancreatic cystic neoplasm. In most cases the correct diagnosis and successful management is based not on a single test but on incorporating data from various sources including patient history, radiologic studies, endoscopic evaluation, in particular EUS, and cyst fluid analysis obtained during fine-needle aspirate. This review focuses on describing the various types of cystic neoplasms of the pancreas and their malignant potential, and provide the clinician with a comprehensive diagnostic approach.

Cystic neoplasms of the pancreas have been recognized for almost 2 centuries, but the principles of management continue to evolve. Clinicians have a better understanding now of the diverse pathologies and behaviors of cystic neoplasms, and can characterize them more precisely into benign, malignant, and of uncertain potential in their manifestations. Treatment is dependent on accurate diagnosis and tailored to the potential aggressiveness of the lesion, the surgical fitness of the patient, and the probability of effecting long-term palliation or survival of the patient. In this article the authors review the classification based on the World Health Organization classification and the latest evidence-based literature of cystic neoplasms, and present their considerations for surgical management of the various lesions. A better understanding of the biologic potential of cystic neoplasms such as intraductal papillary mucinous neoplasms allows for a more patient-specific evidence-based management plan.

Laparoscopic pancreatic resection is performed with increasing frequency for malignant tumors. Data are emerging demonstrating the safety of the laparoscopic approach for distal (left) pancreatectomy, with potential benefits over the standard open approach; however, less information exists as to the effects of laparoscopic resection of cancers of the pancreas. This article reviews and analyzes the existing literature on laparoscopic pancreatectomy for pancreatic malignancies.

THE CLINICS ARE NOW AVAILABLE ONLINE!

Access your subscription at:
www.theclinics.com

Foreword

Evidence-Based Management of Pancreatic Malignancy

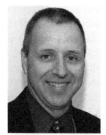

Ronald F. Martin, MD
Consulting Editor

One of the challenging tasks that one faces as a surgical educator is to try to reconcile the difference between the way one learned and the way one should teach. There is the omnipresent temptation to regale learners with stories of "when I was a resident we used to (you supply the story)" or recount how some professor who was larger than life insisted something always be done some way lest one fear for his job and then imply that is justification enough to continue to do it that way. Some of my colleagues refer to this as learning by "eminence based medicine" although it is probably just good survival instinct for some in certain hierarchical environments. To many it is clear that the absolute belief in evidence is far superior to those beliefs held by "eminence" in days gone by, and perhaps rightly so. One, however, does not have to dig too terribly deeply before we find out that "good evidence" can be hard to find and harder to verify. It can also be influenced by eminence, as evidence not disseminated doesn't contribute much to the larger discussion. Also, a lifetime of careful observation may be better evidence than a randomized prospective double-blinded study with a *P* value of .049, but we don't grade them that way.

I have written in past issues of this series about some of the challenges with the dissemination of evidence: who gets to judge the evidence, who decides that it will be disseminated and by what means, who owns the product of inquiry, the open source movement, and possibly even political and system implications. All those issues still persist in some form and still generate debate. Perhaps more important than dissemination is an issue that has not garnered as much attention—how information is received.

Some of you are reading this in print, whereas others are viewing this by electronic media. In fact, odds are that your age is likely to predict which of these formats you are using. My mentors used to tell me about researching information using Index Medicus

doi:10.1016/j.suc.2010.02.001
surgical.theclinics.com

and meeting with librarians in person (the latter is still a good idea, by the way). My generation laughed, under our breath, when we heard such tales, as we used Medline to get our references and then wandered into stacks of journals. My residents laugh, not under their breath, when they hear these stories from me as they sit in conference and download references on G4 networks while I am trying to explain something. The "just-in-time" information is as available to them as their inquiring minds and search engines will allow, and that may just be the biggest problem we face in education.

Our information retrieval processes may be creating a new breed of surgeons who have more mastery of information management than patient management. While I find that thought repellant on most levels, the part that bothers me most is that it might be the desired outcome. Atul Gawande, in his book *The Checklist Manifesto*, has suggested that we have too many pieces of information, in particular critical information, for humans to reliably process safely in patient care. This, of course, becomes even more concerning when the concept is applied to human teams. Furthermore, if we consider that these checklists are rudimentary algorithms with expressed or implied "if-then" instructions then an expansion of these tools beyond simple team and equipment checking to complex diagnostic and treatment drivers is reasonable to expect to some degree. This will as a matter of necessity require our new breed of surgeons to become more facile with information and resource management to successfully care for patients.

My mentors lived in an era of individual mastery leading to institutional greatness, and that is how they taught. Our current focus is shifting, albeit slowly, to systems integration and eliminating basic gaps that degrade large group performance, and that is in large part how we must teach. We must balance fundamental global educational objectives with real-time information access, decision support tools, and collection of data that allows verification and modification of our models. The days of the giants are probably over.

The *Surgical Clinics of North America* counts itself as a believer in the evidence-based movement and has devoted an entire issue of our series to the concept of "Evidence Based Surgery." We try to incorporate those principles to each and every article that we publish. We also strive to maintain that delicate balance between supplying collections of data and expert analysis from people who have achieved mastery of their craft to our readership. Dr Orr and his colleagues have well met that challenge and have given us all a better framework upon which to add our own future insights and observation. I am deeply indebted to him for his efforts. Also, I fervently hope that mastery never goes completely out of style.

Ronald F. Martin, MD
Department of Surgery
Marshfield Clinic
1000 North Oak Avenue
Marshfield, WI 54449, USA

E-mail address:
martin.ronald@marshfieldclinic.org

Preface

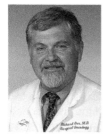

Richard K. Orr, MD, MPH
Guest Editor

When I was a surgical resident in the late 1970s, our chairman, the late Roger T. Sherman MD, frequently said that there were more surgeons who had published papers about Whipple procedures than patients who were long-term survivors of those procedures! Although his admittedly hyperbolic statement was meant to teach the residents about careful analysis of the literature and appropriateness of radical surgery, his numbers were not that far off. At that time, relatively few institutions had extensive experience with pancreaticoduodenectomies, and mortality rates were high. Long-term survivors were rare and far less numerous than those who died from the operation. Since that time many improvements in surgical technique have occurred, and there is now some cautious optimism about pancreatic cancer surgery. Detailed imaging of the pancreas is commonplace, surgical techniques have been standardized, and adjuvant therapies are in place. Pancreaticoduodenectomies are performed at all major institutions with some regularity, and a significant number of "less than major" centers perform the procedure with acceptable results. Perioperative mortality has decreased dramatically, and many feel that further regionalization will save even more lives.

This issue of the *Surgical Clinics of North America* takes a hard look at the available evidence about surgical treatment of pancreatic cancer. The main part of the issue is about adenocarcinoma of the pancreas. Initially, we analyze the literature regarding the critical question, is resectional surgery making a difference, or are we subjecting patients to a futile and expensive operation with little hope of quality survival? Yes, we are making a difference, but not as great as we would hope. There are a limited number of long-term survivors, yet a larger subset receives meaningful palliation with resectional surgery. The "therapeutic ratio" for resectional surgery is slim, and it behooves us to identify the appropriate patients and the appropriate surgical environment. Thus, the first article also looks at the issue of who should be performing these complex operations. Although our earlier hopes of using imaging for early diagnosis of pancreatic cancer have not been fulfilled, surgeons are able to use advanced imaging modalities to define the extent of the malignancy. Careful patient selection is critical in pancreatic cancer surgery, and the next 2 articles provide data regarding the appropriate use of imaging modalities and endoscopic ultrasound, including each

surgical.theclinics.com

modality's expected sensitivities and specificities. The next 3 articles deal with surgical specifics. How is a curative pancreatic resection defined? What technical factors are important to the conduct of the operation? How is resectability defined, and how should we manage the marginally resectable candidate? What is the appropriate usage of vascular resection to extend resectability?

Chemotherapy and radiation therapy are assuming more important roles in the management of operable patients. Several questions need evidence-based answers. When are these modalities appropriate in potentially resectable patients? Can neoadjuvant therapy improve resectability and, ultimately, survival? What is the appropriate sequencing, and does combination therapy offer combined modality benefits or simply combined morbidity? The final 2 articles in the initial part of the issue concern the unfortunately large subset of patients whom we cannot cure with current therapies. What are the therapies that offer the most effective palliation for these unfortunate patients?

The second part of the issue is devoted with a more sanguine outlook to less-common tumors, including intraductal papillary mucinous neoplasms and cystic malignancies. With our better imaging modalities and pathologic subtyping, these have become an ever-increasing part of the pancreatic surgical picture. The final article looks at a cutting-edge technique, laparoscopy. Does it have a role in the management of pancreatic cancer, and if so, when?

I am humbled by the talents of the authors who contributed the individual articles of this issue, and grateful for their prompt article submissions. Each has followed the proposed guidelines of setting forth a thorough review of the available evidence in their particular area. This issue is intended for practicing surgeons to update their knowledge base in a limited area of practice, but it should serve surgical residents as well as surgical oncology and hepatopancreatobiliary fellows as well. I believe that we have created a valid snapshot of the evidence that is available at the time of writing. One hopes that major advances will occur when (and if) more effective adjuvant therapy becomes available.

I would like to thank the editor of the *Surgical Clinics of North America*, Dr Ronald Martin, for inviting me to be guest editor. I would also like to thank my surgical oncology mentors, Drs Walter Lawrence, Jr, Jim Neifeld, and George Parker for getting me started in this wonderful lifetime endeavor. And finally, I wish to acknowledge the great debt I have to Dr Blake Cady, who more than anyone I know, has been constantly critical of established dogma and has practiced "evidence-based" management of individual patients long before that buzzword was commonplace.

Richard K. Orr, MD, MPH
Surgical Oncology at the Gibbs Regional Cancer Center
3rd Floor, 101 East Wood Street
Spartanburg, SC 29303, USA

E-mail address:
Rick1841@yahoo.com

Outcomes in Pancreatic Cancer Surgery

Richard K. Orr, MD, MPH[a,b,*]

KEYWORDS

• Pancreatic cancer • Outcomes • Mortality • Complications

The increase in surgery for pancreatic cancer during the last 3 decades can be correlated with a gradual decline in operative mortality and postoperative complications.[1] Pancreaticoduodenectomy was popularized by Whipple and colleagues[2] in 1935, but mortality remained high until a few surgeons developed significant experience in the 1970s. Several major institutions began developing broader experience and mortality and morbidity decreased dramatically.[3] Although not all surgeons (nor all hospitals) can have equal outcomes, the definition and tabulation of these outcomes have been difficult. Debates about regulating the performance of pancreatic surgery often have been contentious and 1-sided. Few randomized controlled trials exist[4] and most of the existing trials have too few patients for meaningful statistical conclusions. Definition of outcomes in quality-adjusted survival and cost-effectiveness have been even more ephemeral. At the time this article is being written (October 2009), the future of the United States health care system has been the focus of intense debate and proposed legislation. As stated by Tom Russell (Executive Director of the American College of Surgeons): "They will not care about 30-day mortality; they will want to know what is (sic) happened over 5 to 10 years. What is the value? What is the cost/benefit ratio of these high-end operations on very sick patients? …. Given these external forces and the need for comparative effectiveness research… will we even be performing them?"[5] Apropos of this statement, this article asks several pertinent questions: (1) what is the scientific rationale for pancreatic resection? (2) what are the best available results at this time? (3) who should be performing pancreatic resections? For clarity, this article analyzes results of resection for adenocarcinoma of the exocrine pancreas, and excludes duodenal and ampullary cancers, pancreatic endocrine tumors, and tumors of less malignant potential. Various topics including adjuvant

[a] Marsha and Jimmy Gibbs Regional Cancer Center – 3rd Floor, Spartanburg Regional Medical Center, Spartanburg, SC 29303, USA
[b] Medical University of South Carolina, Charleston, SC, USA
* Corresponding author. Marsha and Jimmy Gibbs Regional Cancer Center – 3rd Floor, Spartanburg Regional Medical Center, Spartanburg, SC 29303.
E-mail address: Rick1841@yahoo.com

Surg Clin N Am 90 (2010) 219–234
doi:10.1016/j.suc.2009.12.007
0039-6109/10/$ – see front matter
surgical.theclinics.com

therapy, imaging, and laparoscopy are discussed in detail in other chapters in this issue and are not further reviewed in this article.

SCIENTIFIC RATIONALE FOR PANCREATIC RESECTION

The most important goal of pancreatic cancer surgery is the prolongation of quality life. Comparative studies of survival are fraught with difficulty, and quality-adjusted survival is rarely published. With the exception of operative deaths (discussed later), it is difficult to compare institutional survival curves. Confounding variables, such as patient age, comorbidity, and socioeconomic status exert a huge influence on survival in a disease such as pancreatic cancer. For example, it has been shown that patients who are treated in large referral centers tend to be healthy enough to travel[6,7] and have greater resources available to them (economic resources and family support); they may have better access to postoperative support services also. All of these advantages may translate into better survival. Conversely, it is probable that improved perioperative outcomes may be true markers of extended survival.[8] Patients who have postoperative complications and prolonged convalescences may have shortened survival.[9] The quality of surgery may also make a difference in resectability, positive surgical margins, and blood transfusions, which may be true predictors of survival.[10]

Long-term Survival

Pancreatic cancer has a dismal prognosis. Most patients are not candidates for surgical resection and have median survivals of a few months. The outlook for resected patients may not be much better. Before analyzing the question of who should be performing pancreatic surgery, it is prudent to look at the question posited by Russell (quoted earlier): should anyone be performing resectional surgery for pancreatic cancer? In an earlier era (when operative mortality was higher), Crile[11] showed that palliative bypass was more effective than Whipple operations. He pointed out that the natural history of pancreatic cancer trumped surgical attempts at extirpation. Conversely, Brooks and Culebras[12] was able to show a lower postoperative mortality (12.5% in 1976), and called for a total pancreatectomy as the best method of treating this disease. Wakeman and colleagues[13] analyzed 2 series of patients with pancreatic cancer in New Zealand. Overall median survival for all patients with pancreatic cancer was only 3.1 months, but was improved to 13.9 months in the resected group. Although the median survival for the pancreaticoduodenectomy group was twice that of the bypass group, the authors assert that the procedure is palliative in most patients, as only 21% were alive 3 years postoperatively. Gudjonsson[14] analyzed 340 articles including 80,000 patients and found fewer than 300 resected patients with long-term survival. He concluded that pancreatic resections were wasteful and prohibitively expensive. At about the same time, several other articles carefully analyzed individual institutions' long-term survival data. These articles also attest to the dismal long-term prognosis. The Memorial Sloan-Kettering group[15] reported on 12 patients surviving 5 or more years postresection (10.2% actual 5-year survival). At the time of publication only 6 of 12 were free of pancreatic cancer with follow-ups ranging from 7 to 9 years. There were no clear-cut predictors of survival in this group. For example, 5 of the 12 patients had positive lymph nodes, 3 had tumors larger than 5 cm, 8 had perineural invasion, and 9 had extrapancreatic invasion. The Toronto group[16] showed a 14.6% 5-year survival, but only 4% survived longer than 10 years. In contrast to the Sloan-Kettering data, these investigators felt that tumor stage and grade were independent predictors of survival. Data from the Johns Hopkins[17] group are similar: 5-year survival was 15%, but only 1 of 52 evaluable patients survived 10 years. The Mayo Clinic[18] data were more sanguine, with 5- and 10-year survivals of 18% and 13%.

In the best possible scenario, surgery would be offered only to those patients with a reasonable likelihood of long-term survival. Several recent series have presented careful analyses of factors predictive of poor outcome. Most of these variables are determined only in the resected specimen and few variables discriminate enough to exclude patients from potentially curative surgery. Garcea and colleagues[19] have presented an analysis based on their review of 154 studies detailing outcomes of almost 26,000 patients. They found that several factors were not correlated with prognosis: age, gender, and location of tumor. Several other factors were of questionable prognostic value: ethnicity, socioeconomic status, CA 19-9 levels, C-reactive protein levels, and increased platelet counts. Conversely, advancing tumor size correlates with poorer prognosis. These investigators showed that a tumor larger than 3 cm had a relative hazard (for death) of 3.8, compared with smaller tumors. As expected, patients with negative lymph nodes fared better (median survival 25 months) versus those with positive nodes (median survival 12 months). A few series showed that the ratio of positive to total lymph nodes harvested was also of prognostic value.[20] Tumor grade has been shown to be predictive in many studies and may be almost as important as lymph node status. Histopathologic grade obtained preoperatively may differ from that in the resected specimen and may not be suitable for making preoperative decisions. Perineural invasion was noted in 38% of patients in that cross-sectional study but diminished median survival by only 2.5 months. Blood-vessel invasion was less common (16%) but associated with a clinically significant decrease in median survival (11.9 months vs 20.6 months). The investigators commented on the lack of standardization of pathologic specimens in the literature, and thus difficulty in establishing the true incidence of positive pathologic margins. The median survival for R0 resections (20.3 months) was twice that of R1 resections (10.3%). Several series show that a positive margin does not absolutely imply individual poor prognosis, showing 5-year survival of 5%, 10%, and 12% in the 3 series that reported these data. Intraoperative blood loss or transfusions have been associated with decreased survival in many studies. It is not clear if blood loss is a marker for more extensive tumors or an independent prognosticator.

The precise amount of detriment because of positive margins is debated in the literature. Virtually all studies show that R0 resections are superior to R1 resections, but the definitions of margin status vary. Westgaard and colleagues[21] used a perpendicular sectioning method to clarify the retroperitoneal margin and found involvement in 28% of patients. This method was associated with a hazard ratio of 1.9, and was statistically significant despite the small sample size (114 total patients). These investigators call for standardization of pathologic analysis and caution against conclusions based on studies with high rates of R0 resections. Tumors of the body of the pancreas may be difficult to resect with clear retroperitoneal margins. Strasberg and colleagues[22] has proposed the radical antegrade modular pancreatosplenectomy as an en bloc approach to this problem. Data from 23 patients showed a 21-month median survival and a 91% negative margin rate.

To avoid unhelpful operations, it is hoped that preoperative variables can stratify patients that are not suitable for resection. Garcea and colleagues[19] suggested that patients with tumors greater than 3 cm in cross-sectional diameter on preoperative imaging could be excluded from surgery if they were felt to be reasonably poor operative risks. In an attempt to stratify patients with poor outcomes, Barugola and colleagues[23] suggests that symptom duration greater than 40 days, CA 19-9 greater than 200 U/mL, and pathologic grade 3 or 4 predict dire outcomes and should exclude these patients from surgery. Their series was small (228 patients) and only 43 died within 1 year of surgery. Ideally, these results should be confirmed by other groups before becoming standard practice. Recognizing that the benefit/risk ratio is low for pancreatic resection, the Johns Hopkins group[24] has proposed some biochemical markers that may reliably predict patients at increased risk of complications and perioperative mortality. These markers include increased blood urea nitrogen and low albumin. Postoperatively, increased amylase and aminotransferase values were associated with poor outcomes. Pratt and colleagues[25] used the POSSUM[26] score (Physiologic and Operative Severity Score) to analyze morbidity and mortality retrospectively and found excellent correlation. Although some variables (most notably blood loss) are assigned postoperatively, the POSSUM score uses a series of physiologic and laboratory tests to assign a risk severity score. Use of this score preoperatively may be useful in assessing risk/benefit ratios for individual patients. However, a large European study[27] failed to validate POSSUM as a useful predictor in pancreatic surgery, and another[28] found that the POSSUM score overpredicted mortality.

Laparoscopy has been proposed as a useful adjunct to eliminate potentially incurable patients.[29] There is a general conclusion that laparoscopy eliminates some patients with metastatic disease that is not visualized radiographically, and several contemporary studies have analyzed the usefulness of laparoscopy in an era with better preoperative imaging modalities. The Massachusetts General Hospital group[30] attempted to use multidetector-row computed tomography images to eliminate the need for laparoscopy. Forty-four patients underwent laparotomy after negative imaging. Five of these patients had liver metastases and 3 more had undiagnosed peritoneal metastases. The investigators concluded that high-resolution imaging did not replace laparoscopy. Enestvedt and colleagues[31] studied the cost of laparoscopy and found that that the procedure was cost-effective as an immediate prelude to laparotomy. Mayo and colleagues[32] analyzed data from the Oregon State Cancer Registry (298 patients from 28 hospitals) and found that 27% of patients receiving laparoscopy were found to have signs of incurability and spared a laparotomy. The investigators noted a significant degree of selectivity: 71% of the patients did not have laparoscopy and only 8% of that group was not resected. Because the main reason for unresectability was vascular invasion, it is not likely that laparoscopy would have been helpful in that subgroup. This was a population-based study (without formal guidelines) and there was some variability between institutions. Shah and colleagues[33] have proposed selective criteria for preoperative laparoscopy. They performed laparoscopy in only 39% of their resectable patients, but changed treatment in more than half of these based on laparoscopic findings. Maithel and colleagues[34] proposed adding CA 19-9 as a marker for incurability. Unresectable disease was seen in 26% of 144 patients with CA 19-9 values 130 U/mL or greater, versus 11% of 118 patients with lower values. These investigators suggest that patients with increased CA 19-9 should undergo laparoscopy before attempted resection.

In 2002, Bradley[35] wrote an editorial addressing the concerns of Crile and others regarding the futility of pancreatic resection. Despite improvement in surgical technique, he noted that "recurrence is the rule and not the exception." Locoregional recurrence is a major problem with pancreatic cancer, and several surgeons have attempted increasingly radical operations in hopes of diminishing recurrence. A few studies have looked at the effect of more extensive surgery on short- and long-term outcomes. The Johns Hopkins group analyzed 100 total pancreatectomy patients and compared them with 1286 pancreaticoduodenectomy patients.[36] They found similar 5-year survival in the 2 groups but a higher mortality for total pancreatectomy. They recommend using total pancreatectomy only if oncologically warranted. Nathan and colleagues[37] also analyzed a subset from the SEER (Surveillance Epidemiology and End Results) database and found that patients undergoing total pancreatectomy had similar short- and long-term outcomes when compared with patients undergoing pancreaticoduodenectomy. Schmidt and colleagues[38] analyzed combined series from Johns Hopkins and Indiana and advocate use of total pancreatectomy when necessary to achieve an R0 resection. Thirty-three patients underwent conversion to total pancreatectomy for positive pancreatic neck margins (with clear retroperitoneal and bile duct margins). These patients had an increased median survival (18 months) without increased morbidity or mortality. In contrast, Rosemurgy's[39] group showed no survival benefit for 17 patients requiring extended resections after having a positive frozen section margin.

Pedrazzoli and colleagues[40] reported the results of a multicenter trial comparing standard pancreaticoduodenectomy with standard surgery plus extended lymphadenectomy (hepatic nodes, clearance of the aorta from the diaphragm to the inferior mesenteric artery and including both renal hila). Long-term survival was similar, and the complication rate was also similar. The extended operation took 25 minutes longer and harvested a mean of 6 additional lymph nodes. The investigators commented on a nonsignificant trend for better survival in the node-positive group subjected to the more extensive operation. The Mayo Clinic[41] reported a randomized trial comparing standard pancreaticoduodenectomy versus standard pancreaticoduodenectomy plus extended lymph node resection. Although only 79 patients were randomized, the investigators noted no differences in 1-, 3-, or 5-year survival. The extended lymphadenectomy group suffered more problems with diarrhea, body appearance, and bowel control. The Johns Hopkins group[42] performed another randomized trial comparing standard versus extended pancreaticoduodenectomy and also failed to show a difference in 1- or 5-year survival. An additional randomized trial from Japan[43] showed no difference in survival after extended surgery.

In 1973, Fortner[44] proposed a regional pancreatectomy as a method for increasing the surgical margin and lymph node dissection for adenocarcinoma of the head of the pancreas. Fortner and colleagues[45] published a series of 18 patients (including 5 with arterial resections) in 1977. These procedures were difficult, associated with significant blood loss (mean replacement was 5 units), and prolonged lengths of stay. The 30-day mortality was 17%, but the actuarial survival at 1 year was 62%. Although his theory of regional pancreatectomy has not withstood the test of time, he did prove the feasibility of portal vein resection when required for operative clearance. With modern techniques, mortality has approached that of patients who have not required vascular surgery.[46] Recent series include the Louisville group,[47] who performed arterial or venous resections in 36 patients, with no mortality. Three patients had resection of the common hepatic artery with end-to-end anastomosis and 2 had resection of the superior mesenteric artery (SMA) with vein graft replacement. The median survival of the vascular resection group was 18 months (compared with 19 months for the patients not requiring vascular resections). Although the investigators comment that arterial invasion is not a contraindication to resection, they noted that both patients with SMA involvement had undergone neoadjuvant therapy and the arterial reconstruction had been carefully planned with a vascular surgeon. Similar results were noted from 2 European centers,[48] including 45 patients (6 arterial reconstructions). One patient died postoperatively (2.2%). Median survival was 14 months; overall 1-year survival was 57% and 3-year survival was 19%. Sugiura and colleagues[49] reported on an aggressive series of 107 patients, of whom 62 had vascular reconstruction. Although overall survival was similar in the vascular and nonvascular groups, there were no long-term survivals with SMA or celiac axis resections. Siriwardana and Siriwardena[50] pooled 52 studies of portal/mesenteric vein resection and found an acceptable pooled mortality (5.9%), but only a modest survival. Median survival was 13 months, but only 7% survived 5 years. There was a high rate of nodal metastases (67%) in the pooled series. (See the article by Christians and colleagues elsewhere in this issue for further exploration of this topic.)

Several randomized trials have been published regarding specific questions about pancreatic cancer surgery.[51] These are beyond the scope of this article, but 1 technical area is worth discussing. Pylorus-preserving pancreatectomy was revitalized in the 1970s as an alternative to the standard Whipple procedure. Its proponents argued for shorter operative times and presumably fewer gastrointestinal side effects. Two meta-analyses[52,53] independently surveyed 6 trials (approximately 574 patients) and found that the pylorus-preserving modification was 72 minutes faster and associated with slightly less blood loss and transfusion. Other perioperative and long-term outcomes were not statistically different. Five of these trials assessed delayed gastric emptying. Three of these favored the classic Whipple, but the overall results did not reach statistical significance. The investigators commented that the number of patients enrolled in these trials was too small to exclude small differences in outcome.

To address the potential benefit of pancreatic resection, carefully performed quality-of-life (QOL) studies are necessary. The literature is bereft of such information. The Johns Hopkins group[54] attempted to answer this question by sending QOL questionnaires to patients who had had a pancreaticoduodenectomy, patients who had had a laparoscopic cholecystectomy, and healthy controls. A total of 323 of the questionnaires were sent to patients who had had a pancreaticoduodenectomy who were 6 or more months postoperative, and 192 were returned (59%). Only 28% of those returning surveys had pancreatic adenocarcinoma, 29% had other cancers, and the remainder had benign pathology. For the group as a whole, the investigators found only a slight (and statistically nonsignificant) decrease in QOL compared with controls. Conversely, the patients with pancreatic cancer had decreased (and statistically significant) scores in the physical and psychology domains of the study instrument. Crippa and colleagues[55] followed QOL for patients with pancreatic cancer in various disease states. They found that QOL improved after pancreatic resection for those patients with localized disease and remained higher for 3 to 6 months following surgery.

Trede,[56] an international expert on pancreatic surgery, expressed the notion that pancreatic cancer is an incurable disease when treated exclusively by surgery. He called for randomized trials of chemotherapy, radiotherapy, and other oncologic alternatives to fully assess the potential of nonsurgical treatments to extend survival. Other articles in this issue address chemotherapy and radiotherapy in detail, and the effects of these modalities on survival are not discussed in this article. Because neoadjuvant therapy is of great interest to surgeons, the interested reader is also referred to recently published review articles.[57,58]

BENCHMARK DATA
Short-term Mortality Results in Expert Series

Experienced centers should perform pancreaticoduodenectomies with a mortality less than 5% and major complication rates less than 40%. The Johns Hopkins[59] group recently reported their series spanning nearly 40 years. As their experience increased, mortality dropped from 30% in the 1970s to 1% in 2000 to 2005. Similarly low mortality (<2%) has been reported from other tertiary centers.[60–63] The mortality for total pancreatectomy may be higher, but few recent articles have enough numbers for precise quantification. In most expert series mortality for distal pancreatectomy is similar to or lower than for pancreaticoduodenectomy.

Complication Rates in Expert Series

Complications following pancreatic surgery are common and often associated with mortality. Simons and colleagues[64] reviewed more than 100,000 hospital discharges following pancreatectomy. Complications occurred in 23% and were associated with patient age, type of pancreatectomy, and low hospital volume. Complications were a significant predictor of increased length of hospitalization, transfer to another facility, and death. Complications are also a major source of readmission after discharge and related to a decreased median survival.[65] Nevertheless, complications following pancreatic resection are common in expert centers also. Complication reporting is variable and subject, in many cases, to problems related to retrospective chart review. Two major groups have attempted to clarify this situation, by using standardized reporting. These studies show that complications are extremely common following pancreatectomy. Grobmyer and colleagues[60] reported a 47% complication rate based on a prospective real-time database. Most of these were minor and the median length of stay was only 9 days. However, pancreatic anastomotic leaks occurred in 12% of patients. Nine percent of patients required reoperation within 30 days, and 11% of discharged patients were admitted within 1 month. The Johns Hopkins group[66] developed a complication grading system with the aid of Clavien and colleagues,[67] early proponents of standardized reporting. A total of 58.5% of patients developed at least 1 complication. Infections occurred in 17% of patients and pancreatic fistulas in 9%. About two-thirds of complications were classified as grades 1 and 2, but one-third had more severe complications. The details of specific complications are beyond the scope of this article (and the 2 articles referred to have excellent reference lists).

Pancreatic fistula is 1 of the more frequently discussed complications. The Massachusetts General Hospital group[68] noted 22 fistulas in 66 patients with distal pancreatectomy. They found that this complication tripled mean length of stay from 5.2 to 16.6 days, and doubled the cost of hospitalization. Although pancreatic fistulas are less frequent following pancreaticoduodenectomy, they are associated with increased septic complications and increased length of stay.[69] The literature does not give a clear-cut answer regarding the optimal technique of anastomosis. Adams[70] found more than 1700 publications on a PubMed search for "pancreatic anastomosis." He recommended that surgeons use their own experience, with attention to several principles, including good exposure, a watertight patent anastomosis, preservation of blood supply, tension-free fixation, and coverage of the cut end of the pancreas.

WHO SHOULD PERFORM PANCREATECTOMIES?

In 1979, Luft and colleagues[71] published a landmark article showing a marked difference in mortality recorded at high-volume versus low-volume hospitals for certain high-risk procedures (most notably open-heart surgery, transurethral prostate resections, and vascular surgery). This article has been the impetus for subsequent research analyzing surgical volume versus outcome. Although the adage "practice makes perfect" may be appropriate, Luft's comments are prophetic: "operations are performed and patients are cared for not by hospitals but by surgeons, anesthesiologists, operating-room teams, and nursing staffs." Thus, good (and bad) results are related to many factors. Surgical volume is 1 of the easiest to measure, but may lead to faulty conclusions.[72] Many investigators have shown that high-volume hospitals have better process control, including better intensive care support.[73-76] It is possible that these institutional processes may drive the low mortality, and not simply the case volume. The articles cited in this section are intended to give a balanced view of a difficult subject. In particular, the authors investigate the validity of the "Leapfrog standards," an outcome-based initiative designed to use economic forces to move patients from lower-volume to higher-volume centers.[77]

Birkmeyer and colleagues[78] have published many careful studies relating surgical volume (and other factors) to variability in surgical mortality. In 2002, they analyzed outcomes in 2.5 million cardiovascular and oncologic operations performed from 1994 to 1999. Forty-one percent of pancreatic resections in the United States were performed in low-volume hospitals. Patients in this group suffered a 16.2% mortality. Those in the intermediate volume groups (3–16 procedures per year) experienced a lower mortality (9.4%), and those operated on in the highest-volume hospitals experienced the lowest mortality (3.8%). Although most other operations were associated with some degree of lowered mortality related to increasing volume, only esophagectomy and pneumonectomy showed as wide a difference between the volume groups. Although recognizing that some low-volume hospitals had excellent clinical results, they encouraged referral to high-volume centers. Their follow-up article attempted to address the importance of individual surgeon volume by analyzing 474,000 Medicare claims from 1998 to 1999.[79] They found that surgeon volume was inversely related to operative mortality for several complex operations, including pancreatic resection, esophageal resection, and lung cancer resection. For pancreatectomy, mortality was 14.7% for surgeons performing fewer than 2 procedures annually and 4.6% for surgeons performing greater than 4 procedures annually. As expected, results were related to hospital volume, and individual surgeon volume. Thus, low-volume surgeons in low-volume hospitals experienced the highest mortality (15.7%), whereas low-volume surgeons in higher-volume hospitals had lower mortality (6.1%). Nevertheless, the low-volume surgeons in higher-volume hospitals had mortality that was nearly double their high-volume compatriots (6.1% vs 3.7%). This group noted that in that period, more than half of the Medicare pancreatic resections in the United States were performed by low-volume surgeons in low-volume hospitals. Eppsteiner and colleagues[80] found similar trends from a sample of the Nationwide Inpatient Sample (1998–2005). This study found that surgeon volume was important after controlling for hospital volume, noting that hospital volume accounted for only 19% to 27% of the observed variability. Nathan and colleagues[81] attempted to define the specificity of volume/outcome ratios in hepatopancreaticobiliary surgery. They found that individual surgeon volume had minimal effect on mortality for liver resections, but was as important as hospital volume for pancreatectomy. Furthermore, these investigators found that expertise in 1 area was not transferrable to the other area.

Few articles have analyzed surgical subspecialization and its effect on outcome. Parks and colleagues[82] showed that patients operated on by surgeons professing special interest in pancreatic surgery had a lower operative mortality. As expected, those surgeons classified as specialists also had higher caseloads, so it is impossible to separate the effect of subspecialization from experience. Conversely, Csikesz and colleagues[83] found no effect of specialization on mortality in the United States, but the analysis compared only transplant surgeons with nontransplant surgeons, and did not compare surgical oncologists with general surgeons. The MD Anderson group[84] analyzed surgeon experience using blood loss, operating time, and length of stay as surrogate outcome measures. Because all surgeons began their attending careers at the MD Anderson Cancer Center, University of Texas, Houston, Texas, most of the institutional variability was negated. The investigators noted that there were significant changes between the first 60 and the next 60 cases for each surgeon. They called for integration of newer surgeons into established systems with mentorship during the steep learning curve.

It is probable that volume/experience may equate with better long-term survival also. Birkmeyer and colleagues[85] showed that 3-year survival was significantly higher (37% vs 25%) in the highest- versus lowest-volume hospitals. Although some of this was attributed to hospital deaths in the lower-volume group, the effect persisted after removing postoperative deaths.

Several investigators have warned about overaggressive interpretation of individual data. For example, Dimick and Welch[86] looked at Medicare hospitals with zero mortality for certain high-risk operations during 1997 to 1999. The 383 hospitals with zero mortality for pancreatectomy reported 11.8% mortality in the following year. Their comments are worth noting: (1) mortality is a poor measure of quality when numbers are small, and (2) the statistical phenomenon of regression toward the mean is applicable. In a similar vein, investigators from the University of California, San Francisco noted no changes in their own operative mortality related to year-to-year procedure volume.[87,88]

To end this section, the authors look at the Leapfrog initiative. The Leapfrog group recommends that patients be referred to centers performing at least 11 pancreatectomies per year. Birkmeyer and Dimick[89] estimated that 177 lives per year could be saved by implementing Leapfrog standards, a figure similar to the 2008 estimate (160) prepared by Lwin and Shepard.[90] Although these numbers are not trivial, they are small when compared with the potential gains from in-hospital intensive care unit staffing (55,000 lives saved per year) and computerized patient ordering (>3 million adverse drug reactions averted annually). Coupled with the objections to using volume as the sole criterion for quality,[91] it seems likely that Leapfrog's greatest effect on pancreatic surgery will be the presentation of numerical data to interested consumers (patients and industry). Some smaller-volume hospitals have shown excellent results,[92] and these hospitals will be positioned to present their data and champion their position. The differences in mortality amongst providers are real, and the trend toward outcome-based referrals will almost certainly increase.

CURRENT TRENDS

Gasper and colleagues[93] compared mortality for patients undergoing high-risk operations in the state of California during 1990 to 1994, 1995 to 1999, and 2000 to 2004. They found significant improvements in operative mortality during the last time frame for all types of pancreatectomy. In-hospital mortality decreased from 9.9% in the earliest time period to 7.1% and 6.0% in the later periods. As seen in other studies, mortality was inversely related to hospital procedure volume. In the latest period, the adjusted mortality was only 1.5% in the highest-volume hospitals (>50 pancreatectomies per year), versus 5.6% in the lowest-volume (<6 per year) hospitals. During the earliest time frame, 30% of all pancreatectomies in California were performed in lowest-volume hospitals. By the latest time frame, this number had decreased to 10%. Initially 210 hospitals had performed at least 1 pancreatectomy, but by the later period this number had decreased to 127 hospitals. Because the adjusted mortality had decreased from 14.1% to 5.6% in the lowest-volume hospitals, there is an implied self-selection amongst hospitals or surgeons. The authors posit that the changes in California suggest that modern hospitals "behave as complex, adaptive systems." Thus, they integrate feedback (in this case, mortality data) and make decisions to improve their individual system of care, or in many cases, to cease providing that service. They imply that external regulation (eg, the Leapfrog initiative) may be unnecessary when suitable data are made available to individual hospitals and outside interested parties. Tseng and colleagues[94] analyzed the performance of total pancre-atectomies in the United States. They found that mortality decreased from 14.2% in 1998 to 5.7% in 2006. They noted a higher mortality in low-volume hospitals, but attributed most of that to patient selection. Patients in lower-volume centers were older and had more medical comorbidities.

Conversely, the Florida study by Rosemurgy and colleagues[95] failed to show the sanguine adaptive effects seen in California. They note that in Florida most pancreati-coduodenectomies were performed by surgeons performing fewer than 6 procedures per year. These surgeons experienced increasing mortality (5.5% to 12.3% in 1995–1997 compared with 2003–2005). Because of this, the overall hospital mortality in the state of Florida was similar (5.1% vs 5.9%) during the 2 periods. Attempts in the Netherlands to centralize pancreatic surgery were minimally successful also.[96] Fewer patients were operated on in low-volume hospitals during 2001 to 2004 (57%) than 1994 to 1996 (65%). As expected, differences in survival related to operative volume persisted. The investigators performed a critical review of the literature available at that time including 24 separate studies. All but 1 study favored high-volume centers, and the effect was statistically significant in two-thirds of these.

Ghaferi and colleagues[97] assessed variability of mortality for 84,000 patients under-going general and vascular surgery (2005–2007). Mortality was twice as high in the worst quintile compared with the best quintile. The complication rates were almost identical across quintiles. In an editorial, Jacobs[98] notes that successful hospitals have structures in processes in place to rescue patients who experience complica-tions. Several investigators have been using critical pathways (fast-tracking) as a means of improving efficiency, treating complications, and decreasing costs. Although each institution's pathways are unique, they have several features in common. Most importantly, the pathways combine several disciplines (eg, surgery, nursing, radiology, physical therapy, nutrition) in attempts to optimize individual patient care. As the entire team (including the patient) has a blueprint to work from, the process of care may be streamlined. Specific goals are delineated for ambulation, pain control, and nutritional support.[99] A norm is established and patients deviating from the normal postoperative course are identified and receive more vigorous care according to the protocol. Conversely, diet and ambulation are advanced rapidly in most patients who are within protocol normative guidelines. The MD Anderson group[100] found a 23% reduction in total costs after institution of a clinical pathway for pancreaticoduodenectomies, largely attributed to reduction in mean length of stay. There were no differences in mortality nor readmissions within 1 month of discharge. Whereas the MD Anderson clinical pathway was applied to an experienced team, Kennedy and colleagues[101] implemented their protocol at a time when they were changing from a moderate- to high-volume center. As such, their improvement was more substantial. Their mean costs decreased by 47%, with a reduction in average length of stay by 6 days. Similar improvements have been noted by using critical pathways for distal pancreatectomy also.[102]

Maa and colleagues[103] presented an innovative approach to exporting technology and expertise from a high-volume center to a nearby (20 miles outside the main city) low-volume center, using protocols to improve institutional and surgeon factors. They began by polling high-volume surgeons regarding important features of perioperative care. Subsequently, a single surgeon was appointed as an educator at the secondary hospital, again emphasizing perioperative care protocols. That surgeon participated in all Whipple operations, assisted by 1 of the 4 general surgeons practicing at the secondary hospital. Additional processes were in place to buy needed instrumentation (ultrasound and advanced laparoscopic equipment) and to enable timely operating-room starts. They have shown excellent results in the first 9 patients in their protocol. It remains to be seen whether similar exporting can occur in locations that are not amenable to travel by the experienced surgeon.

REFERENCES

1. McPhee JT, Hill JS, Whalen GF, et al. Perioperative mortality for pancreatectomy–a national perspective. Ann Surg 2007;246:246–53.
2. Whipple AO, Pasons WB, Mullins CR. Treatment of cancer of the ampulla of Vater. Am Surg 1935;102:763–79.
3. Cameron JL, Pitt HA, Yeo CJ, et al. One hundred and forty-five consecutive pancreaticoduodenectomies without mortality. Ann Surg 1993;217:430–8.
4. Traverso LW. The state of the highest level of evidence: an overview of systematic reviews of pancreatobiliary disease customized for the gastroenterologist and GI surgeon. J Gastrointest Surg 2008;12:617–9.
5. Russell TR. Discussion of Gasper WJ, et al. Ann Surg 2009;25:483.
6. Lamont EB, Hayreh D, Pickett KE, et al. Is patient travel distance associated with survival on phase II clinical trials in oncology? J Natl Cancer Inst 2003;95:1370–5.
7. Ballard DJ, Bryant SC, O'Brien PC, et al. Referral selection bias in the Medicare hospital mortality prediction model: are centers of referral for Medicare beneficiaries necessarily centers of excellence? Health Serv Res 1994;28:771–84.
8. Bilimoria KY, Bentrem DJ, Feinglass JM, et al. Directing surgical quality improvement initiatives: comparison of perioperative mortality and long-term survival for cancer surgery. J Clin Oncol 2008;26:4626–33.
9. Kang CM, Kim DH, Choi GH, et al. Detrimental effect of postoperative complications on oncologic efficacy of R0 pancreatectomy in ductal adenocarcinoma of the pancreas. J Gastrointest Surg 2009;13:907–14.
10. Howard TJ, Krug JE, Yu J, et al. A margin-negative R0 resection accomplished with minimal postoperative complications is the surgeon's contribution to long-term survival in pancreatic cancer. J Gastrointest Surg 2006;10:1338–45.
11. Crile G Jr. The advantages of bypass operations over radical pancreaticoduodenectomy in the treatment of pancreatic carcinoma. Surg Gynecol Obstet 1970;130:1049–53.
12. Brooks JR, Culebras JM. Cancer of the pancreas. Palliative operation, Whipple procedure, or total pancreatectomy? Am J Surg 1976;131:516–20.
13. Wakeman CJ, Martin IG, Robertson RW, et al. Pancreatic cancer: management and survival. ANZ J Surg 2004;74:941–4.
14. Gudjonsson B. Carcinoma of the pancreas: critical analysis of costs, results of resections, and the need for standardized reporting. J Am Coll Surg 1995;181:483–503.
15. Conlon KC, Klimstra DS, Brennan MF. Long-term survival after curative resection for pancreatic ductal adenocarcinoma. Clinicopathologic analysis of 5-year survivors. Ann Surg 1996;223:273–9.
16. Cleary SP, Gryfe R, Guindi M, et al. Prognostic factors in resected pancreatic adenocarcinoma: analysis of actual 5-year survivors. J Am Coll Surg 2004;198:722–31.

17. Yeo CJ, Sohn TA, Cameron JL, et al. Periampullary carcinoma – analysis of 5-year survivors. Ann Surg 1998;227:821–31.
18. Schnelldorfer T, Ware AL, Sarr MG, et al. Long-term survival after pancreatoduodenectomy for pancreatic adenocarcinoma: is cure possible? Ann Surg 2008; 247:456–62.
19. Garcea G, Dennison AR, Pattenden CJ, et al. Survival following curative resection for pancreatic ductal adenocarcinoma. A systematic review of the literature. JOP 2008;9:99–132.
20. Riediger H, Keck T, Wellner U, et al. The lymph node ratio is the strongest prognostic factor after resection of pancreatic cancer. J Gastrointest Surg 2009;13: 1337–44.
21. Westgaard A, Tafjord S, Farstad IN, et al. Resectable adenocarcinomas in the pancreatic head: the retroperitoneal margin is an independent prognostic factor. BMC Cancer 2008;8:5.
22. Strasberg SM, Linehan DC, Hawkins WG. Radical antegrade pancreatosplenectomy procedure for adenocarcinoma of the body and tail of the pancreas: ability to obtain negative tangential margins. J Am Coll Surg 2007;204:244–9.
23. Barugola G, Partelli S, Marcucci S, et al. Resectable pancreatic cancer: who really benefits from resection? Ann Surg Oncol 2009. DOI:10.1245/s10434-009-0670-7.
24. Winter JM, Cameron JL, Yeo CJ, et al. Biochemical markers predict morbidity and mortality after pancreaticoduodenectomy. J Am Coll Surg 2007;204:1029–38.
25. Pratt W, Joseph S, Callery MP, et al. POSSUM accurately predicts morbidity for pancreatic resection. Surgery 2008;143:8–19.
26. Copeland GP, Jones D, Walters M. POSSUM: a scoring system for the surgical audit. Br J Surg 1991;78:356–60.
27. De Castro SM, Houwert JT, Lagarde SM, et al. Evaluation of POSSUM for patients undergoing pancreatoduodenectomy. World J Surg 2009;33:1481–7.
28. Khan AW, Shah SR, Agarwal AK, et al. Evaluation of the POSSUM scoring system for comparative audit in pancreatic surgery. Dig Surg 2003;20:539–45.
29. Warshaw AL, Tepper JE, Shipley WU. Laparoscopy in the staging and planning of therapy for pancreatic cancer. Am J Surg 1986;151:76–80.
30. Ellsmere J, Mortele K, Sahani D, et al. Does multidetector-row CT eliminate the role of diagnostic laparoscopy in assessing resectability of pancreatic head adenocarcinoma? Surg Endosc 2005;19:369–73.
31. Ernestvedt CK, Mayo SC, Diggs BS, et al. Diagnostic laparoscopy for patients with potentially resectable pancreatic carcinoma: is it cost-effective in the current era? J Gastrointest Surg 2008;12:1177–84.
32. Mayo SC, Austin DF, Sheppard BC, et al. Evolving preoperative evaluation of patients with pancreatic cancer: does laparoscopy have a role in the current era? J Am Coll Surg 2009;208:87–95.
33. Shah D, Fisher WE, Hodges SE, et al. Preoperative prediction of complete resection in pancreatic cancer. J Surg Res 2008;147:216–20.
34. Maithel SK, Maloney S, Winston C, et al. Preoperative CA 19-9 and the yield of staging laparoscopy in patients with radiographically resectable pancreatic adenocarcinomas. Ann Surg Oncol 2008;15:3512–20.
35. Bradley EL. Pancreatoduodenectomy for pancreatic adenocarcinoma. Triumph, triumphalism, or transition? Arch Surg 2002;137:771–3.
36. Reddy S, Wolfgang CL, Cameron JL, et al. Total pancreatectomy for pancreatic adenocarcinoma: evaluation of morbidity and long-term survival. Ann Surg 2009;250:282–7.

37. Nathan H, Wolfgang CL, Edil BH, et al. Peri-operative mortality and long-term survival after total pancreatectomy for pancreatic adenocarcinoma: a population-based perspective. J Surg Oncol 2009;99:87–92.
38. Schmidt CM, Glant J, Winter JM, et al. Total pancreatectomy (R0 resection) improves survival over subtotal pancreatectomy in isolated neck margin positive pancreatic adenocarcinoma. Surgery 2007;142:572–80.
39. Hernandez J, Mullinax J, Clark W, et al. Survival after pancreaticoduodenectomy is not improved by extending resections to achieve negative margins. Ann Surg 2009;250:76–80.
40. Pedrazzoli S, DiCarlo V, Dionigi R, et al. Standard versus extended lymphadenectomy associated with pancreatoduodenectomy in the surgical treatment of adenocarcinoma of the head of the pancreas: a multicenter, prospective, randomized trial. Ann Surg 1998;228:508–17.
41. Farnell MB, Pearson RK, Sarr MG, et al. A prospective randomized trail comparing standard pancreatoduodenectomy with pancreatoduodenectomy with extended lymphadenectomy in resectable pancreatic head adenocarcinoma. Surgery 2005;138:618–28.
42. Riall TS, Cameron JL, Lillemoe KD, et al. Pancreaticoduodenectomy with or without distal gastrectomy and extended retroperitoneal lymphadenectomy for periampullary adenocarcinoma – part 3: update on 5-year survival. J Gastrointest Surg 2005;9:1191–204.
43. Farnell MB, Aranha GV, Nimura Y, et al. The role of extended lymphadenectomy for adenocarcinoma of the head of the pancreas: strength of the evidence. J Gastrointest Surg 2008;12:651–6.
44. Fortner JG. Regional resection of cancer of the pancreas: a new surgical approach. Surgery 1973;73:307–20.
45. Fortner JG, Fortner JG, Kim DK, et al. Regional pancreatectomy: en bloc pancreatic, portal vein and lymph node resection. Ann Surg 1977;186(1):42–50.
46. Ramacciato G, Mercantini P, Petrucciani N, et al. Does portal-superior mesenteric vein invasion still indicate irresectability for pancreatic carcinoma? Ann Surg Oncol 2009;16:817–25.
47. Martin RCG, Scoggins CR, Egnatashvili V, et al. Arterial and venous reconstruction for pancreatic adenocarcinoma: operative and long-term outcomes. Arch Surg 2009;144:154–9.
48. Adham M, Mirza DF, Chapui F, et al. Results of vascular resections during pancreatectomy from two European centres: an analysis of survival and disease-free survival explicative factors. HPB (Oxford) 2006;8:465–73.
49. Sugiura Y, Horio T, Aiko S, et al. Pancreatectomy for pancreatic cancer with reference to combined resection of the vessels, twenty nine year experience by a single surgeon. Keio J Med 2009;58:103–9.
50. Siriwardana HP, Siriwardena AK. Systematic review of outcome of synchronous portal-superior mesenteric vein resection during pancreatectomy for cancer. Br J Surg 2006;93:662–73.
51. Stojadinovic A, Brooks A, Hoos A, et al. An evidence-based approach to the surgical management of resectable pancreatic adenocarcinoma. J Am Coll Surg 2003;196:954–64.
52. Karanicolas PJ, Davies E, Kunz R, et al. The pylorus: take it or leave it? Systematic review and meta-analysis of pylorus-preserving versus standard Whipple pancreaticoduodenectomy for pancreatic or periampullary cancer. Ann Surg Oncol 2007;14:1825–34.

53. Diener MK, Knaebel HP, Heukaufer C, et al. A systematic review and meta-analysis of pylorus-preserving versus classical pancreaticoduodenectomy for surgical treatment of periampullary and pancreatic carcinoma. Ann Surg 2007; 245:187–200.

54. Huang JJ, Yeo CJ, Sohn TA, et al. Quality of life after pancreaticoduodenectomy. Ann Surg 2000;231:890–8.

55. Crippa S, Dominguez I, Rodriguez JR, et al. Quality of life in pancreatic cancer: analysis by stage and treatment. J Gastrointest Surg 2008;12:783–94.

56. Trede M. Invited critique. Arch Surg 2002;137:773.

57. Vento P, Mustonen H, Joensuu T, et al. Impact of preoperative chemoradiotherapy on survival in patients with resectable pancreatic cancer. World J Gastroenterol 2007;13:2945–51.

58. Morganti AG, Massaccesi M, La Torre G, et al. A systematic review of resectability and survival after concurrent chemoradiation in primarily unresectable pancreatic cancer. Ann Surg Oncol 2009. DOI:10.1245/s10434-009-0762-4.

59. Winter JM, Cameron JL, Campbell KA, et al. 1423 pancreaticoduodenectomies for pancreatic cancer: a single-institution experience. J Gastrointest surg 2006; 10:1199–210.

60. Grobmyer SR, Pieracci FM, Allen PJ, et al. Defining morbidity after pancreaticoduodenectomy: use of a prospective complication grading system. J Am Coll Surg 2007;204:356–64.

61. Pratt WB, Vollmer CM, Callery MP. Outcomes in pancreatic surgery are negatively influenced by pre-operative hospitalization. HPB (Oxford) 2009;11:57–65.

62. Kazanjian KK, Hines OJ, Duffy JP, et al. Improved survival following pancreaticoduodenectomy to treat adenocarcinoma of the pancreas: the influence of operative blood loss. Arch Surg 2008;143:1166–71.

63. Fernandez-del-Castillo C, Rattner DW, Warshaw AL. Standards for pancreatic resection in the 1990s. Arch Surg 1995;130:295–300.

64. Simons JP, Shah SA, Ng SC, et al. National complication rates after pancreatectomy: beyond mere mortality. J Gastrointest Surg 2009;13:1798–805.

65. Reddy DM, Townsend CM Jr, Kuo Y, et al. Readmission after pancreatectomy for pancreatic cancer in Medicare patients. J Gastrointest Surg 2009;13:1963–75.

66. DeOliveira ML, Winter JM, Shafer M, et al. Assessment of complications after pancreatic surgery: a novel grading system applied to 633 patients undergoing pancreaticoduodenectomy. Ann Surg 2006;244:931–9.

67. Clavien PA, Sanabria JR, Strasberg SM. Proposed classification of complications of surgery with examples of utility in cholecystectomy. Surgery 1992;111: 518–26.

68. Rodriguez JB, Soto Germes S, Pandharipande PV, et al. Implications and cost of pancreatic leak following distal pancreatic resection. Arch Surg 2006;141: 361–6.

69. Schmidt CM, Choi J, Powell ES, et al. Pancreatic fistula following pancreaticoduodenectomy: clinical predictors and patient outcomes. HPB Surg 2009; 2009:404520.

70. Adams DB. The pancreatic anastomosis: the danger of a leak, which anastomotic technique is better? J Gastrointest Surg 2009;13:1182–3.

71. Luft HS, Bunker JP, Enthoven AC. Should operations be regionalized? The empirical relationship between surgical volume and mortality. N Engl J Med 1979;301:1364–9.

72. Vollmer CM Jr, Pratt W, Vanounou T, et al. Quality assessment in high-acuity surgery – volume and mortality are not enough. Arch Surg 2007;142:371–80.

73. Joseph B, Morton JM, Hernandez-Boussard T, et al. Relationship between hospital volume, system clinical resources, and mortality in pancreatic resection. J Am Coll Surg 2009;208:520–7.

74. Halm EA, Lee C, Chassin MR. Is volume related to outcome in health care? A systematic review and methodologic critique of the literature. Ann Intern Med 2002;137:511–20.

75. Ihse I. The volume-outcome relationship in cancer surgery: a hard sell. Ann Surg 2003;238:777–81.

76. Khuri SF, Henderson WG. The case against volume as a measure of quality in surgical care. World J Surg 2005;29:1222–9.

77. Leapfrog Group Website. Available at: http://www.leapfroggroup.org/home. Accessed November 1, 2009.

78. Birkmeyer JD, Siwers AE, Finlayson EVA, et al. Hospital volume and surgical mortality in the United States. N Engl J Med 2002;346:1128–37.

79. Birkmeyer JD, Stukel TA, Siewers AE, et al. Surgeon volume and operative mortality in the United States. N Engl J Med 2003;349:2117–27.

80. Eppsteiner RW, Csikesz NG, McPhee JT, et al. Surgeon volume impacts hospital mortality for pancreatic resection. Ann Surg 2009;249:635–40.

81. Nathan H, Cameron JL, Choti MA, et al. The volume-outcome effect in hepato-pancreato-biliary surgery: hospital versus surgeon contributions and the specificity of the relationship. J Am Coll Surg 2009;208:528–38.

82. Parks RW, Bettschart V, Frame S, et al. Benefits of subspecialisation in the management of pancreatic cancer: results of a Scottish population-based study. Br J Cancer 2004;91:459–65.

83. Csikesz NC, Simons JP, Tseng JF, et al. Surgical specialization and operative mortality in hepato-pancreatico-biliary (HPB) surgery. J Gastrointest surg 2008;12:1534–9.

84. Tseng JF, Pisters PWT, Lee JE, et al. The learning curve in pancreatic surgery. Surgery 2007;141:694–701.

85. Birkmeyer JD, Warshae LW, Finlayson SRG, et al. Relationship between hospital volume and late survival after pancreaticoduodenectomy. Surgery 1999;126: 178–83.

86. Dimick JB, Welch HG. The zero mortality paradox in surgery. J Am Coll Surg 2008;206:13–6.

87. Schell MT, Barcia A, Spitzer AL, et al. Pancreaticoduodenectomy: volume is not associated with outcome within an academic health care system. HPB Surg 2008;2008:825940.

88. Mukhtar RA, Kattan OM, Harris HW. Variation in annual volume at a university hospital does not predict mortality for pancreatic resections. HPB Surg 2008;2008:190914.

89. Birkmeyer JD, Dimick JB. Potential benefits of the new Leapfrog standards: effect of process and outcome measures. Surgery 2004;135:569–75.

90. Lwin AK, Shepard DS. Estimating lives saved from universal adoption of the Leapfrog safety and quality standards: 2008 update. Available at: http://www.leapfroggroup.org/about_us/how_and_why. Accessed November 9, 2009.

91. Shahian DM, Normand ST. The volume-outcome relationship: from Luft to Leapfrog. Ann Thorac Surg 2003;75:1048–58.

92. Cunningham JD, O'Donnell N, Starker P. Surgical outcomes following pancreatic resection at a low-volume community hospital: do all patients need to be sent to a regional cancer center? Am J Surg 2009;198:227–30.

93. Gasper WJ, Glidden DV, Chengshi J, et al. Has recognition of the relationship between mortality rates and hospital volume for major cancer surgery in

California made a difference? A follow-up analysis of another decade. Ann Surg 2009;25:472–83.

94. Murphy MM, Knaus WJ, Ng SC, et al. Total pancreatectomy: a national study. HPB (Oxford) 2009;11:476–82.

95. Rosemurgy A, Cowgill S, Coe B, et al. Frequency with which surgeons undertake pancreaticoduodenectomy continues to determine length of stay, hospital charges, and in-hospital mortality. J Gastrointest Surg 2008;12:442–9.

96. Van Heek NT, Kuhlmann KFD, Scholten RJ, et al. Hospital volume and mortality after pancreatic resection. A systematic review and an evaluation of intervention in the Netherlands. Ann Surg 2005;242:781–90.

97. Ghaferi AA, Birkmeyer JD, Dimick JB. Variation in hospital mortality associated with inpatient surgery. N Engl J Med 2009;361:1368–75.

98. Jacobs DO. Variation in hospital mortality associated with inpatient surgery – an S.O.S. N Engl J Med 2009;361:1398–9.

99. Lemmens L, van Zelm R, Borel Rinkes I, et al. Clinical and organizational content of clinical pathways for digestive surgery: a systematic review. Dig Surg 2009; 26:91–9.

100. Porter GA, Pisters PW, Mansyur C, et al. Cost and utilization impact of a clinical pathway for patients undergoing pancreaticoduodenectomy. Ann Surg Oncol 2000;7:484–9.

101. Kennedy EP, Rosato EL, Sauter PK, et al. Initiation of a critical pathway for pancreaticoduodenectomy at an academic institution – the first step in multidisciplinary team building. J Am Coll Surg 2007;204:917–23.

102. Kennedy EP, Grenda TR, Sauter PK, et al. Implementation of a critical pathway for distal pancreatectomy at an academic institution. J Gastrointest Surg 2009; 13:938–44.

103. Maa J, Gosnell JE, Gibbs VC, et al. Exporting excellence for Whipple resection to refine the Leapfrog initiative. J Surg Res 2007;138:189–207.

Evidence-Based Imaging of Pancreatic Malignancies

Timothy Kinney, MD

KEYWORDS

- Pancreatic cancer • Computed tomography
- Endoscopic ultrasound • Cystic neoplasms

Pancreatic cancer is the fourth leading cancer-related cause of death in the United States. Complete surgical resection is the only curative therapy for pancreatic cancer, yet only 20% of patients diagnosed with pancreatic cancer undergo attempted curative surgical resection.[1] Pancreatic malignancies often present with subtle, nonspecific symptoms and have a tendency to invade and metastasize early. Thus, most patients are found to have advanced disease based on imaging criteria at the time of diagnosis.

It is essential for the surgeon to have a thorough understanding of the strengths and weaknesses of the various imaging modalities of the pancreas to make well-informed management decisions. Overstaging a tumor based on inaccuracy or misinterpretation of imaging findings may preclude the possibility of a curative resection, whereas understaging will lead to unnecessary exploratory surgery.

Computed tomography (CT) is the primary method for diagnosing and staging pancreatic malignancy. CT of the pancreas is well complemented by endoscopic ultrasound (EUS), which is more sensitive for detecting early lesions, allows for relatively easy access to the pancreas for tissue diagnosis by fine-needle aspiration (FNA), and provides further important information for tumor staging. Magnetic resonance imaging (MRI) and positron emission tomography (PET) scanning can also play a role under special circumstances when CT and EUS leave questions remaining.

This article reviews the literature supporting the use of various imaging modalities to evaluate pancreatic malignancies. The strengths and weaknesses of each modality for assessing pancreatic neoplasms are discussed, and suggestions as to the best use of each test are made. A final section discussing imaging characteristics that are unique to various cystic neoplasms is included.

Department of Medicine, Division of Gastroenterology, Hennepin County Medical Center, 701 Park Avenue, Minneapolis, MN 55415, USA
E-mail address: kinn0049@umn.edu

Surg Clin N Am 90 (2010) 235–249
doi:10.1016/j.suc.2009.12.003
0039-6109/10/$ – see front matter © 2010 Elsevier Inc. All rights reserved.

surgical.theclinics.com

ULTRASOUND

In most centers, ultrasound is used only as an initial screening test for evaluating suspected pancreaticobiliary disease. Ultrasound is universally available, inexpensive, and noninvasive, and does not carry any risk of iodinated contrast used with CT. Ultrasound is useful for detecting biliary dilation and characterizing cystic lesions of the pancreas when not obscured by body habitus or overlying gas.

Transabdominal ultrasound can provide extraordinary detail for diagnosis and staging of pancreatic malignancies when performed by experts, with results comparable even to CT.[2] Obtaining such results is highly operator dependent, however, and overlying adipose tissue, bowel gas, and patient discomfort often limit the utility of transabdominal ultrasound for evaluating the pancreas.

Newer investigational techniques are in development, such as using carbon dioxide microbubbles as a real-time intravenous contrast agent, using tissue harmonic imaging to improve image quality, and using elastography to provide information about the tissue structure and content. These adjunctive ultrasound technologies may help with vascular staging, help identify malignant lymphadenopathy, or help detect tumor within the setting of inflammation and pancreatitis.[3–8] These techniques are still in their infancy, and further research is required before they are more widely adopted. For the foreseeable future, transabdominal ultrasound will remain an initial screening test for patients with abdominal complaints, who then move on to other imaging modalities.

COMPUTED TOMOGRAPHY

CT remains the most important and useful imaging modality for evaluating pancreatic malignancies. Although other imaging modalities can offer important complementary information, CT provides the most comprehensive evaluation for diagnosis and surgical staging for pancreatic malignancies. CT offers highly accurate T staging, including local invasion and vascular involvement. As with other modalities, CT is less accurate at diagnosing early nodal involvement and metastatic disease. CT technology has advanced significantly over the past several years, and improvements continue in both imaging hardware and software for image processing. Newer multidetector helical CT technology allows for very thin sliced cuts, providing higher image resolution and faster image acquisition. Images can be obtained during both arterial and venous phases of contrast injection. Advanced imaging processing software can provide not only standard multiplanar images but also oblique cuts to highlight anatomic structures, curved planar reformation images, and high-quality volume-rendered 3dimensional (3D) reconstructed images (**Fig. 1**).

Pancreatic Protocol CT

The ideal imaging modality for evaluating pancreatic cancer will not only optimally visualize the pancreatic parenchyma and associated vessels but also evaluate the liver and other organs for metastases. The pancreas is maximally enhanced just after the arterial contrast phase, as contrast travels from the great vessels into the splanchnic arteries and arterioles, and courses through the pancreatic parenchyma.[9] The liver is supplied primarily from the portal venous system and is optimally enhanced later during the venous phase. The typical dual-phase pancreatic protocol CT therefore includes image acquisition just after the arterial phase when the pancreas is maximally enhanced, and then again in the venous phase during peak liver enhancement.[10]

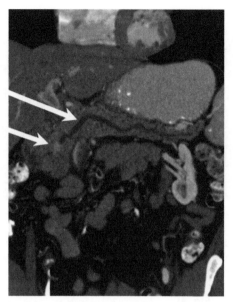

Fig. 1. The entire length of this dilated pancreatic duct is shown in this curved planar reformation image. A hypervascular enhancing neuroendocrine tumor can be seen in the pancreatic head (*arrows*). (*Courtesy of* Dr Gopal Punjabi.)

Diagnosis and Staging of Pancreatic Cancer by CT

The vast majority of solid malignancies of the pancreas are poorly attenuating on CT scan, because of hypovascularization of these tumors. Whereas they can be difficult to see in noncontrast studies, these lesions typically appear as a dark area within the gland during the arterial contrast phase when the rest of the gland is maximally enhanced (**Figs. 2** and **3**).

A much smaller proportion of pancreatic adenocarcinomas are isoattenuating, making diagnosis by CT much more difficult. A series by Prokesh and colleagues[11] reported that 11% of solid pancreatic malignancies were isoattenuating on CT. In this setting, the presence of a mass is suspected by secondary signs such as

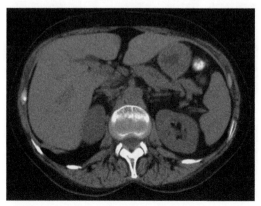

Fig. 2. Precontrast injection showing no evidence of tumor.

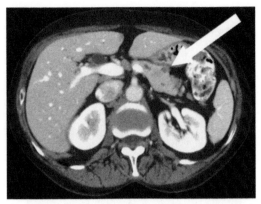

Fig. 3. Postcontrast shows a hypoattenuating adenocarcinoma (*arrow*).

pancreatic or biliary ductal dilatation. Dilatation of either the pancreatic duct or bile duct is a common imaging finding and can be seen in up to two-thirds of patients with pancreatic adenocarcinoma.[12] Pancreatic adenocarcinomas are rarely hyperattenuating. Hypervascular enhancing pancreatic tumors are typically associated with neuroendocrine tumors (**Fig. 4**).

Sensitivity for diagnosing early pancreatic cancer is critically important for any imaging study because of the tendency of pancreatic cancer to metastasize early in the disease course. CT sensitivity is very high for larger pancreatic lesions, but sensitivity drops with lesions less than 1.5 to 2 cm. A study by Leggman and colleagues[13] reported 100% sensitivity for lesions measuring 15 mm or larger, dropping to 67% sensitivity for lesions less than 15 mm in diameter. Another more recent study by Bronstein and colleagues[14] reported only 77% sensitivity for pancreatic lesions less than 20 mm. As CT technology and imaging resolution continues to improve, it is hoped the sensitivity for detecting early lesions of the pancreas will also improve.

CT for Tumor Staging

CT is very accurate for staging pancreatic malignancy. Local tumor extension and vascular invasion can be well delineated on CT. A study by Karmazanovsky and

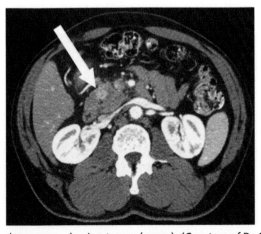

Fig. 4. A hypervascular neuroendocrine tumor (*arrow*). (*Courtesy of* Dr Gopal Punjabi.)

colleagues[15] looking at accuracy of CT for surgical staging found a sensitivity and specificity of 94% for diagnosing vascular invasion. Various grading systems have been suggested to assess vascular invasion by CT imaging. A study by Lu and colleagues[16] showed that the extent of contiguity with the vessels on CT correlated with the likelihood of invasion, with 50% to 75% contiguity associated with 88% likelihood of invasion and greater than 75% with 100% invasion. O'Malley and colleagues[17] suggested that 75% contiguity on CT imaging should be required before denying surgery based on vascular invasion by imaging, to maximize the chance to undergo surgery. Other indicators of vascular invasion include the "teardrop" sign and morphologic deformation of the vessel at the tumor site.[18,19] Dilation of the peripancreatic veins was shown by Hommeyer and colleagues[20] to predict T4 disease with 100% specificity.

CT does not fare nearly as well for assessing nodal metastases. Early micrometastases to lymph nodes can only be detected by histologic evaluation, and early nodal metastases will be missed on imaging if nodal enlargement has not yet occurred. Studies assessing for nodal involvement by CT have primarily used size criteria. Roche and colleagues[21] studied lymph node size criteria to assess for the presence of malignant lymphadenopathy. Using a cutoff nodal diameter of 10 mm in the short access for diagnosing abnormal lymphadenopathy led to a fairly high specificity for tumor invasion of 85%, but sensitivity for invasion was low, at only 14%. When a 5-mm cutoff diameter was used, the sensitivity was increased to 71%; however, specificity dropped to 64%. Lymph node shape or morphologic criteria have generally not been shown in CT studies to be overly helpful in determining malignant status.

Diagnosing metastases to the liver and peritoneum is an important part of preoperative staging. Peritoneal implants and carcinomatosis can be very difficult to diagnose by any imaging modality in early stages.[10] Peritoneal metastases can manifest as ascites, abnormal peritoneal enhancement, and omental thickening on CT.[10,22,23] In the liver, CT performs well for detecting larger metastatic lesions, but small hepatic nodules less than 1 cm can be problematic[10] (**Figs. 5** and **6**). These lesions are common, and typically they are found to be benign. Schwartz and colleagues[24]

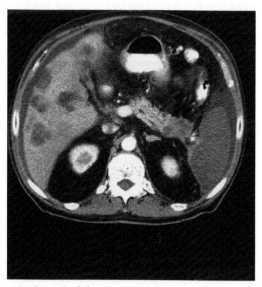

Fig. 5. A mass is seen in the tail of the pancreas with obvious liver metastases.

reported only an 11% incidence of malignancy in small hepatic nodules found on CT during workup of patients with cancer.

Not infrequently, patients are found to have metastases only at the time of surgery. A study by Liu and Traverso[25] found 34% of patients had evidence of metastases on diagnostic laparoscopy despite having no evidence of metastatic disease on CT imaging.

ENDOSCOPIC ULTRASOUND

EUS was developed in the 1980s as a minimally invasive method for imaging and obtaining tissue from the deep-seated organs such as the pancreas and biliary tree. Whereas pancreatic imaging via transabdominal ultrasound can be obstructed by overlying bowel gas and adipose tissue, EUS allows for placement of the ultrasound transducer within close proximity to the pancreas. Very high resolution imaging of the pancreas and associated vascular structures can be obtained, and tissue can be readily sampled using FNA. Interpretation of EUS imaging is somewhat operator dependent, and the steep learning curve for training in EUS has limited the number of well-trained endoscopists in the past. There are now several active training centers around the world, and EUS is becoming much more prevalent.

Diagnosing Pancreatic Malignancy by EUS

EUS is the most sensitive examination for detecting pancreatic tumors. The sensitivity of EUS for the detection of pancreatic cancer is as high as 97%, and compares favorably to CT, particularly with small lesions.[26] Whereas sensitivity of CT begins to decline in pancreatic lesions smaller than 1.5 to 2 cm, EUS can detect lesions measuring 2 to 3 mm.[27,28] In patients with worrisome signs or symptoms for pancreatic malignancy, EUS should be considered for further evaluation despite a negative CT scan.[29]

EUS with FNA offers a relatively easy way of obtaining tissue to establish a cytologic diagnosis (**Fig. 7**). There is debate as to whether patients with early lesions on CT should go straight to surgery without a tissue diagnosis, or whether further staging and tissue sampling should be performed. Diagnostic and therapeutic algorithms differ in various institutions based on local practice patterns and expertise, but it can be argued that in some high-risk patients it may be prudent to obtain as much information as possible to plan surgical intervention so as not to be surprised in the operating room. Especially in

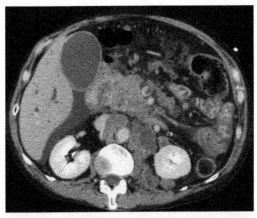

Fig. 6. Retroperitoneal metastases and peritoneal metastases in the setting of pancreatic adenocarcinoma.

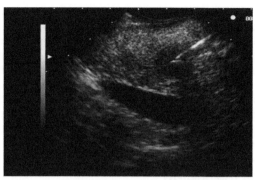

Fig. 7. Fine-needle aspiration performed of a pancreatic adenocarcinoma. (*Courtesy of* Dr Shawn Mallery.)

cases in which resectability may be in question by CT imaging, performing EUS can contribute to preoperative planning. Also in these "borderline" resectable cases, neoadjuvant chemoradiation may be considered and under most circumstances, a tissue diagnosis is needed before initiating adjuvant treatment.[30,31]

EUS for Pancreatic Cancer Staging

EUS is an accurate modality for pancreas cancer staging, comparable and complementary to CT. T-stage accuracy has varied from 64% to 94% in some studies, with N-stage accuracy from 54% to 82%.[32–37] EUS can be very sensitive for detecting vascular invasion and assessing resectability, with sensitivity greater than 90% in some studies,[32,33,38] although more recent studies have not shown such impressive results.[39] EUS provides excellent views of the portal and splenic vein, but it can be difficult to visualize the superior mesenteric vein and artery.[38] An EUS study by Snady and colleagues[40] showed that all patients with dilated peripancreatic collateral vessels, loss of vascular interface, or tumor within the vessel lumen of a major peripancreatic vessel had vascular invasion at the time of surgery. Dewitt and colleagues[41] reviewed 11 studies comparing EUS with CT to assess accuracy for staging of pancreatic cancer. Among the 9 studies comparing tumor detection, all 9 concluded that EUS was superior to CT. With regard to T staging, this review found that more recent studies showed CT was comparable with or even superior to EUS for local T staging and equivalent for N staging. The studies comparing CT and EUS for vascular invasion showed mixed results.

In summary, EUS is more sensitive for detecting early pancreatic malignancies. Whereas CT and EUS are fairly equivalent and perhaps complementary for cancer staging, EUS with FNA allows for tissue diagnosis, which may be important especially when considering neoadjuvant chemoradiation in patients who are "borderline" resectable.

MAGNETIC RESONANCE IMAGING

Although most surgeons are not as comfortable interpreting MR images as they are with CT, MR can be used both to assess the pancreatic parenchyma and to provide high-quality images of fluid-filled structures such as the pancreatic ductal systems and pancreatic cysts. MR can be useful in patients with poor renal function who may be poor candidates for contrast CT. As with CT imaging, adenocarcinoma of the pancreas appears hypointense on T1-weighted images both pre- and postcontrast injection.

MR is likely not as sensitive as CT or EUS for detecting adenocarcinoma. A meta-analysis of 68 studies by Bipat and colleagues[42] showed MR to be less sensitive than CT (84% vs 91%) for detection of pancreatic cancer and about equal to CT for determining resectability. As with CT, newer MR technology and software can obtain excellent 3D reconstructed images with a single breath hold. The addition of secretin stimulation to MR cholangiopancreatography not only can enhance the pancreatic ductal imaging but also may provide information regarding pancreatic function.[43] MR may offer some advantage in visualizing tumor in the setting of pancreatic inflammation, a problem that plagues all imaging technologies.[44,45] MR can also delineate small hepatic nodules that are difficult to characterize on CT.[46]

POSITRON EMISSION TOMOGRAPHY

^{18}F-fluorodeoxyglucose (FDG) is a positron-emitting radiotracer that accumulates and is expressed in cancer cells to a much higher degree than in normal tissue. FDG-PET can be used to diagnose local or metastatic disease, although the limited spacial resolution of FDG-PET makes it a poor test for staging (**Fig. 8**). Like CT, FDG-PET scans have limited sensitivity for lesions smaller than 1 cm. A study by Frolich and colleagues[47] showed 97% detection of lesions greater than 1 cm whereas lesions less than 1 cm were only seen in 43% of cases. PET/CT scans combine tumor affinity of PET scanning with the spatial recognition of CT. Data regarding the utility of PET or PET/CT for the diagnosis or staging of pancreatic cancer are lacking, however. A meta-analysis of several studies comparing PET/CT versus CT alone showed that despite benefit for diagnosis and staging in many individual cases, the data did not support routine use of PET/CT.[48]

IMAGING CYSTIC NEOPLASMS OF THE PANCREAS

Small cystic lesions of the pancreas are often asymptomatic and are found incidentally on cross-sectional imaging. Cystic lesions of the pancreas can represent either benign disease (serous cystadenomas, pseudocysts) or premalignant/malignant mucinous

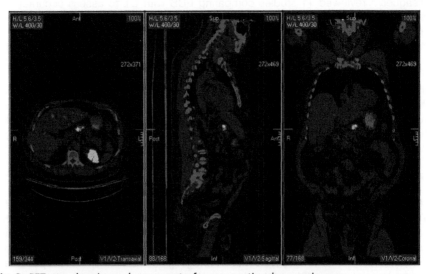

Fig. 8. PET scan showing enhancement of a pancreatic adenocarcinoma.

neoplasms. While mucinous neoplasms can present at advanced stages and act as aggressively as any solid pancreatic adenocarcinoma, cystic neoplasms can also have a more indolent course, taking several years before degenerating into invasive cancer. Using imaging for surveillance has an important role in patients who are not optimal surgical candidates and have neoplasms that lack any invasive features.[49–51]

The same imaging modalities used to evaluate solid pancreatic neoplasms are used to evaluate cystic lesions of the pancreas, although EUS and MR play a greater role in the examination of cystic lesions. Owing to its sensitivity and ability to highlight fluid-filled lesions, MR can provide better resolution than CT for evaluating small cystic lesions less than 3 cm, as well as for defining ductal communication and cyst morphology.[52,53] FDG-PET has not been extensively studied in cystic pancreatic neoplasms, but may provide evidence for malignant transformation in certain settings.[54]

Because of the diverse features of various cystic pancreatic neoplasms, the diagnostic and imaging characteristics of the more common cystic neoplasms are reviewed in the following sections.

Serous Cystadenomas

Serous cystadenomas (SCAs) are benign cystic lesions of the pancreas, and are the most common cystic pancreatic neoplasm.[55] Most SCAs have a classic microcystic or honeycombed appearance on CT scan, and commonly have a central "sunburst" calcification. Less common is the macrocystic variant, with fewer, larger septated cysts (**Fig. 9**). Macrocystic variants of SCA can be more difficult to diagnose by CT criteria alone, with an appearance similar to mucinous neoplasms. SCAs are filled with serous fluid rather than mucin, and EUS plays an important role in establishing the diagnosis not only by imaging features but also by sampling of the cyst contents, which can be analyzed to look for mucin as well as tumor markers such as carcinoembryonic antigen (CEA) and carbohydrate antigen 19-9.[56,57]

Intraductal Papillary Mucinous Neoplasms

Intraductal papillary mucinous neoplasms (IPMNs) are malignant or premalignant mucin-filled cystic lesions associated with pancreatic ductal dilatation. IPMNs can have an appearance ranging from a large irregular polycystic mass to simple dilatation of a small side branch of the pancreatic duct. IPMNs typically arise in elderly patients and can be found in any part of the gland. Imaging features play an important role in

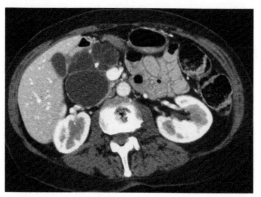

Fig. 9. A macrocystic-variant serous cystadenoma with a central calcification. (*Courtesy of* Dr Gopal Punjabi.)

IPMN, as these lesions frequently occur in elderly patients who may be poor surgical candidates, and certain imaging features suggest a benign course. It is important to differentiate side-branch variant IPMN from main duct IPMN, as main branch IPMN is associated with a higher prevalence of invasive cancer at 57% to 92%. Side-branch variant IPMN has a more indolent course with a 6% to 46% risk of malignant transformation.[58–60]

CT can highlight important features of IPMN such as ductal enhancement, determination of side-branch versus main-branch disease, and a mural nodule within the lesion. Main or side duct dilation greater than 10 mm, mural nodules, solid components within the duct, and calcified intraluminal contents suggest malignancy.[53,61] MR can also be helpful in evaluating IPMN for malignant characteristics. In one MR series of 27 malignant IPMNs, main pancreatic duct wall nodules were observed in 16 carcinomas, and duct wall enhancement was observed in 20 carcinomas.[62]

EUS with FNA is very useful for evaluating IPMN. EUS can help to delineate main branch from side branch involvement, identify and biopsy mural nodules, and aspirate fluid content for mucin evaluation and cytologic markers[63] (**Fig. 10**). Brugge and colleagues[64] used EUS to study 341 patients with pancreatic cysts and showed that CEA levels greater than 192 had a higher incidence of mucinous cysts. The presence of mucin on needle aspiration is specific but not sensitive, and one study showed that special stains for mucin were positive in only 54% of patients with IPMN.[65]

Mucinous Cystic Neoplasms

Mucinous cystic neoplasms (MCNs) are typically round, septated masses that do not communicate with the pancreatic duct. MCNs commonly occur in younger patients and should be considered premalignant, with approximately 25% of patients having cancer at time of diagnosis.[66] CT imaging typically shows a thick cyst wall around a macrocystic, multiloculated lesion.[67,68] Findings of invasive disease on CT include calcification of the cyst wall, mural nodule, a solid component, or size greater than 3 cm in diameter.[69–71] As with IPMNs, EUS with FNA plays an important role in establishing the diagnosis of MCN, and fluid aspiration to assess for mucin and cytologic

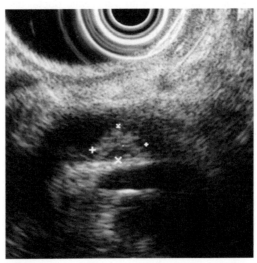

Fig. 10. EUS imaging of a nodule within a dilated pancreatic duct in a patient with IPMN. (*Courtesy of* Dr Shawn Mallery.)

markers can be performed. One pooled analysis found that CEA levels greater than 800 ng/mL was 98% specific for MCN.[72]

Pseudocysts

Pancreatic pseudocysts form after an episode of clinical pancreatitis, either from pancreatic necrosis or a duct leak. High-quality CT with a good clinical history is typically enough to diagnose a pseudocyst. In atypical-appearing lesions, EUS can analyze the fluid content for debris that is more common in pseudocysts, and sampling of the fluid should show a high amylase level with benign cytologic markers.[73,74] Other rare lesions including solid pseudopapillary tumors, lymphoepithelial cysts, and cystadenocarcinomas are evaluated similarly to other pancreatic lesions, starting with CT and followed by EUS or other modalities when further clarification is needed.

SUMMARY

A high-quality pancreatic protocol CT is the primary imaging modality for diagnosing and staging pancreatic malignancy. The main limitation of CT is the lack of sensitivity for early pancreatic lesions. EUS provides an excellent complement to CT for both diagnosis and staging of pancreatic cancer, and allows easy access for needle aspiration and tissue diagnosis. MR can be helpful for evaluating small hepatic nodules or cystic lesions of the pancreas, but in general, the role of MR and PET remains limited to special situations when the results of CT and EUS are equivocal.

REFERENCES

1. Yeo CJ, Cameron JL. Improving results of pancreaticoduodenectomy for pancreatic cancer. World J Surg 1999;23:907–12.
2. Morrin MM, Kruskal JB, Raptopoulos V, et al. State-of-the-art ultrasonography is as accurate as helical computed tomography and computed tomographic angiography for detecting unresectable periampullary cancer. J Ultrasound Med 2001;20:481–90.
3. Kinney TP, Freeman ML. Recent advances and novel methods in pancreatic imaging. Minerva Gastroenterol Dietol 2008;54:85–95.
4. Brambs HJ, Claussen CD. Pancreatic and ampullary carcinoma. Ultrasound, computed tomography, magnetic resonance imaging and angiography. Endoscopy 1993;25:58–68.
5. Uomo G. Ultrasound elastography. A possible improvement into the paraphernalia of pancreatic imaging. JOP 2008;9:666–7.
6. Hohl C, Schmidt T, Haage P, et al. Phase-inversion tissue harmonic imaging compared with conventional B-mode ultrasound in the evaluation of pancreatic lesions. Eur Radiol 2004;14:1109–17.
7. Balci NC, Semelka RC. Radiologic diagnosis and staging of pancreatic ductal adenocarcinoma. Eur J Radiol 2001;38:105–12.
8. Koito K, Namieno T, Nagakawa T, et al. Inflammatory pancreatic masses: differentiation from ductal carcinomas with contrast-enhanced sonography using carbon dioxide microbubbles. AJR Am J Roentgenol 1997;169:1263–7.
9. Lu DS, Vedantham S, Krasny RM, et al. Two-phase helical CT for pancreatic tumors: pancreatic versus hepatic phase enhancement of tumor, pancreas, and vascular structures. Radiology 1996;199:697–701.
10. Wong JC, Lu DS. Staging of pancreatic adenocarcinoma by imaging studies. Clin Gastroenterol Hepatol 2008;6:1301–8.

11. Prokesch RW, Chow LC, Beaulieu CF, et al. Isoattenuating pancreatic adenocarcinoma at multi-detector row CT: secondary signs. Radiology 2002;224:764–8.

12. Fulcher AS, Turner MA. MR pancreatography: a useful tool for evaluating pancreatic disorders. Radiographics 1999;19:5–24 [discussion: 41–4; quiz: 148–9].

13. Legmann P, Vignaux O, Dousset B, et al. Pancreatic tumors: comparison of dual-phase helical CT and endoscopic sonography. AJR Am J Roentgenol 1998;170:1315–22.

14. Bronstein YL, Loyer EM, Kaur H, et al. Detection of small pancreatic tumors with multiphasic helical CT. AJR Am J Roentgenol 2004;182:619–23.

15. Karmazanovsky G, Fedorov V, Kubyshkin V, et al. Pancreatic head cancer: accuracy of CT in determination of resectability. Abdom Imaging 2005;30:488–500.

16. Lu DS, Reber HA, Krasny RM, et al. Local staging of pancreatic cancer: criteria for unresectability of major vessels as revealed by pancreatic-phase, thin-section helical CT. AJR Am J Roentgenol 1997;168:1439–43.

17. O'Malley ME, Boland GW, Wood BJ, et al. Adenocarcinoma of the head of the pancreas: determination of surgical unresectability with thin-section pancreatic-phase helical CT. AJR Am J Roentgenol 1999;173:1513–8.

18. Hough TJ, Raptopoulos V, Siewert B, et al. Teardrop superior mesenteric vein: CT sign for unresectable carcinoma of the pancreas. AJR Am J Roentgenol 1999;173:1509–12.

19. Li H, Zeng MS, Zhou KR, et al. Pancreatic adenocarcinoma: the different CT criteria for peripancreatic major arterial and venous invasion. J Comput Assist Tomogr 2005;29:170–5.

20. Hommeyer SC, Freeny PC, Crabo LG. Carcinoma of the head of the pancreas: evaluation of the pancreaticoduodenal veins with dynamic CT—potential for improved accuracy in staging. Radiology 1995;196:233–8.

21. Roche CJ, Hughes ML, Garvey CJ, et al. CT and pathologic assessment of prospective nodal staging in patients with ductal adenocarcinoma of the head of the pancreas. AJR Am J Roentgenol 2003;180:475–80.

22. Diehl SJ, Lehmann KJ, Sadick M, et al. Pancreatic cancer: value of dual-phase helical CT in assessing resectability. Radiology 1998;206:373–8.

23. Walkey MM, Friedman AC, Sohotra P, et al. CT manifestations of peritoneal carcinomatosis. AJR Am J Roentgenol 1988;150:1035–41.

24. Schwartz LH, Gandras EJ, Colangelo SM, et al. Prevalence and importance of small hepatic lesions found at CT in patients with cancer. Radiology 1999;210:71–4.

25. Liu RC, Traverso LW. Diagnostic laparoscopy improves staging of pancreatic cancer deemed locally unresectable by computed tomography. Surg Endosc 2005;19:638–42.

26. Hunt GC, Faigel DO. Assessment of EUS for diagnosing, staging, and determining resectability of pancreatic cancer: a review. Gastrointest Endosc 2002;55:232–7.

27. Rosch T, Lightdale CJ, Botet JF, et al. Localization of pancreatic endocrine tumors by endoscopic ultrasonography. N Engl J Med 1992;326:1721–6.

28. Rosch T, Lorenz R, Braig C, et al. Endoscopic ultrasound in pancreatic tumor diagnosis. Gastrointest Endosc 1991;37:347–52.

29. Kinney TP, Lai R, Freeman ML. Endoscopic approach to acute pancreatitis. Rev Gastroenterol Disord 2006;6:119–35.

30. Turrini O, Viret F, Moureau-Zabotto L, et al. Neoadjuvant 5 fluorouracil-cisplatin chemoradiation effect on survival in patients with resectable pancreatic head adenocarcinoma: a ten-year single institution experience. Oncology 2009;76:413–9.

31. Satoi S, Yanagimoto H, Toyokawa H, et al. Surgical results after preoperative che-moradiation therapy for patients with pancreatic cancer. Pancreas 2009;38: 282–8.

32. Palazzo L, Roseau G, Gayet B, et al. Endoscopic ultrasonography in the diag-nosis and staging of pancreatic adenocarcinoma. Results of a prospective study with comparison to ultrasonography and CT scan. Endoscopy 1993;25:143–50.

33. Gress FG, Hawes RH, Savides TJ, et al. Role of EUS in the preoperative staging of pancreatic cancer: a large single-center experience. Gastrointest Endosc 1999;50:786–91.

34. Tio TL, Tytgat GN, Cikot RJ, et al. Ampullopancreatic carcinoma: preoperative TNM classification with endosonography. Radiology 1990;175:455–61.

35. Grimm H, Maydeo A, Soehendra N. Endoluminal ultrasound for the diagnosis and staging of pancreatic cancer. Baillieres Clin Gastroenterol 1990;4:869–88.

36. Muller MF, Meyenberger C, Bertschinger P, et al. Pancreatic tumors: evalu-ation with endoscopic US, CT, and MR imaging. Radiology 1994;190: 745–51.

37. Yasuda K, Mukai H, Nakajima M. Endoscopic ultrasonography diagnosis of pancreatic cancer. Gastrointest Endosc Clin N Am 1995;5:699–712.

38. Brugge WR, Lee MJ, Kelsey PB, et al. The use of EUS to diagnose malignant portal venous system invasion by pancreatic cancer. Gastrointest Endosc 1996;43:561–7.

39. Aslanian H, Salem R, Lee J, et al. EUS diagnosis of vascular invasion in pancre-atic cancer: surgical and histologic correlates. Am J Gastroenterol 2005;100: 1381–5.

40. Snady H, Bruckner H, Siegel J, et al. Endoscopic ultrasonographic criteria of vascular invasion by potentially resectable pancreatic tumors. Gastrointest Endosc 1994;40:326–33.

41. DeWitt J, Devereaux B, Chriswell M, et al. Comparison of endoscopic ultrasonog-raphy and multidetector computed tomography for detecting and staging pancreatic cancer. Ann Intern Med 2004;141:753–63.

42. Bipat S, Phoa SS, van Delden OM, et al. Ultrasonography, computed tomography and magnetic resonance imaging for diagnosis and determining resectability of pancreatic adenocarcinoma: a meta-analysis. J Comput Assist Tomogr 2005; 29:438–45.

43. Kinney TP, Punjabi G, Freeman M. Technology insight: applications of MRI for the evaluation of benign disease of the pancreas. Nat Clin Pract Gastroenterol Hep-atol 2007;4:148–59.

44. Ichikawa T, Sou H, Araki T, et al. Duct-penetrating sign at MRCP: usefulness for differentiating inflammatory pancreatic mass from pancreatic carcinomas. Radi-ology 2001;221:107–16.

45. Johnson PT, Outwater EK. Pancreatic carcinoma versus chronic pancreatitis: dynamic MR imaging. Radiology 1999;212:213–8.

46. Sica GT, Ji H, Ros PR. Computed tomography and magnetic resonance imaging of hepatic metastases. Clin Liver Dis 2002;6:165–79, vii.

47. Frohlich A, Diederichs CG, Staib L, et al. Detection of liver metastases from pancreatic cancer using FDG PET. J Nucl Med 1999;40:250–5.

48. Orlando LA, Kulasingam SL, Matchar DB. Meta-analysis: the detection of pancre-atic malignancy with positron emission tomography. Aliment Pharmacol Ther 2004;20:1063–70.

49. Farnell MB. Surgical management of intraductal papillary mucinous neoplasm (IPMN) of the pancreas. J Gastrointest Surg 2008;12:414–6.

50. Fasanella KE, McGrath K. Cystic lesions and intraductal neoplasms of the pancreas. Best Pract Res Clin Gastroenterol 2009;23:35–48.
51. Tanaka M, Chari S, Adsay V, et al. International consensus guidelines for management of intraductal papillary mucinous neoplasms and mucinous cystic neoplasms of the pancreas. Pancreatology 2006;6:17–32.
52. Song SJ, Lee JM, Kim YJ, et al. Differentiation of intraductal papillary mucinous neoplasms from other pancreatic cystic masses: comparison of multirow-detector CT and MR imaging using ROC analysis. J Magn Reson Imaging 2007;26:86–93.
53. Sahani DV, Kadavigere R, Blake M, et al. Intraductal papillary mucinous neoplasm of pancreas: multi-detector row CT with 2D curved reformations—correlation with MRCP. Radiology 2006;238:560–9.
54. Mansour JC, Schwartz L, Pandit-Taskar N, et al. The utility of F-18 fluorodeoxyglucose whole body PET imaging for determining malignancy in cystic lesions of the pancreas. J Gastrointest Surg 2006;10:1354–60.
55. Op de Beeck B, Spinhoven M, Corthouts B, et al. Management of cystic pancreatic masses. JBR-BTR 2007;90:482–6.
56. Bassi C, Salvia R, Gumbs AA, et al. The value of standard serum tumor markers in differentiating mucinous from serous cystic tumors of the pancreas: CEA, Ca 19-9, Ca 125, Ca 15-3. Langenbecks Arch Surg 2002;387:281–5.
57. Fernandez-del Castillo C, Alsfasser G, Targarona J, et al. Serum CA19-9 in the management of cystic lesions of the pancreas. Pancreas 2006;32:220.
58. Agostini S, Choux R, Payan MJ, et al. Mucinous pancreatic duct ectasia in the body of the pancreas. Radiology 1989;170:815–6.
59. Farrell JJ, Brugge WR. Intraductal papillary mucinous tumor of the pancreas. Gastrointest Endosc 2002;55:701–14.
60. McDonald JM, Williard W, Mais D, et al. The incidence of intraductal papillary mucinous tumors of the pancreas(1). Curr Surg 2000;57:610–4.
61. Jang JY, Kim SW, Ahn YJ, et al. Multicenter analysis of clinicopathologic features of intraductal papillary mucinous tumor of the pancreas: is it possible to predict the malignancy before surgery? Ann Surg Oncol 2005;12:124–32.
62. Manfredi R, Graziani R, Motton M, et al. Main pancreatic duct intraductal papillary mucinous neoplasms: accuracy of MR imaging in differentiation between benign and malignant tumors compared with histopathologic analysis. Radiology 2009; 253:106–15.
63. Kubo H, Nakamura K, Itaba S, et al. Differential diagnosis of cystic tumors of the pancreas by endoscopic ultrasonography. Endoscopy 2009;41:684–9.
64. Brugge WR, Lewandrowski K, Lee-Lewandrowski E, et al. Diagnosis of pancreatic cystic neoplasms: a report of the cooperative pancreatic cyst study. Gastroenterology 2004;126:1330–6.
65. Michaels PJ, Brachtel EF, Bounds BC, et al. Intraductal papillary mucinous neoplasm of the pancreas: cytologic features predict histologic grade. Cancer 2006;108:163–73.
66. Levy MJ, Clain JE. Evaluation and management of cystic pancreatic tumors: emphasis on the role of EUS FNA. Clin Gastroenterol Hepatol 2004;2:639–53.
67. Kim SY, Lee JM, Kim SH, et al. Macrocystic neoplasms of the pancreas: CT differentiation of serous oligocystic adenoma from mucinous cystadenoma and intraductal papillary mucinous tumor. AJR Am J Roentgenol 2006;187:1192–8.
68. Sahani DV, Kadavigere R, Saokar A, et al. Cystic pancreatic lesions: a simple imaging-based classification system for guiding management. Radiographics 2005;25:1471–84.

69. Allen PJ, D'Angelica M, Gonen M, et al. A selective approach to the resection of cystic lesions of the pancreas: results from 539 consecutive patients. Ann Surg 2006;244:572–82.
70. Goh BK, Tan YM, Chung YF, et al. A review of mucinous cystic neoplasms of the pancreas defined by ovarian-type stroma: clinicopathological features of 344 patients. World J Surg 2006;30:2236–45.
71. Warshaw AL, Compton CC, Lewandrowski K, et al. Cystic tumors of the pancreas. New clinical, radiologic, and pathologic observations in 67 patients. Ann Surg 1990;212:432–43 [discussion: 444–5].
72. van der Waaij LA, van Dullemen HM, Porte RJ. Cyst fluid analysis in the differential diagnosis of pancreatic cystic lesions: a pooled analysis. Gastrointest Endosc 2005;62:383–9.
73. Frossard JL, Amouyal P, Amouyal G, et al. Performance of endosonography-guided fine needle aspiration and biopsy in the diagnosis of pancreatic cystic lesions. Am J Gastroenterol 2003;98:1516–24.
74. Song MH, Lee SK, Kim MH, et al. EUS in the evaluation of pancreatic cystic lesions. Gastrointest Endosc 2003;57:891–6.

The Role of Endoscopic Ultrasonography in the Evaluation of Pancreatico-Biliary Cancer

Shyam Varadarajulu, MD, Mohamad A. Eloubeidi, MD, MHS*

KEYWORDS

- Endosonography • Endoscopic ultrasound
- Fine needle aspiration • Celiac plexus neurolysis
- Interventional EUS • Pancreatic cancer
- Neuroendocrine tumor • Cancer staging

Pancreatic cancer is the fourth leading cause of cancer-related deaths in the United States and develops in approximately 30,000 people annually. The disease is associated with a high mortality rate and a median survival of approximately 4 months in untreated patients. Data from the National Cancer Database show the 5-year survival rate after surgery to be 3%.[1] If surgery achieves clear margins and negative lymph nodes, the 5-year survival rate approaches 25%. Most patients diagnosed with pancreatic cancer present at an advanced stage of the disease when surgical cure is no longer possible. When the cancer is unresectable, chemotherapy, radiation therapy, or a combination of the two may improve overall survival and quality of life.

The regional anatomy of the pancreas is complex, making procurement of cytologic samples difficult without exploratory laparotomy. Traditionally, CT-guided fine-needle aspiration (FNA) has been used for biopsy of the pancreas. This technique is associated with a risk of peritoneal dissemination of cancer cells and has a false-negative rate of up to 20%.[2,3] Endoscopic retrograde cholangiopancreatography (ERCP) brush cytology has a false-negative rate of nearly 30%.[4]

With endoscopic ultrasonography (EUS), it is possible to position the transducer in direct proximity to the pancreas by means of the stomach and duodenum. The

This article originally appeared in *Gastrointestinal Endoscopy Clinics of North America* Volume 15, Issue 3.
Department of Gastroenterology and Hepatology and the Pancreatico-biliary Center, the University of Alabama at Birmingham, 1530 3rd Avenue, South - ZRB 636, Birmingham, AL 35294-0007, USA
* Corresponding author.
E-mail address: meloubeidi@uabmc.edu

high-frequency transducer enables production of detailed high-resolution images of the pancreas that far surpass those of CT or MRI. The high resolution of these images allows identification of lesions as small as 2 to 3 mm and their relationship to adjacent blood vessels, such as the portal vein and mesenteric vasculature (**Fig. 1**). An added advantage of EUS is the ability to perform FNA. Compared with other imaging modalities, the results of EUS-FNA of pancreatic masses are excellent, with a sensitivity of 85% to 90% and a specificity of virtually 100%.[5–7] The procedure is safe, with reported complication rates being <1%.[8] EUS-guided therapies, such as celiac plexus neurolysis for pain control and direct injection of cytotoxins into malignant lesions, are becoming important adjuncts in the management of patients with surgically unresectable disease. This article focuses on the role of EUS in the diagnosis and staging of malignant pancreatic lesions.

PANCREATIC ADENOCARCINOMA
Accuracy of Staging by Endoscopic Ultrasonography

EUS staging of pancreatic and other tumors follows the (T)umor, (N)ode (M)etastasis system of the American Joint Committee on Cancer (AJCC). In 2002, the AJCC modified the T staging system for pancreatic cancer to classify tumors invading the portal venous (superior mesenteric vein or portal vein) (see **Fig. 1**) system as T3 (these were previously staged as T4) and tumors invading the celiac or superior mesenteric artery as T4 (**Fig. 2**). Although this change is likely to result in decreased reported accuracy for EUS, it remains unclear if surgical therapy is beneficial compared with radiochemotherapy for tumors invading the portal venous system. Most literature is based on the previous AJCC staging system, in which all mesenteric vascular invasion (venous or arterial) were staged T4.

Many large series have found T-stage accuracy to range from approximately 78% to 94% and nodal (N)-stage accuracy to range from 64% to 82%.[9–12] Lower accuracy has also been described. In a study of 89 patients in whom EUS was compared with surgical and histopathologic TNM staging,[13] the overall accuracy of EUS for

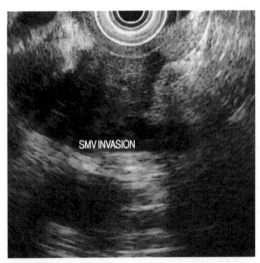

Fig. 1. Radial EUS image (Olympus GF-UM 130; range 6 cm, frequency 7.5 Mhz) of a patient with pancreatic head mass invading the superior mesenteric vein (SMV).

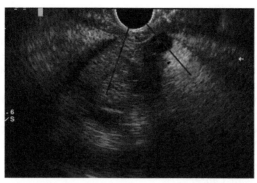

Fig. 2. Curvilinear echoendoscope image (Olympus UC-30 P, scanning at 5 Mhz) with Doppler reveals mass in pancreatic body with splenic artery invasion.

T and N staging was 69% and 54%, respectively. Only 46% of tumors believed to be resectable by EUS were found to be resectable during laparotomy. Staging accuracy of EUS can be influenced by several factors, including the experience level of the endosonographer, imaging artifacts, and the endosonographer's knowledge of the results of previous imaging tests. In general, T-stage accuracy for EUS is highest in patients with smaller tumors, whereas helical CT is more accurate in staging larger tumors.[14–16] The accuracy of EUS for detecting invasion into the superior mesenteric artery and vein is lower than that for detecting portal or splenic vein invasion.[17,18]

A recent review[19] that pooled data from four studies comparing the accuracy of EUS with helical CT in the evaluation of pancreatic cancer found that EUS detected more tumors (97% vs 73%), was more accurate for determining tumor resectability (91% vs 83%), and was more sensitive for detecting vascular invasion (91% vs 64%). When the data were interpreted individually, two of the reports concluded that CT and EUS were approximately equivalent in detecting the primary tumors,[14,20] whereas the other two found EUS to be superior.[21,22] Several features of the individual reports may account for these variable conclusions, including differences in the gold standards, variations in the specific techniques used for helical CT, and the proportion of patients with advanced disease in each study. A reasonable conclusion from these data and from clinical experience is that EUS and helical CT are complementary for staging pancreatic cancer. EUS is a more accurate modality for local T staging and for predicting vascular invasion, especially in tumors <3 cm, whereas helical CT is better for the evaluation of distant metastasis and for staging larger tumors. Similar to CT, studies comparing MRI with EUS suggest that EUS may be more sensitive for detecting small tumors while providing complementary information regarding resectability.[23]

Recent advances in CT technology, including the development of spiral scanners and more recently multidetector CT (MDCT) scanners, and the development of three-dimensional (3D) imaging software have improved the ability of CT to image the pancreas and to evaluate a wide range of pancreatic pathology. In most of the published series, older dynamic scanners or single-row spiral scanners were used, and 3D imaging was not included. With the narrow collimation and faster scanning possibilities with new MDCT scanners, it is likely that the CT accuracy for detecting pancreatic tumor will improve. In a recently published study by McNulty and colleagues[24] using MDCT, 27 of 28 pancreatic cancers were detected. This progress will continue as manufacturers introduce the next generation of scanners, which can acquire up to 32 slices per second with faster scan times. The impact of these new scanners on diagnostic accuracy will need to be carefully evaluated.

Several studies have compared the accuracy of angiography and EUS for determining vascular invasion.[17,18,25] Although the results varied, a general conclusion is that EUS is as accurate or more accurate for determining vascular invasion, with the exception of some tumors that invade the superior mesenteric artery. In a study of 21 patients with pancreatic cancer who underwent EUS and angiography before an attempt at curative resection, EUS was more sensitive than angiography for detecting vascular invasion (86% vs 21%). The specificity and accuracy of EUS were 71% and 81%, respectively, compared with 71% and 38% for angiography.[23]

Role of Endoscopic Ultrasonography-guided Fine-needle Aspiration in Pancreatic Cancer

EUS has an important role in guiding a biopsy needle into lesions that are too small to be identified by CT or MRI or too well encased by surrounding vascular structures to safely allow percutaneous biopsy (**Figs. 3** and **4**).[26] The impact of EUS-FNA was studied by Chang and colleagues[27] in a series of 44 patients. EUS-FNA had an accuracy rate of 95% for pancreatic lesions and 88% for lymph nodes. Three patients had enlarged celiac nodes on EUS that showed malignancy on FNA. FNA precluded surgery in 41% of the patients, avoided the need for further diagnostic tests in 57%, and influenced clinical decisions in 68% of the patients, thus providing substantial cost savings. Gress and colleagues[26] examined the role of EUS-FNA in patients with suspected pancreatic cancer after a negative CT-guided FNA or ERCP brush cytology. Of 102 patients, 57 had positive cytology on EUS-FNA, and 37 had negative cytology. The examination was inconclusive in eight patients. After a median follow-up of 24 months, all 57 patients with positive cytology on EUS-FNA had verification of the diagnosis of pancreatic cancer. Of the 45 patients with negative or inconclusive cytology on EUS-FNA, 41 had no evidence of pancreatic malignancy at follow-up. One important application of EUS-FNA is the detection of malignant lymph nodes. FNA has been demonstrated to increase the accuracy of lymph node staging and thereby reduce the number of unnecessary surgical explorations by identifying patients with surgically incurable disease.[27]

Lesions located in the uncinate process of the pancreas are the most difficult to puncture. To access a mass in the uncinate process, the echoendoscope must be advanced into the duodenal C-loop in the "long" position. This exerts substantial angulation and torque on the FNA needle. The needle is more difficult to advance,

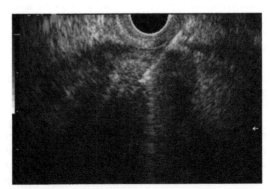

Fig. 3. Linear EUS image (Olympus UC-30 P, scanning at 5 Mhz) of a patient with pancreatic head mass undergoing EUS-FNA.

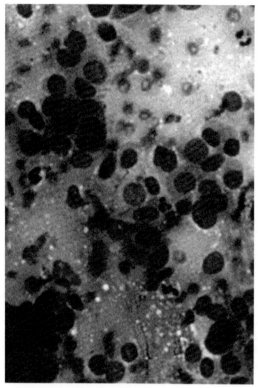

Fig. 4. Cytologic features consistent with malignancy (Papanicoulou stain 40×).

and the procedure causes a "bowed shape" in the needle. This altered shape can result in mistargeting. Lesions in the pancreatic isthmus pose a similar challenge in that the echoendoscope is usually in the "long" scope position with the tip in the gastric antrum.

A transgastric approach can be more difficult than the transduodenal approach due to the laxity and redundancy of the gastric wall and the capaciousness of the stomach. Lacking anchorage, the echoendoscope tends to displace during advancement of the FNA needle.

A controversial issue is identifying who should undergo EUS-FNA **(Box 1)**. There is general consensus that it is reasonable to obtain a tissue diagnosis in patients suspected of having pancreatic cancer who are poor surgical candidates. Histologic confirmation in such patients can be helpful in deciding on chemotherapy or radiotherapy. More controversial is the role of EUS-FNA in patients suspected of having pancreatic cancer who seem to be resectable on other imaging studies. One view is that a tissue diagnosis does not alter management and is therefore unnecessary. This argument is supported by the recognition that the sensitivity of EUS-FNA is in the range of 85% to 90%, thereby potentially leading to false-negative results in up to 15% of patients. An argument can be made for EUS-FNA in such patients when the establishment of a histologic diagnosis before surgery may alter management because other types of malignancy involving the pancreas can mimic adenocarcinoma (eg, lymphoma). Therapy for these tumors may not include surgery. Some patients and physicians want to know definitively whether cancer is present before

---

Box 1
Indications for the use of EUS-FNA

- To document a diagnosis of malignancy in a patient with an unresectable mass as a prerequisite for adjuvant chemotherapy or radiation therapy

- To exclude other tumor types, such as lymphoma, small-cell metastasis, or neuroendocrine cancer, that may require a different management strategy

- To determine a diagnosis in patients who are reluctant to undergo major surgery without a definitive diagnosis

- To document the absence of malignancy when the pretest probability of malignancy is low

---

undergoing a surgical resection. When the FNA is negative, some patients may be willing to accept the 15% chance of missing a diagnosis of cancer rather than undergoing surgery. This is especially true when there is concurrent acute or chronic pancreatitis that may mimic a focal pancreatic cancer.

Role of Endoscopic Ultrasonography in Metastatic Pancreatic Cancer

An emerging role for EUS is the detection of small, occult liver metastases in patients with pancreatic tumors. Although EUS is best suited for loco-regional staging, its high resolution and proximity to the left lobe and inferior right lobe of the liver has led to detection of small liver metastases.[28,29] The ability to perform immediate EUS-FNA allows accurate distinction of benign from malignant lesions. A recent study reported the results of EUS-FNA of liver lesions in 167 patients (including 62 with pancreatic cancer), all of whom had negative or equivocal CT or ultrasound (US) of the liver. EUS-FNA was highly accurate, with a complication rate of 4%. One death occurred when EUS-FNA of a liver lesion was performed in the setting of an obstructed biliary stent, leading to cholangitis. Antibiotic prophylaxis and biliary drainage should be used in conjunction with EUS-FNA of liver lesions in the setting of obstructing pancreatic tumors.[29]

Another emerging role of EUS is the identification of small, occult pancreatic tumors in the patients with liver metastases of "unknown" primary. In the report by ten-Berge and colleagues,[29] EUS identified a pancreatic tumor in 17 of 33 patients whose CT showed only metastatic tumor of unknown primary. The identification of a pancreas primary allowed pancreas-specific chemotherapy to be administered in each of these cases.

Safety and Complications of Endoscopic Ultrasonography-guided Fine-needle Aspiration

The safety of EUS-FNA for evaluating pancreatic lesions is well established.[30,31] Rare complications include pancreatitis, infection, and bleeding. In a multicenter study evaluating the safety of EUS-FNA of solid pancreatic masses, 14 of 4958 patients developed pancreatitis.[30] In another study involving EUS-FNA of pancreatic cystic lesions, 1 of 81 patients developed an infected cystadenoma after EUS-FNA.[31] This patient did not receive prophylactic antibiotics before the procedure. The current standard of care includes routine administration of antibiotics for patients undergoing FNA of pancreatic cystic lesions.

Management of Pancreatic Focal Solid Masses

Accurate staging of patients with pancreatic cancer is critical to avoid the expense, morbidity, and mortality related to unnecessary surgery. Although several tests are available for assessing such patients, consensus has not been achieved on the optimal approach. Thus, the role of EUS and EUS-FNA varies among treatment centers. EUS has a more prominent role at our institution (**Fig. 5**). We recommend that helical CT be performed initially to evaluate for the presence of a pancreatic mass. EUS is most clearly indicated when no clear tumor or only equivocal changes are seen on CT. If metastatic disease is evident, EUS or CT-guided biopsy can establish the diagnosis. If the helical CT is negative for metastatic disease or an obvious mass, EUS should be performed to further evaluate the pancreas (if the clinical suspicion is high for pancreatic cancer) followed by EUS-FNA of any apparent mass noted.

Neuroendocrine Tumors

Pancreatic endocrine tumors are often small and hard to detect by radiologic techniques. Since the original description of gastrinomas in 1955 by Zollinger and Ellison,[32] multiple imaging modalities have been evaluated to localize pancreatic neuroendocrine lesions for surgical resection. Studies have shown that CT, MRI, and conventional US detect tumors in less than 50% of patients.[33] Somatostatin receptor scintigraphy (SRS) is reported to have the highest sensitivity for gastrinomas but is less accurate for detecting insulinomas.[34] The optimal algorithm for staging pancreatic neuroendocrine tumors is unknown. Issues important for clinical management include (1) Is the tumor localized to the region of the pancreas (including gastrinoma triangle) or metastatic? (2) Is the tumor unifocal or multifocal within the pancreas? and (3) Is it functional or nonfunctional, benign or malignant?

To determine whether a tumor is localized or metastatic, cross-sectional imaging and SRS are likely more accurate than EUS due to their ability to image broad areas.[35] For imaging within the pancreas, EUS provides superior resolution and accuracy compared with CT scan. In a study of 82 patients, Anderson and colleagues[35] identified 100 tumors in 54 patients, emphasizing the frequency of multifocal tumors. EUS accurately localized the tumor in 93% of patients and had a specificity of 95%, which was higher than CT or transabdominal US. EUS was not reliable for detection of extrapancreatic tumors. Zimmer and colleagues[36] compared EUS with CT, SRS, US, and MRI in 40 patients with neuroendocrine tumors. EUS had the highest overall accuracy for gastrinomas and insulinomas but missed 50% of extra pancreatic tumors. In a report of patients who had negative ultrasonography and CT scans, EUS detected endocrine tumors in the pancreas with high sensitivity (82%) and specificity (95%).[37]

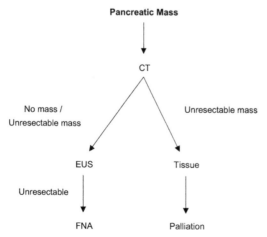

Fig. 5. Algorithm for management of pancreatic cancer.

In patients with nonfunctioning neuroendocrine tumors where the risk of surgery is high, it is useful to distinguish benign from malignant neuroendocrine tumors. In two studies, EUS was able to accurately distinguish malignant lesions based on the presence of an irregular inhomogeneous hypoechoic mass or on invasion and obstruction of the pancreatic duct.[38,39] Tumors without these features were almost always benign.

Intraductal Ultrasonography and Neuroendocrine Tumors

Intraductal endoscopic ultrasonography (IDUS) involves the insertion of an ultra-thin (2 mm) US probe directly into the pancreatic duct during ERCP. Preliminary experience suggests that it may be more accurate than standard EUS for the detection of neuroendocrine tumors. Although experience with IDUS is limited, initial data suggest that IDUS may improve the evaluation of these patients and lead to the identification of tumors arising within the pancreas that have gone unrecognized by other techniques.[40,41] In one study, IDUS was able to identify the presence of an islet cell tumor in seven of seven patients.[41] In one of these patients who had multifocal disease, IDUS accurately determined the number of tumors, whereas EUS failed to detect all lesions. The distance from the tumors to the main pancreatic duct was accurately determined, thus aiding preoperative planning of wedge resection, which was possible in two patients.

EUS can be useful for preoperative localization of pancreatic endocrine tumors by its ability to tattoo lesions by fine-needle injection using India ink.[42] This may shorten operative time because it obviates the need to localize the tumor by palpation and intraoperative US. This technique may have the potential to facilitate tumor resection by less invasive methods, such as laparoscopic enucleation.

These data suggest that EUS serves an important role in localizing tumors within the pancreas, detecting multifocal tumors, and distinguishing benign from malignant tumors. In addition, EUS should be used with cross-sectional imaging and SRS to identify extra-pancreatic tumors or metastases.

CHOLANGIOCARCINOMA

Cholangiocarcinoma is a difficult neoplasm to diagnose non-operatively. Although ERCP remains the modality of choice for characterizing common bile duct strictures, a definitive histologic diagnosis of a neoplastic stricture is not made in many patients despite aggressive endoscopic techniques, including the combination of brushings, biopsy, and FNA.[43–46] Without a histologic or cytologic diagnosis of cancer, potentially beneficial therapy may be inappropriately withheld. Left untreated, more than 95% of afflicted patients die within 1 to 2 years. To achieve the best survival rates, complete radical tumor resections, including major partial hepatectomies, are usually required. These procedures remain challenging, with a mortality rate of 8% to 10% and a complication rate of 37% to 64%.[47–49] Because of the therapeutic dilemma and technical challenges of radical surgery, patients need to be chosen carefully because only 20% to 49% fulfill the criteria for resectability to undergo radical surgery and because about 20% may have diagnoses other than cholangiocarcinoma, and surgery might not be the first choice for therapy in these patients.[50,51] Therefore, it seems preferable to have a histologic diagnosis available before attempting curative surgical resection so that individualized treatment can be provided.

Accuracy of Endoscopic Ultrasonography-guided Fine-needle Aspiration in Cholangiocarcinoma

Although EUS can identify biliary strictures, tissue diagnosis is crucial for differentiation of malignant versus benign lesions. Two prospective studies have evaluated the role of EUS-FNA in biliary strictures (**Fig. 6**). In the first study, 44 patients with strictures at the liver hilum underwent EUS-FNA. The accuracy, sensitivity, and specificity for diagnosis of cholangiocarcinoma were 91%, 89%, and 100%, respectively. EUS and EUS-FNA changed the pre-planned surgical approach in 27 of 44 patients.[52] In the second study, 28 patients with previously failed tissues diagnosis underwent EUS-FNA of biliary strictures.[53] The sensitivity, specificity, positive predictive value, negative predictive value, and accuracy of EUS-FNA were 86%, 100%, 100%, 57%, and 88%, respectively. EUS-FNA had a positive impact on patient management in 84% of patients: preventing surgery for tissue diagnosis in patients with inoperable disease ($n = 10$), facilitating surgery in patients with unidentifiable cancer by other modalities ($n = 8$), and avoiding surgery in benign disease ($n = 4$). No major complications were reported in either study. Both studies were done at tertiary referral centers by expert endosonographers. It remains to be seen whether these results can be replicated and reproduced in other settings. EUS is most optimal for lesions in the mid- or distal bile duct. Hilar lesions, when not visualized by EUS, can usually be seen using the IDUS probes with the caveat that tissue procurement is not possible.

Technique of Endoscopic Ultrasonography-guided Fine-needle Aspiration

The technique of EUS-FNA of biliary lesions is more difficult and slightly different from FNA of pancreatic mass lesions. Evaluation of the bile duct is usually started with the echo endoscope positioned at the papilla. By gradually withdrawing and rotating the instrument cephalad into the duodenal bulb and pylorus region, the common bile duct up to the proximal part can be visualized. A stent, when present, serves as a guide to follow the bile duct. When the tip of the scope is placed and bent posteriorly just beyond the pylorus, the hepatic hilum can be well identified, with the tumor appearing as an echo-poor transductal lesion. This enables assessment of the biliary lesion, its spread in the liver and relation to portal vein and hepatic arteries, and the presence and status of lymph nodes. Color Doppler US is useful to verify the different vessels in or in relation to the liver because the anatomy of the hepatic arteries can vary. While the hilar area is imaged, the echoendoscope often tends to slip back into the stomach and needs frequent repositioning; this is of concern, particularly when performing FNA of hilar lesions. To circumvent the problem, the scope can be brought into a "long

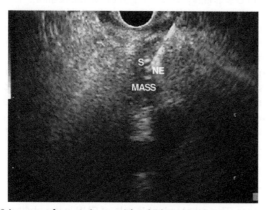

Fig. 6. Linear EUS-image of a patient with cholangiocarcinoma undergoing EUS-FNA (Olympus UC-140T, scanning at 5 Mhz). FNA needle (NE) is advanced into a hypoechoic mass that is associated with the bile duct containing a biliary stent (S).

position" to allow the wall of the greater curve to provide support for the force exerted when the needle is advanced into the tumor.

Intraductal Ultrasound
The IDUS probe used for local staging of biliary strictures can be inserted into the bile duct at ERCP over a guide wire. Although initial studies suggested a need for biliary sphincterotomy, a new small-diameter IDUS probe has been developed that obviates the need for sphincterotomy.[54] Its small diameter and monorail design allows insertion over a 0.035-inch guidewire and greatly simplifies IDUS. The IDUS image of the normal bile duct wall comprises two or three sonographic layers: An outer hyperechoic layer represents the adipose layer of the subserosa, the serosa, and the interface echo between serosa and surrounding organs. Occasionally a third inner hyperechoic layer is identified and represents an interface echo.

IDUS criteria that suggest malignancy include a hypoechoic mass, especially if it is infiltrating surrounding tissues, heterogeneity of the internal echo pattern, notching or irregularity of the outer border, a papillary surface, and disruption of the normal sonographic structure of the duct.[55,56] In a study by Menzel and colleagues[56] that included 56 consecutive patients with bile duct strictures and obstructive jaundice, IDUS was more accurate than EUS (89% vs 76%, $P<0.002$) for determining the nature of the bile duct strictures. IDUS was also better for determining the resectability of bile duct tumors (82% vs 76%, $P<0.0002$) and T stage (78% vs 54%, $P<0.001$). Although IDUS does not reliably determine the nature of a stricture in all cases, the findings may be useful in directing management. As suggested by Tamada and colleagues,[55] when IDUS identifies disruption of the wall layers by a protruding tumor, surgical exploration is indicated, even in the absence of tissue confirmation of malignancy. When IDUS demonstrates a localized tumor or polypoid lesion in the presence of a normal-appearing wall, directed biopsy specimens should be obtained. If a polypoid mass identified by IDUS is >8 mm in diameter, even when the wall layers are preserved, malignancy is likely. When IDUS fails to identify a localized intraductal lesion, even if cholangiography suggests irregularity of the duct, the need for further diagnostic evaluation becomes less certain.

IDUS improves the accuracy of local tumor staging of bile duct carcinomas. One study found that local tumor staging by IDUS was accurate in 77% of patients compared with 54% for staging by EUS.[56] The benefit of IDUS over EUS may be even greater for tumors arising from mid-duct to bifurcation. The limited depth of penetration restricts the value of IDUS for assessing tumor extension outside the hepatoduodenal ligament and precludes assessment of distant metastasis (M-stage). The utility of IDUS for lymph node assessment (N-stage) is uncertain and likely limited by the inability to perform FNA.

Bile duct wall thickening may result from tumor spread or inflammation, and IDUS cannot reliably distinguish both in all instances. This is relevant in patients with prior biliary stents. One study found that the presence of a bile duct stent for at least 14 days correlated with the development of wall thickening, possibly as the result of inflammation.[57] Hence, a better understanding of the factors that influence bile duct wall thickening would be helpful.

SUMMARY

EUS is now established as an accurate method for staging malignancies of the pancreatico-biliary system. The most valuable role of EUS is the ability to identify patients unlikely to be cured from surgical excision due to vascular invasion or regional nodal metastasis. The ability to obtain tissue confirmation plays a critical role in identifying those patients unsuitable for surgical therapy but would benefit from palliation. EUS and EUS-FNA are invaluable additions to our armamentarium for the management of pancreatico-bilary cancers.

REFERENCES

1. Stephens J, Kuhn J, O'Brien J, et al. Surgical morbidity, mortality, and long-term survival in patients with peripancreatic cancer following pancreaticoduodenectomy. Am J Surg 1997;174:600–4.
2. Murr MM, Sarr MG, Oishi AJ, van Heerden JA. Pancreatic cancer. CA Cancer J Clin 1994;44:304–18.
3. Bret PM, Nicolet V, Labadie M. Percutaneous fine-needle aspiration biopsy of the pancreas. Diagn Cytopathol 1986;2:221–7.
4. Lee JG, Leung J. Tissue sampling at ERCP in suspected pancreatic cancer. Gastrointest Endosc Clin North Am 1998;8:221–35.
5. Eloubeidi MA, Jhala D, Chhieng DC, et al. Yield of endoscopic ultrasound-guided fine-needle aspiration biopsy in patients with suspected pancreatic carcinoma. Cancer 2003;99:285–92.
6. Gress F, Gottlieb K, Sherman S, et al. Endoscopic ultrasonography- guided fine-needle aspiration biopsy of suspected pancreatic cancer. Ann Intern Med 2001; 134:459–64.
7. Harewood GC, Wiersema MJ. Endosonography-guided fine needle aspiration biopsy in the evaluation of pancreatic masses. Am J Gastroenterol 2002;97:1386–91.
8. Wiersema MJ, Vilmann P, Giovannini M, et al. Endosonography guided fine-needle aspiration biopsy: diagnostic accuracy and complication assessment. Gastroenterology 1997;112:1087–95.
9. Rosch T, Lorenz R, Braig C, et al. Endoscopic ultrasound in pancreatic tumor diagnosis. Gastrointest Endosc 1991;37:347–52.
10. Palazzo L, Roseau G, Gayet B, et al. Endoscopic ultrasonography in the diagnosis and staging of pancreatic adenocarcinoma: results of a prospective study with comparison to ultrasonography and CT scan. Endoscopy 1993;25:143–50.
11. Gress FG, Hawes RH, Savides TJ, et al. Role of EUS in the preoperative staging of pancreatic cancer: a large single-center experience. Gastrointest Endosc 1999;50:786–91.
12. Yasuda K, Mukai H, Nakajima M, et al. Staging of pancreatic carcinoma by endoscopic ultrasonography. Endoscopy 1993;25:151–5.
13. Ahmad NA, Lewis JD, Ginsberg GG, et al. EUS in preoperative staging of pancreatic cancer. Gastrointest Endosc 2000;52:463–8.
14. Legmann P, Vignaux O, Dousset B, et al. Pancreatic tumors: comparison of dual phase helical CT and endoscopic sonography. Am J Roentgenol 1998;170: 1315–22.
15. Yasuda K, Mukai H, Fujimoto S, et al. The diagnosis of pancreatic cancer by endoscopic ultrasonography. Gastrointest Endosc 1988;34:1–8.
16. Nakaizumi A, Uehara H, Iishi H, et al. Endoscopic ultrasonography in diagnosis and staging of pancreatic cancer. Dig Dis Sci 1995;40:696–700.
17. Rosch T, Dittler HJ, Strobel K, et al. Endoscopic ultrasound criteria for vascular invasion in the staging of cancer of the head of the pancreas: a blind reevaluation of videotapes. Gastrointest Endosc 2000;52:469–77.
18. Brugge WR, Lee MJ, Kelsey PB, et al. The use of EUS to diagnose malignant portal venous system invasion by pancreatic cancer. Gastrointest Endosc 1996;43:561–7.

19. Hunt GC, Faigel DO. Assessment of EUS for diagnosing, staging, and determining resectability of pancreatic cancer: a review. Gastrointest Endosc 2002; 55:232–7.
20. Midwinter MJ, Beveridge CJ, Wilsdon JB, et al. Correlation between spiral computed tomography, endoscopic ultrasonography and findings at operation in pancreatic and ampullary tumours. Br J Surg 1999;86:189–93.
21. Mertz HR, Sechopoulos P, Delbeke D, et al. EUS, PET, and CT scanning for evaluation of pancreatic adenocarcinoma. Gastrointest Endosc 2000;52:367–71.
22. Harewood GC, Wiersema MJ. Endosonography-guided fine needle aspiration biopsy in the evaluation of pancreatic masses. Am J Gastroenterol 2002;97: 1386–91.
23. Ahmad NA, Lewis JD, Siegelman ES, et al. Role of endoscopic ultrasound and magnetic resonance imaging in the preoperative staging of pancreatic adenocarcinoma. Am J Gastroenterol 2000;95:1926–31.
24. McNulty NJ, Francis IR, Platt JF, et al. A multi-detector row helical CT of the pancreas: effect of contrast-enhanced multiphasic imaging on enhancement of the pancreas, peri-pancreatic vasculature, and pancreatic adenocarcinoma. Radiology 2001;220:97–102.
25. Ahmad NA, Kochman ML, Lewis JD, et al. Endosonography is superior to angiography in the preoperative assessment of vascular involvement among patients with pancreatic carcinoma. J Clin Gastroenterol 2001;32:54–8.
26. Gress F, Gottlieb K, Sherman S, et al. Endoscopic ultrasonography- guided fine-needle aspiration biopsy of suspected pancreatic cancer. Ann Intern Med 2001; 134:459–64.
27. Chang KJ, Nguyen P, Erickson RA, et al. The clinical utility of endoscopic ultrasound-guided fine-needle aspiration in the diagnosis and staging of pancreatic carcinoma. Gastrointest Endosc 1997;45:387–93.
28. Prasad P, Schmulewitz N, Patel A, et al. Detection of occult liver metastases during EUS for staging of malignancies. Gastrointest Endosc 2004;59:49–53.
29. tenBerge J, Hoffman BJ, Hawes RH, et al. EUS-guided fine needle aspiration of the liver: indications, yield, and safety based on an international survey of 167 cases. Gastrointest Endosc 2002;55:859–62.
30. Eloubeidi M, Gress FG, Savides TJ, et al. Acute pancreatitis after EUS-guided FNA of solid pancreatic masses: a pooled analysis from (EUS) centers in the United States. Gastrointest Endosc 2004;60:385–9.
31. Fickling W, Madani N, Hoffman B, et al. Endoscopic ultrasound fine-needle aspiration of cystic lesions of the pancreas: a safe procedure? [abstract]. Gastrointest Endosc 2002;56:S150.
32. Zollinger RM, Ellison EH. Primary peptic ulcerations of the jejunum associated with islet cell tumors of the pancreas. Ann Surg 1955;142:709–23.
33. Prinz RA. Localization of gastrinomas. Int J Pancreatol 1996;19:79–91.
34. Jensen RT, Gibril F, Termanini B. Definition of the role of somatostatin receptor scintigraphy in gastrointestinal neuroendocrine tumor localization. Yale J Biol Med 1997;70:481–500.
35. Anderson MA, Carpenter S, Thompson NW, et al. Endoscopic ultrasound is highly accurate and directs management in patients with neuroendocrine tumors of the pancreas. Am J Gastroenterol 2000;95:2271–7.
36. Zimmer T, Scherubl H, Faiss S, et al. Endoscopic ultrasonography of neuroendocrine tumors. Digestion 2000;62(Suppl 1):45–50.
37. Rosch T, Lightdale CJ, Botet JF, et al. Localization of pancreatic endocrine tumors by endoscopic ultrasonography. N Engl J Med 1992;326:1721–6.

38. Sugiyama M, Abe N, Izumisato Y, et al. Differential diagnosis of benign versus malignant nonfunctioning islet cell tumors of the pancreas: the role of EUS and ERCP. Gastrointest Endosc 2002;55:115–9.
39. Kann P, Bittinger F, Engelbach M, et al. Endosonography of insulin-secreting and clinically non-functioning neuroendocrine tumors of the pancreas: criteria of benignancy and malignancy. Eur J Med Res 2001;6:385–90.
40. Furukawa T, Oohashi K, Yamao K, et al. Intraductal ultrasonography of the pancreas: development and clinical potential. Endoscopy 1997;29:561–9.
41. Menzel J, Domschke W. Intraductal ultrasonography may localize islet cell tumours negative on endoscopic ultrasound. Scand J Gastroenterol 1998;33:109–12.
42. Gress FG, Barawi M, Kim D, et al. Preoperative localization of a neuroendocrine tumor of the pancreas with EUS-guided fine needle tattooing. Gastrointest Endosc 2002;55:594–7.
43. Howell DA, Beveridge RP, Bosco J, et al. Endoscopic needle aspiration biopsy at ERCP in the diagnosis of biliary strictures. Gastrointest Endosc 1992;38:531–5.
44. Howell DA, Parsons WG, Jones MA, et al. Complete tissue sampling of biliary strictures at ERCP using a new device. Gastrointest Endos 1996;43:498–502.
45. Jailwala J, Fogel EL, Sherman S, et al. Triple-tissue sampling at ERCP in malignant biliary obstruction. Gastrointest Endosc 2000;51:383–90.
46. Kurzawinski T, Deery A, Davidson BR. Diagnostic value of cytology for biliary stricture. Br J Surg 1993;80:414–21.
47. Kosuge T, Yamamoto J, Shimada K, et al. Improved surgical results for hilar cholangiocarcinoma with procedures including major hepatic resection. Ann Surg 1999;230:663–71.
48. Neuhaus P, Jonas S, Bechstein WO, et al. Extended resections for hilar cholangiocarcinoma. Ann Surg 1999;230:808–18.
49. Ortner MA, Liebetruth J, Schreiber S, et al. Photodynamic therapy of nonresectable cholangiocarcinoma. Gastroenterology 1998;114:536–42.
50. Chamberlain RS, Blumgart LH. Hilar cholangiocarcinoma: a review and commentary. Ann Surg Oncol 2000;7:55–66.
51. Launois B, Reding R, Lebeau G, et al. Surgery for hilar cholangiocarcinoma: French experience in collective survey of 552 extrahepatic bile duct cancers. J Hepato-Biliary-Pancreatic Surg 2000;7:128–34.
52. Fritscher-Ravens A, Broering DC, Knoefel WT, et al. EUS-guided fine-needle aspiration of suspected hilar cholangiocarcinoma in potentially operable patients with negative brush cytology. Am J Gastroenterol 2004;99:45–51.
53. Eloubeidi MA, Chen VK, Jhala NC, et al. Endoscopic ultrasound-guided fine needle aspiration biopsy of suspected cholangiocarcinoma. Clin Gastroenterol Hepatol 2004;2:209–13.
54. Ascher SM, Evans SR, Goldberg JA, et al. Intraoperative bile duct sonography during laparoscopic cholecystectomy: experience with a 12.5 MHz catheter-based US probe. Radiology 1992;185:493–6.
55. Tamada K, Ueno N, Tomiyama T, et al. Characterization of biliary strictures using intraductal ultrasonography: comparison with percutaneous cholangioscopic biopsy. Gastrointest Endosc 1998;47:341–9.
56. Menzel J, Poremba C, Dietl KH, et al. Preoperative diagnosis of bile duct strictures comparison of intraductal ultrasonography with conventional endosonography. Scand J Gastroenterol 2000;35:77–82.
57. Tamada K, Nagai H, Yasuda Y, et al. Transpapillary intraductal US prior to biliary drainage in the assessment of longitudinal spread of extrahepatic bile duct carcinoma. Gastrointest Endosc 2001;53:300–7.

The Evidence for Technical Considerations in Pancreatic Resections for Malignancy

Ronald F. Martin, MD[a,b,*], Kashif A. Zuberi, MD[a]

KEYWORDS

• Pancreas • Resection • Malignant • Surgery

Pancreatic resections for malignancy represent some of the great surgical challenges. These operations are performed more commonly now than in the past, largely because many more operations are being performed by surgeons who have dedicated much time and effort to learning the nuances of these operations and have focused their practice development in an attempt to master many of these procedures. Despite these efforts, even the best of surgeons can be easily humbled by a challenging patient with a complex pancreatic problem. Some of these operations have become almost mystical in their stature, but, like so many other complicated problems, the truth is that much is known about the choices that are made whenever these surgical challenges are addressed and little depends on wizardry. Much is left to learn, as some dilemmas are not well understood.

This article focuses on what evidence is available to us when the usual decision points are encountered when considering pancreatic resection for malignancy. The article is organized into components based on the major technical decision branch points: type of resection, extent of resection, extended operations, vascular considerations, and reconstructive options. The sections on vascular considerations and distal pancreatic resections are brief as they are discussed in greater detail elsewhere in this issue.

As Dr Blake Cady once said, "When it comes to cancer, biology is king, patient selection is queen and the techniques are the princes and princesses of the realm."

[a] Department of Surgery, Marshfield Clinic and Saint Joseph's Hospital, 1000 North Oak Avenue, Marshfield, WI 54449, USA
[b] University of Wisconsin School of Medicine and Public Health, Madison, WI, USA
* Corresponding author. Department of Surgery, Marshfield Clinic and Saint Joseph's Hospital, 1000 North Oak Avenue, Marshfield, WI 54449.
E-mail address: martin.ronald@marshfieldclinic.org

Surg Clin N Am 90 (2010) 265–285
doi:10.1016/j.suc.2010.01.001
0039-6109/10/$ – see front matter © 2010 Elsevier Inc. All rights reserved.

surgical.theclinics.com

The authors make no effort to describe the king, we leave it you to acquaint yourselves with the queen, and we give you our assessment of the princes and princesses.

PANCREATICODUODENECTOMY WITH PYLORUS PRESERVATION VERSUS PANCREATICODUODENECTOMY WITH HEMIGASTRECTOMY

The 2 most commonly performed operations for the resection of periampullary carcinoma or carcinoma of the head of the pancreas are pancreaticoduodenectomy (PD) with hemigastrectomy (PDhG) or pylorus-preserving pancreaticoduodenectomy (PPPD). The collected evidence for the efficacy of either procedure suggests that both are comparable for the treatment of pancreatic head and periampullary cancers. The focus of this section is on overall survival, oncologic clearance, metabolic consequence, return of normal motility, and ulcerogenesis.

OVERALL SURVIVAL

Many studies have been published in the last several decades describing patient survival following PD with hemigastrectomy versus PD with pylorus preservation. Randomized, controlled, clinical trials and larger retrospective reviews have shown that for pancreatic ductal adenocarcinoma, short-term mortality ranges from 0% to 8%, and 5-year survival ranges from 6% to 11%, irrespective of whether pylorus preservation or hemigastrectomy is performed with PD. Five-year survival rates of 40% to 70% are reported for PD for other periampullary tumors, depending on tumor cell origin, and are not influenced by subchoice of procedure. Neither short-term nor long-term survival rates are reported as statistically significant comparing PPPD and PDhG (**Table 1**).

Lin and colleagues[1,2] conducted a prospective, randomized, controlled trial (RCT) from 1994 to 1997, subsequently extended until 2002. Thirty-one patients were included in the initial group and 36 in the extended group. Low mortality and operative morbidity rates were reported in analyses for PPPD or PDhG. Five-year survival rates for PPPD versus PDhG were 0% versus 7.5%, respectively, and were not statistically significant. In 2 large RCTs by Seiler and colleagues,[3] and Tran and colleagues,[4] with 214 and 170 patients, respectively, perioperative mortality, cumulative overall morbidity, and specific surgical and medical perioperative complications were similar for patients undergoing PPPD or PDhG. Both groups also found that overall 5-year survival was similar for the treatment of pancreatic cancer and periampullary cancers for the 2 procedures at 20% to 40%, but was influenced by the histologic subtype of carcinoma. A meta-analysis of 6 randomized controlled clinical trials recently published by Diener and colleagues[5] included 4 studies that provided survival data. Pooled survival data as well as each individual trial's data showed no statistically significant difference in overall survival between the 2 procedure groups. Median survival was reported in months; 12 to 34 (PPPD) versus 11 to 27 (PDhG).

Tsao and colleagues[6] conducted a retrospective review of 106 patients undergoing PPPD. The overall hospital mortality was 5.7%. Their review revealed 5-year actuarial survival rates that differed greatly based on cell type of origin: 45.1% ($\pm$9.0%) for ampullary adenocarcinoma, 6.6% ($\pm$6.1%) for pancreatic ductal adenocarcinoma, 33.3% ($\pm$10.7%) for distal bile duct adenocarcinoma, and 60.6% ($\pm$15.7%) for duodenal carcinoma.[6] Their results, compared with existing published data from 1985 to 1992, were similar to long-term survival rates reported for PDhG. A larger retrospective analysis conducted by Mosca and colleagues,[7] which included 221 patients, found that the type of surgical procedure did not affect the survival rate for pancreatic ductal adenocarcinoma or ampullary carcinoma. Five-year survival was

Table 1
PPPD versus PDhG

Citations	Level of Evidence	Patient Groups	Overall Survival (5 y)	Hospital Mortality	Comments
Lin et al[1] Br J Surg 1999	I	PPPD n = 16 PDhG n = 15		3% overall	PPPD had higher delayed gastric emptying
Tran et al[4] Ann Surg 2004	I	PPPD n = 87 PDhG n = 83	12 mo vs 11 mo (median)	3.4% vs 7.2%	No difference overall
Lin et al[2] Hepatogastroenterology 2005	I	PPPD n = 14 PDhG n = 22	9.4% overall	8% overall	No difference in overall survival at 5 y
Seiler et al[3] Br J Surg 2005	I	PPPD n = 64 PDhG n = 66	49 mo vs 39 mo node negative	2% vs 3%	Earlier return to work with PPPD
Tsao et al[6] Arch Surg 1994	II-2	PPPD n = 95	45.4% periampullary cancer 6.6% ductal adenocarcinoma	5.7% overall	PPPD as the procedure of choice for locally resectable periampullary cancer provided the duodenal margin is viable and tumor free
Patel et al[14] Arch Surg 1995	II-2	PPPD n = 15 PDhG n = 52		0% vs 1.55%	The data provided no evidence of any advantage for the PPPD in patients with malignant periampullary tumors
Mosca et al[7] Surgery 1997	II-2	PPPD n = 50 PDhG n = 14	19.1% vs 21.6% ductal adenocarcinoma 40% vs 28.5% periampullary cancer	7.0% vs 8.2%	PPPD was as successful as PDhG in the treatment of ductal adenocarcinoma and periampullary cancer of the pancreas. Long-term survival was not influenced by the type of resection
Diener et al[5] Ann Surg 2007	II-2	6 randomized controlled trials	0.74 hazard ratio ($P = .11$)	0.49 odds ratio ($P = .18$)	In the absence of relevant differences in mortality, morbidity, and survival, the PPPD seems to be as effective as the PDhG

lower in patients with pancreatic ductal adenocarcinoma, 6.2% (PDhG) versus 11.2% (PPPD), compared with those with other periampullary carcinomas (69.2% [PDhG] vs 61.8% [PPPD]). However, the differences were not statistically significant between operative groups.

ONCOLOGIC CONTROL

The 2 main technical issues of immediate oncologic concern when comparing PPPD with PDhG are margin positivity and nodal clearance. One postulated concern about PPPD as an oncologic operation is that the proximal duodenal resection margin may be compromised by sparing the pylorus. Another concern is whether preservation of the pylorus and antrum compromises the clinical effectiveness of the lymph node clearance. An RCT, prospective case series, and retrospective reviews have shown that lymph node involvement reduces survival up to eightfold,[6,8–11] and positive margin status[4,6] reduces survival up to fivefold.

Positive resection margins were noted in 17% of patients undergoing PDhG and 26% of patients in the PPPD in a study reported by Tran and colleagues.[4] Most of the positive margins were located at or near the pancreatic resection area, defined as the posterior resection margin or the margin beyond the pancreatic parenchyma anteriorly and exclusive of the distal pancreatic remnant. No difference in survival between the 2 procedural groups was shown and locoregional tumor-positive lymph nodes were equally noted in both groups. In the report by Tsao and colleagues[6] of 106 patients (ampullary adenocarcinoma in 32%, pancreatic ductal adenocarcinoma in 25%, distal cholangiocarcinoma in 23%, duodenal carcinoma in 10%, pancreatic islet cell carcinoma in 6%, and pancreatic cystadenocarcinoma in 4%) the duodenal resection margin was free of tumor in all 106 patients, peripancreatic and retroperitoneal extension of the tumor was found in 20%. Eleven of the original 106 patients required conversion to a total pancreatectomy (TP); 3 of these had ampullary carcinoma, 4 had pancreatic ductal adenocarcinoma with 1 requiring portal vein resection, and 1 had cystadenocarcinoma. Factors associated with decreased survival were regional nodal metastasis and tumor involvement of the resection margin. Five-year survival rates of 6% in patients with positive resection margins compared with 44% in patients without margin involvement ($P<.0001$) were reported, leading them to conclude that the potential benefits of hemigastrectomy are frequently obviated by the presence of positive margins or lymph node involvement.[6] Similar results were reported by Klinkenbijl and colleagues[12] who concluded that PPPD had similar survival, locoregional recurrence, and distant metastases to PDhG. Neoptolemos and colleagues[13] reported that resection margin status (R0/R1) was not as powerful as tumor grade and lymph node status as a prognostic indicator of survival.

Cubilla and colleagues[8] and Cooperman[9] have described the distribution of lymph node involvement in various types of periampullary cancer. Eighty-six percent of patients with pancreatic ductal adenocarcinoma had regional lymph node metastasis, compared with 33% of patients with ampullary carcinoma. Their reports detail the specific location and node stations of tumor spread to lymph nodes. Cubilla and colleagues[8] also noted that in 21 patients with pancreatic ductal adenocarcinoma only 1 of the second tier node groups was found to have tumor involvement, and none of the second tier node groups were found to be involved with tumor in the patients with other types of periampullary carcinoma.[8] Cooperman's[9] report confirmed this finding, as has a report of autopsy specimens by Nagai and colleagues.[10] Tsao and colleagues[6] reported 5-year survival rates of 12% for patients with regional nodal metastasis, compared with 49% for those patients without nodal involvement. In a review by Cameron and colleagues[11] of 89 patients, no positive duodenal margins were present in 37 patients with pancreatic ductal adenocarcinoma and factors influencing long-term survival were negative lymph nodes and the absence of blood vessel invasion. Patel and colleagues[14] suggested that lymph node clearance was slightly improved by PDhG compared with PPPD (10 nodes vs 5 nodes, respectively) and reported that there was no evidence of any advantage for PPPD in patients with malignant periampullary tumors.

METABOLIC CONSEQUENCES

Metabolic consequences following PD result from possible alterations in endocrine or exocrine functions of the pancreas, gut motility, or absorption. Of considerable importance are the changes in glucose metabolism and pancreatic exocrine function.

Kozuschek and colleagues[15] studied 43 patients treated with PPPD for malignant disease, compared with 25 patients treated by PDhG, and evaluated extensive functional studies including nutritional state and weight change, blood glucose levels, pyloric function, orocecal transit time, and pancreatic exocrine function. They found that digestion was described as normal in 86% of the PPPD group, but 50% in the PDhG group. They noted increased weight gain in the PPPD group compared with the PDhG group. Glucose tolerance was not changed after PPPD, but was impaired in the PDhG group.[15] In a retrospective, multicenter Japanese study of 1066 patients undergoing PPPD reported by Yamaguchi and colleagues,[16] glucose intolerance developed in 61 patients, resolved in 15, showed no change in 170, was absent in 695, and was ameliorated in 17. Litwin and colleagues[17] published a prospective case series involving 20 patients who had undergone a PDhG during a period of a year, studying glucose metabolism pre- and postoperatively. Their study did not focus on comparing the differences between PPPD and PDhG, but did show an improvement in glucose tolerance among patients who had undergone PDhG for neoplastic disease, from 15% at the time of operation to 45% at 6 months. Jang and colleagues[18] studied the effect of PG versus PJ in 34 patients undergoing PPPD who survived for more than 1 year without clinical evidence of recurrence. They found no statistically significant difference in general nutritional status and quality of life (QoL) among the 2 groups.[18] There were 4 mild and 15 severe cases of pancreatic exocrine insufficiency among those who underwent PJ, whereas all of the patients who underwent PG showed severe pancreatic insufficiency. On glucose tolerance testing (GTT), excluding preoperative diabetic patients, 43.8% (7/16) of the PJ group had abnormal results after surgery, whereas 75.0% (9/12) of the PG group had an abnormal postoperative GTT.

Yamaguchi and colleagues[19] studied 60 Japanese patients with 3 different types of pancreatic head resection: PDhG, PPPD, and duodenum preserving pancreatic head resection for benign (n = 30) and malignant disease (n = 30). Fasting blood sugar concentrations were not different among the 3 groups at short- and long-term intervals after the operation.[19]

RETURN OF GASTROINTESTINAL FUNCTION

The most frequent complication of PD (PDhG or PPPD) is delayed gastric emptying (DGE), occurring in up to 40% of patients. Most of the time, this may be the hallmark feature of an undiagnosed pancreatic leak/fistula or intra-abdominal collection or abscess. Some retrospective reviews have concluded that PPPD is more frequently associated with DGE (20%–60%) than with PDhG (0%–40%).[6,14] Subsequent randomized controlled clinical trials have shown no difference between either procedure[3,4] regarding DGE, whereas others suggest that DGE is more common following PPPD.[1,2] Pooled results from meta-analyses have shown no statistical difference between DGE rates following PPPD (20%–30%) and PDhG (20%–40%).[5]

ULCEROGENIC POTENTIAL

PD leads to a significant change in upper gastrointestinal physiology and alters normal upper gastrointestinal protective mechanisms. The degree to which PPPD and PDhG result in marginal ulceration has only been studied retrospectively. Some series suggest that a higher rate of peptic ulceration is associated with PPPD (4%–14%) than with PDhG (0%–11%).[7,14,20]

TP VERSUS PARTIAL PANCREATECTOMY

TP may be considered for select patients with chronic pancreatitis, multifocal islet cell tumors, and diffuse intraductal papillary mucinous neoplasms (IPMNs). The role for TP in pancreatic ductal adenocarcinoma is more controversial. Total gland removal avoids the risk of pancreaticoenteric leaks and removes all pancreatic tissue at risk for synchronous disease in the gland.[21,22] However, TP has endocrine and exocrine consequences. Some investigators argue that pancreatic ductal adenocarcinoma necessitating a TP is associated with a worse tumor biology and poorer outcome.[22] There is a lack of RCTs addressing this question. This article reviews the role of total or partial pancreatectomy (PP) (**Table 2**) with respect to the extent of resection and positive neck margin status. Reports on the effects of extended lymph node resection and vascular resection and reconstruction are summarized in **Table 3**.

EXTENT OF RESECTION

The intent of pancreatic resection when a malignancy is suspected is to achieve an R0 resection. Whether a PP or TP is indicated depends on intraoperative findings and the resources of the surgical team. Much of the evidence on extended resection or TP comes from high-volume centers with significant experience and large patient databases. In an analysis of 100 total pancreatectomies for pancreatic ductal adenocarcinoma performed by Reddy and colleagues,[21] it was noted that, in 58 patients, planned partial pancreaticoduodenectomies were converted to total pancreatectomies because of microscopic (n = 45) or macroscopic (n = 13) disease at the transected pancreatic neck margin. These results revealed an increased 30-day postoperative mortality compared with standard PD (8.0% vs 1.5%). Operative morbidity was higher in the TP group (69% vs 38.6% P<.0001) and 1-year survival was worse for patients who had undergone a TP (52.7%) versus PD (66.9%).

Nathan and colleagues[23] studied the Surveillance, Epidemiology, and End Results (SEER) database for patients undergoing total and PP with curative intent for pancreatic adenocarcinoma from 1998 to 2004. They excluded patients with benign disease, IPMNs, and metastatic disease from their analysis. Kaplan-Meier survival estimates were similar following TP and PP. They concluded that perioperative mortality and long-term survival were similar for TP and PP, which supported the role for TP when oncologically appropriate.

Muller and colleagues[22] studied 147 patients undergoing TP prospectively for perioperative and follow-up data including QoL assessment using the European Organisation for Research and Treatment of Cancer (EORTC) QLQ-C30 questionnaire. In addition to finding 1- and 3-year survival rates of 64% and 36%, respectively, their QoL analysis for

Table 2
TP versus PP

Citations	Level of Evidence	Patient Population	Hospital Mortality	Median Survival	Comments
Schmidt et al[25] Surgery 2007	II-1	TP = 33 PP = 28	6% (TP) vs 7% (PP)	18 mo (TP) vs 10 mo (PP)	Conversion of PP to TP to achieve an R0 resection in patients with pancreatic adenocarcinoma is associated with a survival benefit
Muller et al[22] Ann Surg 2007	II-2	TP = 147	4.8%	21.9 mo	In this cohort study, mortality and morbidity after elective TP are not significantly different from the PP. Because of improvements in postoperative management, QoL is acceptable, and is almost comparable to that of PP patients
Reddy et al[21] Ann Surg 2009	II-2	TP = 100 PP = 1286	8% (TP) vs 1.5% (PP)	5-year survival 18.9% (TP) vs 18.5% (PP)	TP should be performed when oncologically appropriate
Nathan et al[23] J Surg Oncol 2009	II-2	Head tumor TP = 292 PD = 2988 Body/tail TP = 32 DP = 283 Unspecified TP = 52 PP = 374	Head tumor TP = 9.0% PD = 6.5% Body/tail TP = 9.3% DP = 3.9% Unspecified TP = 5.8% PP = 6.5%	Hazard ratio between TP and PP Head = 1.06 Body/tail =0.84 Unspecified = 1.06	Perioperative mortality and long-term survival are similar following TP vs PP for pancreatic adenocarcinoma, supporting the use of TP when oncologically appropriate

Table 3
Survival evidence regarding superior mesenteric-portal venous resection (SMPVR) and or extended lymph node dissection (LND)

Citations	Level of Evidence	Postoperative Morbidity/Mortality SMPVR vs No-SMPVR	Survival After Extended LND vs None at 1 y[a]	Margin-negative Resection	2-, 3-Year Survival[b]	Comments
Pedrazzoli et al[36] Ann Surg 1998	I	NA	50.6%*	72.5% vs 78%	22%*	No survival difference found between standard group and extended LND groups
Yeo et al[37] Ann Surg 1999	I	NA	83%* vs 77%*	88% vs 95%	47%* vs 56%*	Radical PD can be safely performed but are data not mature enough to establish survival benefit
Yeo et al[38] Ann Surg 2002	I	NA	80%* vs 77%*	88% vs 93%	44% both groups	Fails to show any added benefit to extended LND
Farnell et al[39] Surgery 2005	I	NA	71%* vs 82%*	76% vs 82%	25% vs 41%	No benefit gained from extended LND
Capussotti et al[40] Arch Surg 2003	II-1	33.3%/0% vs 37.6%/6.4%	68.5% overall	16.7% vs 79.2%	16.3% overall	Extended lymphadenectomy and vein resection did not result in significant prognostic factors

Study						Comment
Bachellier et al[42] Am J Surg 2001	II-2	48.4%/3.2% vs 47.1%/2.5%	NA	62% vs 73%	22%* vs 24%*	Survival rates higher for patients undergoing SMPVR with margin-negative resection
Tseng et al[45] J Gastrointest Surg 2004	II-2	NA	NA		Median survival 23.4 mo vs 26.5 mo	Properly selected patients with adenocarcinoma of the pancreatic head who require vascular resection have a median survival of approximately 2 y, which does not differ from those who undergo standard PD and is superior to historical patients believed to have locally advanced disease treated nonoperatively
Roder et al[41] Am J Surg 1996	II-3	41.9% overall	NA	31.8% overall	20%*	Portal vein resection does not prolong survival

a Figures marked with an asterisk indicate there were no survivors after 1 year.
b Two-year survival figures are marked with as asterisk.

patients undergoing TP revealed significantly lower functional scale, role functioning, social functioning, and a worse symptom scale and financial strain score.

POSITIVE PANCREATIC NECK MARGIN STATUS

There is level 2 evidence to suggest that overall survival is significantly reduced by an R1 resection versus an R0 resection, suggesting a significant role for conversion to TP in patients with positive pancreatic neck margin status at PD.[21,24,25] This is predicated on the notion that, by extending the degree of pancreatic resection, one will eventually achieve an R0 resection; the basis of the old adage that your operation is only as good as your worst margin.

Raut and colleagues[24] evaluated 360 consecutive patients in whom PD was performed for pancreatic adenocarcinoma. Patients who underwent an R1 resection had a median overall survival of 21.5 months compared with 27.8 months in patients who underwent an R0 resection. After controlling for other variables on multivariate analysis, resection status did not independently affect survival. Recurrent disease was identified in 41 (68.3%) of 60 patients who underwent an R1 resection and in 199 (66.3%) of 300 patients who underwent an R0 resection ($P = .83$). Asiyanbola and colleagues[26] also reported that surgical margin status was not independently associated with survival.

In a multi-institutional review conducted by Schmidt and colleagues[25] for pancreatic adenocarcinoma, 28 patients who had undergone a PD with R1 resection were compared with 33 patients who underwent conversion to TP to achieve an R0 resection. Median survival (Kaplan-Meier method) was 17.9 months for the TP group, compared with 9.7 months for the PD group.

METASTATIC DISEASE

Eighty percent of resections reported for metastases to the pancreas result from 4 primary cancer types: renal cell cancer, colorectal cancer, sarcoma, and melanoma.[27–33] Currently the data are limited to level 2 and level 3 evidence.

The usefulness of pancreatic metastasectomy can only be assessed by evaluating long-term survival in retrospective analyses. Pancreatic metastasectomy is usually performed as a partial pancreatic resection such as PD or distal pancreatectomy (DP). Less often, pancreatic metastasectomy is done by enucleation or a pancreas-sparing operation such as a central pancreatectomy.[27] The largest study of pancreatic metastasectomy includes only 49 patients,[28] and others include from 16 to 29 patients.[29–32] All have found that long-term survival can be achieved with pancreatic metastasectomy under selected conditions. In a review of data from the Endocrine Registry of the Armed Forces Institute of Pathology, Thompson and Heffess[33] identified 21 patients with isolated renal cell cancer metastatic to pancreas and suggested that resection may be associated with prolonged patient survival. Renal cell carcinoma is associated with the best outcome following pancreatic resection for metastatic disease, whereas lung cancer was associated with the worst outcome.[28]

ADJACENT ORGAN INVOLVEMENT

There are limited data, retrospective or prospective, that evaluate outcomes, survival, complications, or morbidity associated with adjacent organ involvement with pancreatic ductal adenocarcinoma. Nikfarjam and colleagues[34] evaluated 105 patients who underwent PD with multivisceral resection performed in 19 patients. Despite a complication rate of 60%, including DGE (39%) and pancreatic fistula (16%), they felt that multivisceral resection and PD can be performed without significant added morbidity compared with PD alone. Many investigators, the authors among them, would take exception to this analysis.

LYMPH NODE INVOLVEMENT AND LYMPHADENECTOMY

A retrospective review published by Henne-Bruns and colleagues[35] found no survival advantage to extended retroperitoneal lymphadenectomy. However, a prospective, randomized multicenter study conducted by Pedrazzoli and colleagues[36] suggested a survival advantage treated with an extended rather than a standard lymphadenectomy. They also found that the addition of an extended lymphadenectomy and retroperitoneal soft-tissue clearance to a pancreaticoduodenal resection does not significantly increase morbidity and mortality. Subsequent prospective studies by Yeo and colleagues[37,38] showed no survival difference at 1-, 3-, and 5-year survival compared with the standard versus radical lymphadenectomy groups, nor did a randomized controlled clinical trial by Farnell and colleagues[39] comparing standard PD and PD with extended lymphadenectomy in patients with resectable pancreatic head adenocarcinoma.

Capussotti and colleagues[40] conducted a non-RCT of 149 consecutive patients undergoing PD for macroscopically curative periampullary carcinoma (122 patients underwent a standard PD, 37 underwent an extended lymphadenectomy, and 20 patients underwent a vein resection) in which no statistically significant difference was found in morbidity, mortality, or postoperative stay when extended lymphadenectomy and vein resection were performed. In the 100 patients with ductal adenocarcinoma, extended resection permitted better pathologic staging and was associated with an early survival advantage, but long-term survival was possible only in patients with favorable prognostic factors.

VASCULAR RECONSTRUCTION

The addition of vascular resection to PD for achieving an R0 resection can be accomplished safely and effectively with low perioperative morbidity and mortality. However, most retrospective case series have shown poor 5-year survival with a median survival of 16 months to 20 months despite careful patient selection. Some of the evidence for venous and arterial resection and reconstruction in combination with PD is discussed here.[41-46]

In a retrospective review, Roder and colleagues[41] analyzed 31 patients who underwent a tangential (n = 9) or segmental (n = 22) resection of the portal or superior mesenteric vein in an attempt to achieve an R0 resection with PD. The overall complication rate was 41.9%. Seventy-one percent of the patients had pancreatic ductal adenocarcinoma and successful R0 resection was achieved in 31.8% of this subset. Tumor infiltration of the resected vein was documented in 61.3% of cases.[41] Median survival for all patients undergoing PD with vein resection was 8 months. They found that the prognosis was significantly better for patients without histologically documented portal or superior mesenteric vein invasion than for those with histologic tumor invasion. Bachellier and colleagues[42] also showed that final resection status was an important determinant of survival, whereas vascular resection in itself was not a contributing factor to survival.

Siriwardana and Siriwardena[43] performed a systematic review of 52 studies involving 1646 patients who were treated with venous resection as part of pancreatectomy for cancer. Postoperative morbidity ranged from 9% to 78% (median 42%). Mortality data were available for 1235 patients with a reported overall 5.9%

perioperative mortality. Median survival was 13 months, and 1-, 3-, and 5-year survivals were 50%, 16%, and 7% respectively. In a more recent retrospective review of 593 patients undergoing consecutive pancreatic resections for pancreatic adenocarcinoma, Martin and colleagues[44] identified 36 patients who underwent concomitant vascular resection: 88% underwent venous resection only, 8% combined arterial and venous resection, and 6% underwent arterial resection only (superior mesenteric artery). Perioperative morbidity and mortality at 90 days were 0% and 35%, respectively, compared with 2% and 39% for the group who had not undergone vascular resection.[44] Median survival of 18 months and 19 months were reported for the groups with and without vascular resection, respectively. Tseng and colleagues[45] showed no significant difference in survival for those patients undergoing vascular resection or PD alone, but did report and improvement compared with historical results for patients who were not operated on. In a review of 12 patients undergoing arterial resection only, Stitzenberg and colleagues[46] found that the 60-day mortality was 17%. Median survival after resection was 17 months, and 3-year survival was 17%. There were no 5-year survivors.

PANCREATICOJEJUNOSTOMY VERSUS PANCREATICOGASTROSTOMY

One of the most dreaded complications in pancreatic surgery is anastomotic leak or fistula formation. The management of the pancreatic stump after resection has been the source of much debate. The role of reconstruction by various forms of pancreaticojejunostomy (PJ) and pancreaticogastrostomy (PG) is discussed in this section. The reports reviewed are listed in **Table 4**. The use of pancreatic duct stents, types of anastomosis, including duct-to-mucosa and invagination techniques, the use of optical magnification when performing the anastomosis, and the role of duct occlusion and anastomotic sealants are reviewed.

Recently reported retrospective reviews have suggested that PD with PG reconstruction is superior to PJ reconstruction regarding postoperative fistula rate and hospital mortality. In 3 retrospective studies, 2 showed similar mortality for PG compared with PJ,[47,48] and 1 showed a lesser mortality with PG compared with PJ.[49] Pancreatic fistula rates were similar with the 2 techniques in 2 of the reports,[48,49] and were less common with PG in 1 report.[47] Need for reoperation was similar when comparing PG and PJ in 1 study.[47] Similar results were seen with a nonrandomized prospective study conducted by Takano and colleagues,[50] who reported pancreatic fistula rates of 0% and 13% for PG and PJ, respectively.

The results of the current level 1 data have shown that PG or PJ reconstruction are equally effective after PD and that the pancreatic fistula rates of 12% to 16% (PG) and 11% to 20% (PJ) are not statistically significant.[51–54] One study randomized 151 patients with soft residual pancreatic tissue and a pancreatic duct size of less than 5 mm to receive a PG (n = 69) or end-to-side PJ (n = 82). The PG was created using a single layer of interrupted nonabsorbable sutures. The PJ was created using a single layer duct-to-mucosa technique. Clinically significant pancreatic fistulas were observed in 22 patients; 9 (13%) in the PG group versus 13 (16%) in the PJ group, which was not statistically significant. Furthermore, no significant difference in overall postoperative complications was noted, although DGE, biliary fistula, and postoperative fluid collections were significantly less common in patients treated with PG.[51] In a single-blind, randomized, controlled, multicenter trial enrolling 149 patients, 81 patients underwent PG and 68 patients underwent a PJ; pancreatic fistula rates of 16% were reported in the PG group and 20% in the PJ group. The difference was not statistically significant.[52] In a prospective RCT conducted by Yeo and

Table 4 PG versus PJ				
Citations	Level of Evidence	Pancreatic Fistula PJ vs PG	Hospital Mortality	Comments
Yeo et al[53] Ann Surg 1995	I	11.1% vs 12.3%	NA	No difference between PG and PJ in postoperative outcomes
Bassi et al[51] Ann Surg 2005	I	16% vs 13%	NA	No significant difference in postoperative complications and pancreatic fistula
Duffas et al[52] Am J Surg 2005	I	20% vs 16%	11%	No difference in outcomes between PJ and PG
Aranha et al[49] J Gastrointest Surg 2003	II-2	14% vs 12% $P =$ nonsignificant	4 vs 0	Found that PG was associated with fewer complications
Oussoultzoglou et al[47] Arch Surg 2004	II-2	53% vs 38.3%	2.4% (PJ) vs 2.9% (PG)	Found that PG is superior to PJ
Nakao et al[48] J Hepatobiliary Pancreat Surg 2006	II-2	12.2% vs 20.7%	0%	No difference in outcome
Wente et al[54] Am J Surg 2007	II-2	$P =$ nonsignificant	NA	Meta-analysis revealed no difference between PG and PJ

colleagues,[53] 145 patients were assigned to receiving a PG (n = 73) or PJ (n = 72) after undergoing a PD. The pancreaticoenteric anastomosis was performed in a double-layer fashion without the use of pancreatic stents and as an end-to-end (n = 48) anastomosis or end-to-side (n = 24) anastomosis at the surgeons discretion. The overall rate of complications did not differ between the 2 groups and no overall difference in operative outcome with the use of either pancreaticoenteric anastomosis.

A meta-analysis of 16 articles, including the 3 RCTs and 13 nonrandomized observational studies described earlier, revealed no statistically significant difference between PG and PJ with respect to overall complications, pancreatic fistula, intra-abdominal fluid collections, or mortality.[54] The 13 nonrandomized observational studies showed significant results in favor of PG, which may suggest a publication bias.

STENTED VERSUS NONSTENTED

Several RCTs, and several retrospective reviews, have suggested that stenting of the pancreaticojejunal anastomosis with external drainage decreases the pancreatic fistula rate. A prospective RCT with 120 patients showed a significant decrease in their pancreatic fistula rate, from 20% to 6.7%, with the use of external stenting. The type of surgical procedure performed was otherwise similar between the 2 groups. The overall morbidity rates for the stented and nonstented groups were 31.7% and 38.3%, respectively, and hospital mortality were 1.7% and 5%, respectively. Neither was reported to be statistically significant. Univariate analysis identified only pancreatic duct diameter of less than or equal to 3 mm ($P = .032$) and the use of a pancreatic duct stent ($P = .0302$) as significant in affecting the pancreatic fistula rate.[55] Another prospective study of 85 patients undergoing a PP compared 44 patients having a temporary stent and external drainage of the pancreatic duct with 41 controls. Pancreatic fistula was diagnosed in 6.8% of patients with a stent and 29.3% of patients without a stent. The analysis suggested that temporary external drainage of the pancreatic duct after PD may reduce the leakage rate of the PJ.[56]

One recent RCT of 238 patients, evaluating internal stenting of the pancreatic duct with PJ reconstruction, showed no significant difference in fistula rate with stenting.[57] In this trial, patients were stratified according to gland texture and the use of stents. Fistula rates were similar with or without the use of stents, but were more frequently observed in the group of patients with soft-textured pancreata.[57]

DUCT-TO-MUCOSA TECHNIQUE VERSUS INVAGINATION TECHNIQUE

Many retrospective reviews evaluating different anastamotic techniques have shown no significant difference in fistula rates between duct-to-mucosa and invagination reconstruction techniques.[56,58–61] One study showed fistula rates of 25% for end-to-end invagination technique and 10% for end-to-side duct-to-mucosa techniques.[56] Bartoli and colleagues[58] observed a higher incidence of fistulas (16.5%) after end-to-side anastomosis than after end-to-end (11.7%) or duct-to-mucosa (11.5%) anastomosis. Crist and Cameron[59] observed no difference in the incidence of fistulas between invagination (13%) and duct-to-mucosa (16%) anastomosis. Similar data have been reported by Grace and colleagues[60] and Braasch and colleagues,[61] with fistula rates of 6% to 13% after invagination anastomosis and 11% to 14% after duct-to-mucosa anastomosis.

A recent prospective RCT evaluated 144 patients undergoing PD who were randomly assigned to receive a duct-to-mucosa anastomosis using fine prolene sutures or a 1-layer end-to-side PJ using nonabsorbable sutures. The incidence of intra-abdominal complications was 35% in the prolene group and 38% in the absorbable suture group. Pancreatic fistulas were seen in 13% and 15% of the 2 respective groups.[62] No statistically significant difference was seen between the 2 groups. In a dual-institutional prospective randomized trial, 197 patients were stratified by pancreatic texture and randomized to an end-to-side invagination (n = 100) or a duct-to-mucosa (n = 97) PJ anastomosis. There was a 24% pancreatic fistula rate in the duct-to-mucosa cohort and a 12% pancreatic fistula rate in the invagination cohort ($P<.05$).[63] The investigators suggested that the greatest risk factor for pancreatic fistula was soft gland texture.

DUCT OCCLUSION VERSUS ANASTAMOTIC SEALANTS

Anastamotic sealants have not been shown in retrospective or prospective randomized trials to reduce pancreatic fistula rates. Pancreatic fistula rates in these reports remain in the 20% to 30% range even with application of sealants.[64–66] Duct occlusion has not been shown to be superior to PJ anastomosis in reducing fistula rates. In a prospective trial of 169 patients, 86 patients were randomized to undergo pancreatic duct occlusion without anastomosis and 83 patients underwent PJ reconstruction after PD. Pancreatic duct occlusion was obtained by injection of Ethibloc (n = 18), neoprene (n = 45), or Tissucol (n = 23).[66] This study noted no significant difference in postoperative complications (P = .069), mortality (P = .536), or exocrine insufficiency. There was a significantly higher incidence of diabetes mellitus (P = .001) in patients with duct occlusion and pancreatic fistula (P = .013).[66] In another prospective, randomized, single-blinded, multicenter study, 182 patients undergoing PD or DP there was no statistically significant difference between the 2 groups for intra-abdominal complications or pancreatic fistula (15% vs 17%).[67] However, there were significantly more patients in the ductal occlusion group who received octreotide (53% vs 26%, P<.001), who had reinforcement of their anastomosis by fibrin glue (59% vs 10%, P<.001), or who had a fibrotic pancreatic stump (46% vs 30%, P = .02).

BILIARY DRAINAGE AND STENTING

A retrospective review of 240 consecutive cases of PD showed that preoperative biliary drainage may be associated with an increase in infectious complications[68] and smaller retrospective case series, suggesting that internal (nonstented) drainage also reduces infectious complications.[69]

INTRAOPERATIVE PLACEMENT OF DRAINS

Conlon and colleagues[70] conducted a RCT of closed suction drains placed intraoperatively after pancreatic resection versus no drains. There was no significant difference in the overall complication rate or the absolute number of complications between the drain and no-drain groups. However, a significantly increased incidence of intra-abdominal abscesses/collections and fistulas was noted in the drained group (P<.02).[70] The data suggested that the presence of drains failed to reduce the need for interventional radiologic drainage or surgical exploration for intra-abdominal sepsis. Based on these results, the investigators suggested that closed suction drainage should not be considered mandatory or standard after pancreatic resection. This study further validated the results obtained in an earlier retrospective report by Jeekel and colleagues,[71] who suggested that drainage could be omitted without producing clinically significant complications.

ALIMENTARY RECONSTRUCTION

The alimentary reconstruction is the last anastomosis usually performed during a PD. The configuration of the anastomosis has been shown in prospective randomized trials and retrospective reviews to influence the incidence of DGE. DGE has been reported to occur in approximately 30% of patients in whom the duodenojejunostomy is placed in the retrocolic position, versus 5% in the antecolic position.[72–74]

A small observational study compared the Imanaga technique (enteric anastomosis, pancreatic anastomosis, biliary anastomosis in sequence; n = 8) and Child technique (pancreatic anastomosis, biliary anastomosis, enteric anastomosis in sequence; n = 10) reconstructions after PD with a control group of 7 normal healthy volunteers. Patients who underwent the Imanaga reconstruction showed a "more physiologic" pattern than those patients who underwent a Child reconstruction by biliary scintigraphy.[75] Kotoura and colleagues[76] showed similar results. A retrospective review of 55 cases of pylorus-preserving PD with Imanaga reconstruction found that DGE, pancreatic leak, and marginal ulceration occurred in 45%, 5%, and 5% of patients respectively. This study concluded that the Imanaga method could be performed with acceptable complication rates.[77] Hishinuma and colleagues[78] further studied the Imanaga reconstruction after PPPD with hepatobiliary and gastrointestinal dual scintigraphy in 24 patients and found that most of the patients had adequate food and bile mixing at 2 hours. The clinical relevance of this is unclear.

POSTOPERATIVE FEEDING

Clinical trials and retrospective reviews in patients undergoing PD for pancreatic ductal adenocarcinoma or other periampullary tumors have shown that enteral feeding is superior to total parenteral nutrition (TPN) in reducing septic complications and shortening hospital length of stay,[79,80] and that nasojejunal tubes are superior to gastrojejunal tubes because of a reduced incidence of tube-related complications.[81] In a 3-arm randomized trial of 212 patients, outcomes were compared after PD. The first arm received standard a enteral formula through a feeding jejunostomy; the second received an enteral diet enriched with arginine, omega-3 fatty acids, and ribonucleic acid; and the third arm received TPN. The overall and septic complications were significantly fewer in the enterally fed groups.[79] Another retrospective study of 1873 patients undergoing PD for pancreatic ductal adenocarcinoma reported 14% of patients received TPN, 23% had enteral feeding, and 63% received no supplementation. The study showed that TPN use led to a prolonged hospital stay (P<.0001).[80] In another review, 180 consecutive patients undergoing pancreaticoduodenectomies were studied in 2 nonrandomized groups: those with early postoperative tube feeding (n = 98) and those with no planned feeding (n = 82). Jejunal tube feeding was delivered via a bridled nasojejunal tube in 56% and a gastrojejunal tube in 44%. Vomiting, use of TPN, readmission rates, early and late complications, and infections occurred less in the jejunal feeding group. Tube-related complications were seen more frequently in the gastrojejunal group.[81] However, these results must be interpreted cautiously because those patients who require supplemental enteral feeding or parental support may represent a subset of patients who have had other perioperative complications.

DP

DP has been developed in the past decade for laparoscopic surgical resection and splenic preservation. Open and laparoscopic procedures seem to be equally effective in managing premalignant and benign conditions of the body and tail of the pancreas.[82–84] Most of the data on treating malignant lesions with DP are retrospective, and no RCTs exist to address its effectiveness. Splenic preservation has also been reviewed retrospectively, and prospective trials are lacking to address the value of splenic preservation.

One large retrospective review found patients undergoing laparoscopic DP to have fewer postoperative complications and shorter hospital stays compared with patients undergoing open DP.[83] In this report of 103 consecutive patients undergoing laparoscopic pancreatic resection, 82 patients underwent laparoscopic DP (52 with splenic preservation and en bloc splenopancreatectomy in 30), and laparoscopic enucleation was performed in 20 patients. Of the 52 patients undergoing laparoscopic DP with splenic preservation, the splenic vessels were preserved 18 patients and sacrificed in 64 patients. The conversion rate from laparoscopic to open technique was 7%. No mortalities were reported. Overall complication rates were highest in the enucleation group and were increased when splenic vessels were not preserved in the DP with the splenic preservation group. Of the 103 patients, 26.2% had malignant disease. R0 resection was achieved in 90% of patients with ductal adenocarcinoma and 100% of patients with other malignant tumors. Median survival for patients with ductal adenocarcinoma was 14 months.[83]

Another large review comparing splenectomy with splenic preservation showed that patients undergoing splenectomy had shorter operative times, less blood loss, and shorter hospital stays.[84] In this review of 259 patients who underwent DP with (n = 75) or without (n = 184) splenic preservation during a 10-year period, splenic preservation was not a significant predictor of complications in univariate analysis ($P = .445$) or adjusted analysis ($P = .543$).[84]

A prospectively conducted study compared distal pancreatectomies performed by open or laparoscopic techniques in 112 patients. Baker and colleagues[82] concluded that laparoscopic DP was comparable with open DP for managing premalignant neoplasms of the pancreatic body and tail in terms of morbidity rates, but patients undergoing laparoscopic DP had shorter hospital stays. They also noted that laparoscopic DP was less effective at nodal clearance than open DP.

SUMMARY

The surgeon who wishes to perform successful resections for malignant processes involving the pancreas has to be conversant with a broad range of topics. There are extensive collections of data that usually give excellent guidance, but sometimes also provide conflicting advice. No matter what the data suggest might work best, the surgeon and local collaborators must be able to deliver the quality care cited in some of these reports; usually it is the best results that are published. There is a difference between results that are statistically significant, clinically significant, and important to the patient, and these concepts should never be confused.

REFERENCES

1. Lin PW, Lin YJ. Prospective randomized comparison between pylorus-preserving and standard pancreaticoduodenectomy. Br J Surg 1999;86:603–7.
2. Lin PW, Shan YS, Lin YJ, et al. Pancreaticoduodenectomy for pancreatic head cancer: PPPD versus Whipple procedure. Hepatogastroenterology 2005;52:1601–4.
3. Seiler CA, Wagner M, Bachmann T, et al. Randomized clinical trial of pylorus-preserving duodenopancreatectomy versus classical Whipple resection-long term results. Br J Surg 2005;92:547–56.
4. Tran KTC, Smeenk HG, van Eijck CH, et al. Pylorus preserving pancreaticoduodenectomy versus standard Whipple procedure: a prospective, randomized, multicenter analysis of 170 patients with pancreatic and periampullary tumors. Ann Surg 2004;240(5):738–45.
5. Diener MK, Knaebel HP, Heukaufer C, et al. A systematic review and meta-analysis of pylorus-preserving versus classical pancreaticoduodenectomy for surgical treatment of periampullary and pancreatic carcinoma. Ann Surg 2007; 245(2):187–200.
6. Tsao JI, Rossi RL, Lowell JA. Pylorus-preserving pancreaticoduodenectomy: Is it an adequate cancer operation. Arch Surg 1994;129:405–12.
7. Mosca F, Giulianotti PC, Balestracci T, et al. Long-term survival in pancreatic cancer: pylorus-preserving versus Whipple pancreaticoduodenectomy. Surgery 1997;122(3):553–66.
8. Cubilla AL, Fortner J, Fitzgerald PJ. Lymph node involvement in carcinoma of the head of the pancreas area. Cancer 1978;4:880–7.
9. Cooperman AM. Cancer of the pancreas: a dilemma in treatment. Surg Clin North Am 1981;61:107–15.

10. Nagai H, Kuroda A, Morioka Y. Lymphatic and local spread of T1 and T2 pancreatic cancer. Ann Surg 1986;204:65–71.
11. Cameron JL, Crist DW, Sitzmann JV, et al. Factors influencing survival after pancreaticoduodenectomy for pancreatic cancer. Am J Surg 1991;161:120–5.
12. Klinkenbijl JHG, van der Schelling GP, Hop WC, et al. The advantages of pylorus-preserving pancreaticoduodenectomy in malignant disease of the pancreas and periampullary region. Ann Surg 1992;216:142–5.
13. Neoptolemos JP, Talbot IC, Carr-Locke DL, et al. Treatment and outcome in 52 consecutive cases of ampullary carcinoma. Br J Surg 1987;74:957–61.
14. Patel AG, Toyama MT, Kusske AM, et al. Pylorus preserving Whipple resection for pancreatic cancer: is it any better? Arch Surg 1995;130:838–43.
15. Kozuschek W, Reith HB, Waleczek H, et al. A comparison of long-term results of the standard Whipple procedure and the pylorus preserving pancreaticoduodenectomy. J Am Coll Surg 1994;178:443–53.
16. Yamaguchi K, Tanaka M, Chijiiwa K, et al. Early and late complications of pylorus-preserving pancreaticoduodenectomy in Japan 1998. J Hepatobiliary Pancreat Surg 1999;6(3):303–11.
17. Litwin J, Dobrowolski S, Orłowska-Kunikowska E, et al. Changes in glucose metabolism after Kausch-Whipple pancreatectomy in pancreatic cancer and chronic pancreatitis patients. Pancreas 2008;36:26–30.
18. Jang JY, Kim SW, Park SJ, et al. Comparison of the functional outcome after pylorus-preserving pancreatoduodenectomy: pancreatogastrostomy and pancreatojejunostomy. World J Surg 2002;26(3):366–71.
19. Yamaguchi K, Yokohata K, Nakano K, et al. Which is a less invasive pancreatic head resection: PD, PPPD, or DPPHR? Dig Dis Sci 2001;46(2):282–8.
20. Sakaguchi T, Nakamura S, Suzuki S, et al. Marginal ulceration after pylorus-preserving pancreaticoduodenectomy. J Hepatobiliary Pancreat Surg 2000;7(2):193–7.
21. Reddy S, Wolfgang CL, Cameron JL, et al. Total pancreatectomy for pancreatic adenocarcinoma: evaluation of morbidity and long term survival. Ann Surg 2009;250:282–7.
22. Muller MW, Friess H, Kleeff J, et al. Is there still a role for total pancreatectomy? Ann Surg 2007;246:966–75.
23. Nathan H, Wolfgang CL, Edil BH, et al. Peri-operative mortality and long-term survival after total pancreatectomy for pancreatic adenocarcinoma: a population-based perspective. J Surg Oncol 2009;99:87–92.
24. Raut CP, Tseng JF, Sun CC, et al. Impact of resection status on pattern of failure and survival after pancreaticoduodenectomy for pancreatic adenocarcinoma. Ann Surg 2007;246:52–60.
25. Schmidt CM, Glant J, Winter JM, et al. Total pancreatectomy (R0 resection) improves survival over subtotal pancreatectomy in isolated neck margin positive pancreatic adenocarcinoma. Surgery 2007;142:572–80.
26. Asiyanbola B, Gleisner A, Herman JM, et al. Determining pattern of recurrence following pancreaticoduodenectomy and adjuvant 5-flurouracil-based chemoradiation therapy: effect of number of metastatic lymph nodes and lymph node ratio. J Gastrointest Surg 2009;13:752–9.
27. Reddy S, Wolfgang CL. The role of surgery in the management of isolated metastases to the pancreas. Lancet Oncol 2009;10(3):287–93.
28. Reddy S, Edil BH, Cameron JL, et al. Pancreatic resection of isolated metastases from non-pancreatic primary cancers. Ann Surg Oncol 2008;15:3199–206.

29. Varker KA, Muscarella P, Wall K, et al. Pancreatectomy for non-pancreatic malignancies results in improved survival after R0 resection. World J Surg Oncol 2007;5:145.
30. Zerbi A, Ortolano E, Balzano G, et al. Pancreatic metastasis from renal cell carcinoma: which patients benefit from surgical resection? Ann Surg Oncol 2008;15: 1161–8.
31. Bahra M, Jacob D, Langrehr JM, et al. Metastatic lesions to the pancreas. When is resection reasonable? Chirurg 2008;79:241–8.
32. Hiotis SP, Klimstra DS, Conlon KC, et al. Results after pancreatic resection for metastatic lesions. Ann Surg Oncol 2002;9:675–9.
33. Thompson LD, Heffess CS. Renal cell carcinoma to the pancreas in surgical pathology material. Cancer 2000;89(5):1076–88.
34. Nikfarjam M, Sehmbey M, Kimchi ET, et al. Additional organ resection combined with pancreaticoduodenectomy does not increase postoperative morbidity and mortality. J Gastrointest Surg 2009;13(5):915–21.
35. Henne-Bruns D, Vogel I, Lüttges J, et al. Ductal adenocarcinoma of the pancreas head: survival after regional versus extended lymphadenectomy. Hepatogastroenterology 1998;45:855–66.
36. Pedrazzoli S, DiCarlo V, Dionigi R, et al. Standard versus extended lymphadenectomy associated with pancreaticoduodenectomy in the surgical treatment of adenocarcinoma of the head of the pancreas: A multicenter, prospective, randomized study. Ann Surg 1998;228(4):508–17.
37. Yeo CJ, Cameron JL, Sohn TA, et al. Pancreaticoduodenectomy with or without extended retroperitoneal lymphadenectomy for periampullary adenocarcinoma: Comparison of morbidity and mortality and short-term outcome. Ann Surg 1999;229(5):613–24.
38. Yeo CJ, Cameron JL, Lillemoe KD, et al. Pancreaticoduodenectomy with or without distal gastrectomy and extended retroperitoneal lymphadenectomy for periampullary adenocarcinoma, part 2: randomized controlled trial evaluating survival, morbidity and mortality. Ann Surg 2002;236(3):355–68.
39. Farnell MB, Pearson RK, Sarr MG, et al. A prospective randomized trial comparing standard pancreaticoduodenectomy with extended lymphadenectomy in resectable pancreatic head adenocarcinoma. Surgery 2005;138(4):618–30.
40. Capussotti L, Massucco P, Ribero D, et al. Extended lymphadenectomy and vein resection for pancreatic head cancer: outcomes and implications for therapy. Arch Surg 2003;138:1316–22.
41. Roder JD, Stein HJ, Siewert JR. Carcinoma of the periampullary region: who benefits from portal vein resection? Ann Surg 1996;170:171–6.
42. Bachellier P, Nakano H, Oussoultzoglou PD, et al. Is pancreaticoduodenectomy with mesentericoportal venous resection safe and worthwhile? Am J Surg 2001; 182:120–9.
43. Siriwardana HP, Siriwardena AK. Systematic review of outcome of synchronous portal-superior mesenteric vein resection during pancreatectomy for cancer. Br J Surg 2006;93(6):662–73.
44. Martin RC II, Scoggins CR, Egnatashvili V, et al. Arterial and venous resection for pancreatic adenocarcinoma: operative and long-term outcomes. Arch Surg 2009;144(2):154–9.
45. Tseng JF, Raut CP, Lee JE, et al. Pancreaticoduodenectomy with vascular resection: margin status and survival duration. J Gastrointest Surg 2004;8(8):935–50.
46. Stitzenberg KB, Watson JC, Roberts A, et al. Survival after pancreatectomy with major arterial resection and reconstruction. Ann Surg Oncol 2008;15(5): 1399–406.

47. Oussoultzoglou E, Bachellier P, Bigourdan JM, et al. Pancreaticogastrostomy decreased relaparotomy caused by pancreatic fistula after pancreaticoduodenectomy compared with pancreaticojejunostomy. Arch Surg 2004;139:327–35.
48. Nakao A, Fujii T, Sugimoto H, et al. Is pancreaticogastrostomy safer than pancreaticojejunostomy? J Hepatobiliary Pancreat Surg 2006;13:202–6.
49. Aranha G, Hodul P, Golts E, et al. A comparison of pancreaticogastrostomy and pancreaticojejunostomy following pancreaticoduodenectomy. J Gastrointest Surg 2003;7(5):672–82.
50. Takana S, Ito Y, Watanabe Y, et al. Pancreaticojejunostomy versus pancreaticogastrostomy in reconstruction following pancreaticoduodenectomy. Br J Surg 2000;87(4):423–7.
51. Bassi C, Falconi M, Molinari E, et al. Reconstruction by pancreaticojejunostomy versus pancreaticogastrostomy following pancreatectomy: results of a comparative study. Ann Surg 2005;242:767–73.
52. Duffas JP, Suc B, Msika S, et al. A controlled randomized multicenter trial of pancreaticogastrostomy or pancreaticojejunostomy after pancreaticoduodenectomy. Am J Surg 2005;189:720–9.
53. Yeo CJ, Cameron JL, Maher MM, et al. A prospective randomized trial of pancreaticogastrostomy versus pancreaticojejunostomy after pancreaticoduodenectomy. Ann Surg 1995;222(4):580–92.
54. Wente MN, Shrikhande SV, Müller MW, et al. Pancreaticojejunostomy versus pancreaticogastrostomy: systematic review and meta-analysis. Am J Surg 2007;193:171–83.
55. Poon RTP, Fan ST, Lo CM, et al. External drainage of pancreatic duct with a stent to reduce leakage rate of pancreaticojejunostomy after pancreaticoduodenectomy: a prospective randomized trial. Ann Surg 2007;246:425–35.
56. Roder JD, Stein HJ, Böttcher KA, et al. Stented versus nonstented pancreaticojejunostomy after pancreaticoduodenectomy: a prospective study. Ann Surg 1999;229(1):41–8.
57. Winter JM, Cameron JL, Campbell KA, et al. Does pancreatic duct stenting decrease the rate of pancreatic fistula following pancreaticoduodenectomy? Results of a prospective randomized trial. J Gastrointest Surg 2006;10(9):1280–90.
58. Bartoli FG, Arnone GB, Ravera G, et al. Pancreatic fistula and relative mortality in malignant disease after pancreaticoduodenectomy. Review and statistical meta-analysis regarding 15 years of literature. Anticancer Res 1991;11:1831–48.
59. Crist DW, Cameron JL. Current status of pancreaticoduodenectomy for periampullary carcinoma. Hepatogastroenterology 1989;36:478–85.
60. Grace PA, Pitt HA, Longmire WP. Pancreaticoduodenectomy with pylorus preservation for adenocarcinoma of the head of the pancreas. Br J Surg 1986;73:647–50.
61. Braasch JW, Rossi RL, Watkins E Jr, et al. Pyloric and gastric preserving pancreatic resection. Experience with 87 patients. Ann Surg 1986;204:411–8.
62. Bassi C, Falconi M, Molinari E, et al. Duct-to-mucosa versus end-to-side pancreaticojejunostomy reconstruction after pancreaticoduodenectomy: Results of a prospective randomized trial. Surgery 2003;134:766–71.
63. Beger AC, Howard TJ, Kennedy EP, et al. Does type of pancreaticojejunostomy after pancreaticoduodenectomy decrease rate of pancreatic fistula? A randomized, prospective, dual-institution trial. J Am Coll Surg 2009;208:738–49.
64. Fischer WE, Chai C, Hodges SE, et al. Effect of BioGlue on the incidence of pancreatic fistula following pancreatic resection. J Gastrointest Surg 2008;12:882–90.
65. Lillemoe KD, Cameron JL, Kim MP, et al. Does fibrin glue sealant decrease the rate of pancreatic fistula after pancreaticoduodenectomy? Results of a prospective randomized trial. J Gastrointest Surg 2004;8(7):766–72.

66. Tran K, Van Eijck C, Di Carlo V, et al. Occlusion of the pancreatic duct versus pancreaticojejunostomy: a prospective randomized trial. Ann Surg 2002;236(4):422–8.
67. Suc B, Msika S, Fingerhut A, et al. Temporary fibrin glue occlusion of the main pancreatic duct in the prevention of intra-abdominal complications after pancreatic resection: prospective randomized trial. Ann Surg 2003;237(1):57–65.
68. Povoski SP, Karpeh MS Jr, Conlon KC, et al. Association of preoperative biliary drainage with postoperative outcome following pancreaticoduodenectomy. Ann Surg 1999;230(2):131–42.
69. Fujino Y, Matsumoto I, Shinzeki M, et al. Impact of internal biliary drainage after pancreaticoduodenectomy. J Hepatobiliary Pancreat Surg 2009;16(2):160–4.
70. Conlon KC, Labow D, Leung D, et al. Prospective randomized clinical trial of the value of intraperitoneal drainage after pancreatic resection. Ann Surg 2001; 234(4):487–94.
71. Jeekel J. No abdominal drainage after Whipple's procedure. Br J Surg 1992; 79:182.
72. Tani M, Terasawa H, Kawai M, et al. Improvement of delayed gastric emptying in pylorus-preserving pancreaticoduodenectomy: results of a prospective, randomized, controlled trial. Ann Surg 2006;243:316–20.
73. Park YC, Kim SW, Jang JY, et al. Factors influencing delayed gastric emptying after pylorus-preserving pancreatoduodenectomy. J Am Coll Surg 2003;196:859–65.
74. Horstmann O, Markus PM, Ghadimi MB, et al. Pylorus preservation has no impact on delayed gastric emptying after pancreatic head resection. Pancreas 2004;28: 69–74.
75. Hashimoto N. Hepatobiliary imaging after pancreaticoduodenectomy – a comparative study on Billroth I and Billroth II reconstruction. Hepatogastroenterology 2005;52(64):1023–5.
76. Kotoura Y, Takahashi T, Ishikawa Y, et al. Hepatobiliary and gastrointestinal imaging after pancreaticoduodenectomy – a comparative study on Billroth I and Billroth II reconstructions. Jpn J Surg 1990;20(3):294–9.
77. Hishinuma S, Ogata Y, Matsui J, et al. Complications after pylorus-preserving pancreaticoduodenectomy with gastrointestinal reconstruction by the Imanaga method. J Am Coll Surg 1998;186(1):10–6.
78. Hishinuma S, Ogata Y, Matsui J, et al. Evaluation of pylorus-preserving pancreaticoduodenectomy with the Imanaga reconstruction by hepatobiliary and gastrointestinal dual scintigraphy. Br J Surg 1999;86(10):1306–11.
79. Gianotti L, Braga M, Gentilini O, et al. Artificial nutrition after pancreaticoduodenectomy. Pancreas 2000;21(4):344–51.
80. Yermilov I, Jain S, Sekeris E, et al. Utilization of parenteral nutrition following pancreaticoduodenectomy: is routine jejunostomy tube placement warranted? Dig Dis Sci 2009;54(7):1582–8.
81. Baradi H, Walsh RM, Henderson JM, et al. Postoperative jejunal feeding and outcome of pancreaticoduodenectomy. J Gastrointest Surg 2004;8(4):428–33.
82. Baker MS, Bentrem DJ, Ujiki MB, et al. A prospective single institution comparison of peri-operative outcomes for laparoscopic and open distal pancreatectomy. Surgery 2009;146(4):635–43.
83. Frenandez-Cruz L, Cosa R, Blanco L, et al. Curative laparoscopic resection for pancreatic neoplasms: a critical analysis from a single institution. J Gastrointest Surg 2007;11(12):1607–22.
84. Rodriguez JR, Madanat MG, Healy BC, et al. Distal pancreatectomy with splenic preservation revisited. Surgery 2007;141(5):619–25.

Solid Tumors of the Body and Tail of the Pancreas

Katherine A. Morgan, MD*, David B. Adams, MD

KEYWORDS

- Neuroendocrine tumors • Laparoscopic surgery
- Pancreatic adenocarcinoma • Surgical resection

There was a time when the diagnosis and surgical treatment of solid tumors of the body and tail of the pancreas began in pessimism and ended in futility. Identifying resectable malignancies of the pancreas was much less common than identifying tumors that were unresectable or frequently margin-positive, with associated patient survival that rarely exceeded 6 months. Patients with long-term survival of pancreatic ductal cancer were so few that many questioned whether distal pancreatectomy for adenocarcinoma was an indicated procedure. Patients with Whipple's triad and a small insulinoma in the tail of the pancreas were few. Autoimmune pancreatitis was unknown. Computed tomography (CT) scanning was not used so freely by emergency room and primary care physicians; thus small, asymptomatic tumors were rarely discovered. The precise identification and biopsy of small lesions in the tail and body of the pancreas by a flexible endoscope with an ultrasonic probe were unheard of. However, with widespread use of CT and magnetic resonance imaging (MRI) scanning for patients with gastrointestinal and nongastrointestinal disorders, the identification of benign and malignant conditions of the pancreas that are favorable surgical challenges with excellent long-term outcomes has instilled new interest and enthusiasm in the diagnosis and management of solid tumors of the body and tail of the pancreas. The practice of abandoning pancreatic resection for unexpected celiac axis tumor invasion has largely been replaced by a laparoscopic spleen-preserving distal pancreatectomy for an early cancer or a benign tumor.

Solid tumors of the body and tail of the pancreas continue to represent a relatively uncommon clinical entity. The most likely diagnosis of a solid tumor remains ductal adenocarcinoma, which holds a poor prognosis similar to cancer in the head of the pancreas but is not incurable when discovered at a favorable stage. Many other potential diagnoses occur and may follow a benign course with excellent long-term survival rates.

Section of Gastrointestinal and Laparoscopic Surgery, Medical University of South Carolina, 25 Courtenay Drive Suite 7018, MSC 290, Charleston, SC 29425, USA
* Corresponding author.
E-mail address: morganka@musc.edu

Surg Clin N Am 90 (2010) 287–307
doi:10.1016/j.suc.2009.12.009   surgical.theclinics.com

Management of these tumors has progressed notably over the past decade, paralleling advances in technology and surgical technique. Improvements in radiographic imaging modalities have enabled diagnosis with a good degree of certainty. Minimally invasive surgery is an exciting and dynamic tool in the approach to these patients.

RADIOGRAPHY

Evaluation of a patient with a solid tumor of the body and tail of the pancreas includes an attempt to obtain diagnosis to help guide management. Various radiographic studies are valuable in this differentiation. Beyond diagnosis, preoperative staging with radiography help is essential to guide management.

COMPUTED TOMOGRAPHY

CT is the premier imaging test for diagnosing and staging solid pancreatic tumors. The modern CT capability (multiphase contrast-enhanced, thin section, spiral, or multidetector) has maintained this modality's utility in the face of other developing technologies (ie, MRI and endoscopic ultrasound [EUS]). CT can detect small lesions (>1 cm diameter) and give clues to diagnosis based on enhancement (hypovascular, hypervascular) and behavioral (invasion of nearby structures) characteristics. CT gives valuable information about vascular involvement, local invasion, and metastatic disease to help guide management decisions including resectability (**Fig. 1**). In a recent meta-analysis, modern CT has been shown to have a sensitivity and specificity of 91% and 85%, respectively, for diagnosis of pancreatic cancer, and a sensitivity and specificity of 81% and 82%, respectively, for resectability. The primary limitation of CT is in the ability to detect small peritoneal and liver metastases.[1]

MAGNETIC RESONANCE

MR shows excellent results in terms of tumor detection and staging in evaluation of solid tumors of the pancreas. There have been multiple studies comparing MR with

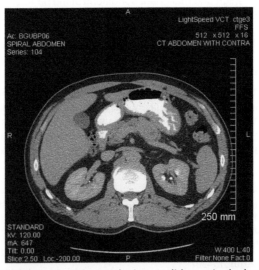

Fig. 1. Axial contrasted dynamic CT image depicts a solid mass in the body of the pancreas, consistent with a pancreatic adenocarcinoma.

CT in the assessment of pancreatic masses, but none has shown significant benefit of MR over CT. MR has been shown to have a sensitivity and specificity of 84% and 82%, respectively, for diagnosis of pancreatic cancer, and a sensitivity and specificity of 82% and 78%, respectively, for resectability.[1] MR may have better differentiation of the characteristics of liver lesions, and magnetic resonance cholangiopancreatography (MRCP) allows for important specifics in the evaluation of cystic masses but confers no clear benefit in solid masses.

ENDOSCOPIC ULTRASOUND

EUS was introduced approximately 25 years ago, with the goal of improved visualization of the pancreas as compared with conventional imaging. EUS can be useful in the diagnosis and localization of solid tumors of the body and tail of the pancreas.

Functional neuroendocrine tumors of the pancreas are often diagnosed based on the associated clinical syndrome and confirmatory laboratory evidence of functional hormone hypersecretion. EUS is useful for localization of small tumors. In a prospective study of 82 patients with functional pancreatic neuroendocrine tumors, EUS was found to have a sensitivity and accuracy of 93%, with a specificity of 95%.[2]

In solid tumors of the body and tail of the pancreas, including nonfunctional neuroendocrine tumors, pancreatic adenocarcinoma, and metastatic lesions, EUS can be useful in detecting and better characterizing small tumors (sensitivity 95%–100%) and, particularly with the aid of fine-needle aspiration (FNA), can help in diagnosis (sensitivity 80%–90%, specificity 100%). The differentiation of pancreatic adenocarcinoma arising in the setting of chronic pancreatitis is a primary cause for a false negative test.[3] Because of the potential for complications (overall 2.2%, pancreatitis 2%, tumor seeding <0.5%), EUS-FNA should only be used when the results are likely to alter therapy.[4–7]

EUS has an overall accuracy of 85% for tumor staging in pancreatic adenocarcinoma and 72% for nodal staging.[8] Comparative studies of EUS and contrast-enhanced helical CT are inconsistent, with no consistent advantage to EUS.[6] EUS is an excellent complementary test to CT in staging of solid tumors of the body and tail of the pancreas.[9]

SURGICAL APPROACH

Left-sided pancreatectomy is the most commonly indicated procedure for solid tumors of the body and tail of the pancreas. The pancreas is approached through the gastrocolic ligament into the lesser sac. The short gastric vessels are taken down to fully retract the stomach. The splenic flexure of the colon also is taken down. The retroperitoneum overlying the inferior border of the pancreas is divided with careful preservation of the superior mesenteric vein. The inferior mesenteric vein is identified and ligated. The splenic artery is identified and ligated securely near its origin from the celiac trunk, as is the splenic vein, with caution taken to avoid narrowing the portal vein. The pancreatic tissue can be divided with a surgical stapler or with an energy modality, depending on surgeon preference and tissue consistency.[10] In general, at least a 2-cm gross margin is sought from the tumor, although frozen section confirmation of microscopically negative margins should be confirmed intraoperatively. In cases with malignant tumors, a proper regional lymphadenectomy that includes the lymph nodes along the celiac trunk and splenic artery should be done. In these cases, the spleen is generally taken en bloc with the pancreas so as to include the associated lymph node basin. In the treatment of benign diseases, the spleen may be spared either by preservation of the splenic artery and vein or in the manner of

Warshaw by maintaining splenic perfusion off of the short gastric vessels.[11,12] Alternatively, enucleation of the tumor may be appropriate in benign tumors such as insulinoma, as long as there is no involvement of the main pancreatic duct.

Distal pancreatectomy for adenocarcinoma carries a 23% to 47% morbidity rate. Pancreatic fistula is the most common complication, occurring in 5% to 29% of cases.[13-20] Pancreatic fistulae are best graded by the classification system defined by the international study group on pancreatic fistula.[21] Most pancreatic fistulae are of minimal clinical consequence, although rarely they may require reoperation and may result in mortality. Technical factors in the prevention of pancreatic fistulae have been studied by many groups, without a consistent identified factor that seems to confer an advantage in large studies. Specifically, staplers, staple line reinforcement, direct duct ligation, a falciform patch, and fibrin glue have not consistently shown an advantage.[10,22] Rather, patient-related factors such as elevated body mass index, male gender, an additional concomitant procedure, tobacco use, and indication for surgery have been found to be predictive.[10,23]

LAPAROSCOPIC SURGERY

The use of laparoscopy in the management of solid tumors of the body and tail of the pancreas has expanded over the past 2 decades and warrants careful consideration.

Initially, laparoscopy was used in the management of pancreatic cancer primarily for diagnostic purposes. In 1911, Bernkeim[24] reported that cystoscopy of the abdominal cavity could potentially identify patients with metastatic pancreatic cancer. In 1978, Cuschieri and colleagues[25] described the use of diagnostic laparoscopy to aid in identifying patients with advanced pancreatic cancer. In 1986, Warshaw and colleagues[26] proposed a benefit of diagnostic laparoscopy for these patients. In patients with malignant tumors of the body and tail of the pancreas without metastatic disease by preoperative imaging, diagnostic laparoscopy identifies patients with occult metastatic disease in a proportion of patients, particularly in patients with locally advanced disease (34%–37%), aiding in decision making for therapy.[27,28]

In 1994, Soper and colleagues[29] showed the feasibility of laparoscopic stapling techniques in pancreatectomy in the porcine model, thus opening the door for more complex laparoscopic pancreatic surgeries.

In 1996, Gagner and colleagues[30] reported on a series of 12 patients undergoing laparoscopic procedures for pancreatic neuroendocrine tumors. Eight underwent attempted laparoscopic distal pancreatectomy (3 conversions to open), whereas 4 underwent attempted enucleation (1 successful). Thus, resective procedures for benign and low-grade neoplasms of the pancreas were found to be feasible.

In 2007, Melotti and colleagues[31] in Verona reported the largest single institution series of patients undergoing laparoscopic distal pancreatectomy. Fifty out of 58 patients had benign or low-grade neoplasms, 1 had pancreatitis, and the remaining 7 had adenocarcinoma. The investigators reported a pancreas-related morbidity of 43% and a pancreatic fistula rate of 27.5%.

In 2008, Kooby and colleagues[32] reported on the largest multicenter series to date, with 667 total cases of left sided pancreatectomy, 159 (24%) of which were performed laparoscopically. The primary indication for surgery was a benign neoplasm (102, 64%). Fourteen (9%) were for chronic pancreatitis; 16 (10%) were for adenocarcinoma of the pancreas. The morbidity was 40%, with pancreatic fistula in 11%. In comparison with the open pancreatectomy group, the laparoscopic patients had less morbidity, less intraoperative blood loss, and a shorter length of hospital stay. They found no difference in margin status, operative times, or fistula rates.

Laparoscopic distal pancreatectomy may be the surgery of choice for patients with benign and low-grade neoplasms of the body and tail of the pancreas. There are no randomized controlled trials that evaluate the essential outcomes, including tumor recurrence and disease-specific survival rates, in understanding the role of laparoscopic distal pancreatectomy for malignant neoplasms. Given the excellent visualization, lymphadenectomy is technically achievable and the procedure is safe. It is, therefore, likely an appropriate operative approach for cancer. In theory, the blunted stress response and therefore the lessened immunosuppressive effects of laparoscopy as compared with open surgery may confer some advantage to the laparoscopic approach in terms of tumor biology.

ADENOCARCINOMA OF THE PANCREAS

Adenocarcinoma of the body and tail of the pancreas is the most common solid tumor of this region of the pancreas, representing approximately 15% to 25% of cases of pancreatic adenocarcinoma.[19,33,34] Patients present in the seventh decade of life, median age 65 to 68 years of age, and the genders are equally affected.[20,27,34]

Presenting symptoms are caused by tumor growth and mass effect and include abdominal pain (87%), weight loss (55%), and new onset diabetes.[20] Tumors are generally large on presentation, median size 4.9 to 5.5 cm.[19,20] Patients typically present with advanced disease, with 80% of patients presenting with metastases and only 10% to 16% ultimately determined to be resectable at surgery.[15,19,20,34,35] Median survival for those patients who are unable to undergo resection because of advanced disease is 5.8 months.[16]

The surgical approach is distal pancreatectomy with splenectomy to include an adequate lymphadenectomy. Mortality rates are reported at 0% to 4%. Morbidity is reported at to 23% to 49%.[13–20,34] In 35% to 39% of patients, an en bloc resection to include locally involved structures may be necessary (including portal venous confluence, stomach, colon, left kidney, or left adrenal gland). This more extended resection has been shown to be effective, with equivalent survival rates, although short-term morbidity is potentially greater.[16,20,34]

Median survival after resection for pancreatic adenocarcinoma is 12 to 15.9 months, with 5-year actuarial survival of 9 to 22 months.[15,16,19,20] Several variables have been identified as potential prognostic indicators, although the evidence for this varies between studies. Several investigators have found the presence of lymph node disease to predict poor outcome,[16,34] whereas others have found them to be without correlation.[19,20] The presence of microscopically positive margins has been found to be important by some investigators,[19,34] but nonpredictive by others.[16,20] Tumor size,[19,20] histologic grade,[16,19] and age[19,20] have all been found to be predictive of outcome in various reports.

Adenocarcinoma of the body and tail of the pancreas is an aggressive disease. Surgical management with resection should be considered in all patients without distant metastatic disease, with local resectability.

NEUROENDOCRINE TUMORS

Neuroendocrine tumors of the pancreas (PNETs), which are neoplasms of the family of amine precursor uptake decarboxylase cells, are uncommon tumors, representing 2% to 4% of all pancreatic neoplasms. These tumors are much less common than pancreatic adenocarcinoma by a ratio of 125 to 1, although PNETs have been reported in up to 1.5% of autopsies.[36] PNETs affect women and men approximately equally, and present at a mean age of 51.7 to 56.8 years.[37–43] PNETs may occur sporadically or in the setting of a genetic syndrome such as multiple endocrine neoplasia I (MEN I), von Hippel Lindau disease, neurofibromatosis type I, or tuberous sclerosis.

Radiographically, PNETs can be detected by contrast-enhanced CT scan as hypervascular tumors. Sensitivity of CT for PNETs is directly related to size, with tumors less than 1 cm detected with a sensitivity of 10%, and larger tumors much more easily detected, with a sensitivity as high as 82%[44–46] (Fig. 2A). On MRI, PNETs demonstrate low signal intensity on T1-weighted imaging and high signal intensity on T2-weighted images. Like CT, the sensitivity improves with increased size of the tumor, with tumors smaller than 1 cm poorly detected and those larger than 2 cm very well visualized, with a sensitivity of 85% to 90% and specificity approaching 100%.[46,47] Somatostatin receptor scintigraphy (SRS) takes advantage of tumor expression of somatostatin receptor subtype 2. Sensitivity for SRS is at least 80% for all PNETs except insulinomas (only about two-thirds of which express the somatostatin receptor), and SRS is currently essential as the most sensitive noninvasive test for tumor localization and postoperative surveillance for most PNETs. SRS has been shown to change management in 19% to 47% of patients with PNETs.[48–50] Endoscopic ultrasound (EUS) has evolved over the past two decades to become the test of choice in localizing small PNETs of all types. EUS can detect very small lesions, as small as 0.2 to 0.5 cm. EUS has a sensitivity of 93% for detecting PNETs, particularly in the head and body of the pancreas.[51,52] EUS-FNA can add the ability for diagnostic testing.[53] Positron emission tomography (PET) scanning using ^{18}F-fluorodeoxyglucose is insensitive for PNETs given their slow growth rate. More recently, PET scans using ^{11}C-labeled DOPA or 5-hydroxytryptophan show excellent sensitivity for PNETs, perhaps even better than SRS.[54]

PNETs arise from pluripotent cells in the pancreatic ductal epithelium. Histologically, PNETs appear as uniform patterns of cells with scant mitoses (see Fig. 2B). Immunohistochemistry is typified by positive staining for chromogranin A, cytokeratin, synaptophysin, and neuron-specific enolase, all demonstrating the neuroendocrine differentiation of these tumors.

PNETs are generally divided into functional and nonfunctional neuroendocrine tumors. Functional neuroendocrine tumors (F-PNETs) secrete hormonal peptides that lead to defined clinical syndromes related to the hypersecreted peptide. Nonfunctional tumors (NF-PNETs) are not associated with a clinical syndrome, due either to secretion of a peptide without evident or easily measurable clinical effect (ie, pancreatic polypeptide, chromogranin A) or to peptide nonsecretion. Because functional and

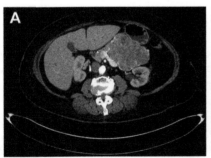
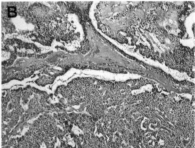

Fig. 2. (A) Axial contrasted dynamic CT image reveals a large heterogeneous mass in the body of the pancreas, demonstrating mass effect. This image is consistent with a nonfunctional pancreatic neuroendocrine tumor. (B) Histologic section at magnification ×10 demonstrating a pancreatic neuroendocrine tumor with uniform small blue cells.

nonfunctional neuroendocrine tumors represent very different clinical entities with important distinguishing characteristics in management and prognosis, they are considered separately.

Functional Neuroendocrine Tumors

F-PNETs are islet cell tumors that are associated with a defined clinical syndrome due to the hypersecretion of a hormonal peptide. F-PNETs are often detected at small sizes due to their biochemical activity and resultant symptomatology. F-PNETs represent 28% to 85% of all PNETs, with decreasing proportional frequency as more asymptomatic NF-PNETs are discovered incidentally by imaging for another indication.[37–43] The most common F-PNETs are insulinomas, followed by gastrinomas. Together they represent 95% of these tumors, with less common functional tumors including glucagonomas, tumors of excess vasoactive intestinal peptide secretion (VIPomas), somatostatinomas, and corticotropinomas.

Insulinoma

In 1926, Wilder and colleagues[55] reported a patient with severe hypoglycemic attacks who was explored by William Mayo and found to have an insulinoma metastatic to the liver. In 1929, Graham successfully resected an insulinoma, curing his patient of hypoglycemic events.[56] Insulinoma is the most common type of F-PNET. Insulinomas are generally benign, with 5% to 8% demonstrating malignant behavior on diagnosis.[41,57,58]

In 1935 Whipple[59] described his classic triad of symptoms attributable to hypoglycemia, low serum glucose measured at the time of symptoms, and relief of symptoms with administration of glucose. Insulinoma is characterized clinically by fasting hypoglycemia and neuroglycopenia. Up to 15% of patients present with sympathoadrenal mediated cardiovascular symptoms such as palpitations or tachycardia.[36,57]

The diagnosis of insulinoma can be made with a 72-hour fast, with measured insulin and glucose levels. In patients with insulinoma, the dysregulation between insulin and glucose becomes apparent as inappropriately elevated serum insulin in the face of low serum glucose (insulin to glucose ratio greater than 0.4). The sensitivity for this test is 75% at 24 hours and 98% at 72 hours.[36]

Insulinomas are typically small, with 90% less than 2 cm. Therefore, localization can be challenging. In the modern era of multiphase technique, the sensitivity of contrast-enhanced CT is at best 64%.[44,60] EUS should be performed, with a sensitivity of 75% to 93%.[51,52,60] EUS is less sensitive for tumors of the body and tail of the pancreas (closer to 40%).[60] In addition, calcium-stimulated angiography with portal venous sampling can be useful, with a sensitivity of 67% to 88%.[36,61] Many tumors, however, cannot be localized preoperatively and are discovered instead on operative exploration.[62] Intraoperative ultrasound is an important tool for identification of insulinomas, with a sensitivity of 92% to 97%.[57,60] Several investigators have proposed that elaborate preoperative imaging is not necessary for localization because of the efficacy of intraoperative ultrasound.[62,63]

The treatment of insulinoma is by complete surgical resection. An organ-sparing technique should be employed, including enucleation. Often these tumors are ideally suited to a laparoscopic approach.[30,64,65]

The vast majority of insulinomas are benign (92%–97%) and the diagnosis does not shorten long-term survival compared with the general population.[57,58,66] In the Mayo series of 224 patients older than 60 years, 87% of patients were asymptomatic 6 months after surgery. Among patients who had initial response at surgery, 6% developed recurrent hypoglycemia at 10 years.[58] In a recent series of 61 patients from the Massachusetts General Hospital, the investigators found a 10-year disease-specific survival of 100%. Malignant disease with lymph node involvement was found to be a predictor for recurrence of disease but not for mortality. In those patients with positive surgical margins after resection, no recurrences were seen at follow-up.[57]

Gastrinoma

In 1955, Zollinger and Ellison[67] described a syndrome of upper jejunal ulceration, gastric acid hypersecretion, and an islet cell tumor of the pancreas. In 1964, Gregory and Tracy[68] implicated gastrin as the gut hormone in excess. Gastrinoma is the second most common F-PNET. The incidence is estimated to be 1% of patients with peptic ulcer disease.[36] Gastrinoma should be investigated in any patient with peptic ulcer disease and diarrhea, with peptic ulcer disease without *Helicobacter pylori*, with complicated peptic ulcer disease, or with prominent gastric rugae on endoscopy.[69] Whereas most gastrinomas are sporadic, 16% to 35% are associated with MEN I.[36]

Diagnosis of gastrinoma begins with a serum gastrin level, with the upper limit of normal being 100 pg/mL. A serum gastrin level greater than 1000 pg/mL is generally considered diagnostic of gastrinoma. Other causes of hypergastrinemia (generally between 100 and 1000 pg/mL) include achlorhydria (particularly secondary to proton pump inhibitor use), gastric outlet obstruction, renal insufficiency, and retained gastric antrum. The secretin stimulation test can help differentiate gastrinoma from other causes of hypergastrinemia. This test hinges on the fact that secretin inhibits gastrin release from normal G cells but stimulates gastrin release from gastrinoma cells. An increase in serum gastrin greater than 200 pg/mL with administration of secretin is considered a positive test. The secretin stimulation test is 90% sensitive (and specific) in the diagnosis of gastrinoma.[36]

Localization of gastrinomas can be challenging, as most tumors are small and 30% to 50% are located in the duodenum.[70,71] The gastrinoma triangle, where greater than 90% of gastrinomas are located, is well described (marked by the neck of the pancreas, the border of the second and third portions of the duodenum, and the cystic duct). SRS is somewhat useful for localization, with a sensitivity of 58%.[49] EUS is the diagnostic test of choice, with sensitivity reported between 82% and 93%.[2]

The treatment of gastrinoma is by complete surgical resection. The principles of exploration for gastrinoma include a Kocher maneuver to permit careful examination of the head and uncinate process of the pancreas; mobilization of the body and tail of the pancreas to allow manual palpation and ultrasound evaluation; and duodenotomy for thorough assessment.

At the time of diagnosis, 50% to 60% of tumors are malignant. Postoperative cure rates with gastrinoma approximate 60%, while disease-free survival at 5 years is 40% and at 10 years is 34%.[72] In a study evaluating outcomes in 195 gastrinoma patients (160 surgery, 35 without surgery) followed for 12 years, Norton and colleagues[73] at Stanford demonstrated that surgery increases survival, as 21% of patients who underwent surgery died versus 54% who did not (P<.002). Disease-specific survival was much improved with surgery (98% vs 74% at 15 years, P<.0002). Surgery seems to extend disease-related survival through its intervention on the natural history of gastrinoma. During follow-up, 16% of patients who underwent surgery had developed new metastatic lesions versus 37% of patients who did not. Ellison and colleagues[74] at Ohio State University reported that R0 (normal postoperative gastrin) or R1 (hypergastrinemia with no measurable disease) resection improves survival in gastrinoma patients while R2 resection (gross residual disease) does not improve survival

(P<.0001). Given these outcomes, it seems prudent that routine surgical exploration with intent for resection should be performed in all patients without extensive metastatic disease. Those patients with extensive and unresectable disease burden presumably will not benefit from surgical exploration.

Hepatic metastases occur in nearly 40% of patients at a median of 7 years. Ten-year survival of metastatic gastrinoma is approximately 35%.[74] Surgical resection improves survival in patients with metastatic neuroendocrine tumors, including gastrinoma.[75,76]

Glucagonoma

In 1942, Becker and Kahn[77] reported a patient with diabetes, weight loss, a distinct rash, and an islet cell tumor of the pancreas. Glucagonomas are typically found in the body or tail of the pancreas. Glucagonomas differ from the other F-PNETs in that they are often large on diagnosis (>4 cm). In tumors larger than 5 cm, the rate of malignancy is 60% to 80%. Hepatic metastases have been reported in more than 50% of patients on diagnosis.

The clinical presentation is marked by diabetes, a characteristic rash, necrolytic migratory erythema, anemia, and deep venous thrombosis. The diabetes, present in 75% to 95% of patients, is typically mild and easy to manage. The rash is present in 70% of patients; it develops over several weeks and consists of erythematous plaques that coalesce into larger areas that then have central clearing and peripheral blistering. The rash is resolved with amino acid supplementation. A normocytic anemia is seen in 90% of patients on presentation. Up to 30% of patients with glucagonoma develop deep venous thrombosis.[78]

Diagnosis of glucagonoma is best determined with a serum glucagon level. CT scan can localize these tumors, with greater than 85% sensitivity (as they are large).

After nutritional supplementation, complete surgical resection is ideal. Only 30% of patients who are resected have no residual or recurrent tumor. Glucagonomas typically present at an advanced stage but demonstrate indolent behavior.

VIPoma

In 1958, Verner and Morrison[79] described a syndrome consisting of refractory watery diarrhea, hypokalemia, achlorhydria, and an islet cell tumor. VIPomas are rare tumors, occurring in 1 per 10,000,000 population. Vasoactive intestinal peptide (VIP) normally functions as a neurotransmitter. VIP activates enteric smooth muscle and stimulates pancreatic exocrine and intestinal secretion. Specifically, with pathologically elevated serum levels, VIP stimulates the secretion and inhibits the reabsorption of sodium, chloride, potassium, and water in the gut, resulting in profound secretory diarrhea.

Diagnosis of VIPoma is confirmed with serum hormone measurement. VIPomas are median 5 cm on diagnosis, with 72% located in the tail of the pancreas. Given the typically large size of these tumors, contrast-enhanced CT scan is the modality of choice for localization. Fifty-nine percent are metastatic on presentation.

Treatment begins with correcting the metabolic aberrations associated with the secretory diarrhea. Octreotide is very effective in stopping the diarrhea to allow for electrolyte resuscitation, although with time tachyphylaxis may develop. Complete surgical resection is the definitive treatment of choice. In patients with extensive local or metastatic disease, debulking is warranted to ameliorate symptoms.

In a review of reported cases in the literature, Ghaferi and colleagues[80] reported that 59% of patients at a median follow-up of 15 months were reported as alive with no evidence of disease, 23% had died of their disease, and 18% were alive with disease.

Somatostatinoma

In 1977, Ganda[81] described a syndrome of diabetes, gallstones, elevated serum somatostatin, and an islet cell tumor. Somatostatinomas are rare tumors, accounting for less than 1% of all F-PNETs, which arise from the delta cells of the endocrine pancreas. Somatostatinomas are often large (>5 cm) at diagnosis. Two-thirds of tumors are located in the pancreas and one-third of these are located in the body or tail of the pancreas. Sixty percent to 70% are metastatic on presentation.

Somatostatin is an inhibitor of insulin, glucagon, gastrin, and growth hormone secretion; it is also a cholecystokinin inhibitor. Many somatostatinomas are discovered incidentally. Symptoms include diabetes mellitus (60%), gallstones (70%), and steatorrhea. Diagnosis is confirmed with a serum somatostatin level. Given their large size, contrast-enhanced CT is an excellent means of tumor localization.

Complete surgical resection is the treatment of choice, although debulking is warranted in highly symptomatic patients to ameliorate diarrheal symptoms.[82]

Nonfunctional Neuroendocrine Tumors

NF-PNETs are islet cell tumors that are not associated with a clinical syndrome secondary to hormone hypersecretion. NF-PNETs constitute 15% to 72% of all endocrine tumors of the pancreas.[37–43] NF-PNETs are generally larger than functional tumors, a median 4.4 to 4.6 cm diameter on presentation.[37,38,40] NF-PNETs typically present with symptoms of tumor growth such as abdominal pain, abdominal fullness, or weight loss, although 16% to 88% are asymptomatic. Incidentally discovered tumors have become more frequent over the past two decades because of more frequent use of noninvasive imaging for other indications.[37,38,41,43] Incidentally discovered NF-PNETs tend to be smaller, are less likely to be malignant, and have a better overall survival than their symptomatic counterparts.[37,43]

NF-PNETs are evenly distributed through the pancreas. The surgical approach is dictated by tumor extent and location. Surgical treatment is complete resection with negative margins when possible. With well-differentiated tumors, margin status does not appear to be prognostic, whereas in patients with malignant tumors, a positive surgical margin is a predictor of poor outcome.[43,83,84]

The disease-specific 5-year survival for patients with NF-PNETs is 60% to 77%. Prognostic indicators for improved survival include lack of tumor symptoms, resection of primary tumor, absence of liver metastases, and small tumor size.[37–40,43,84] In those patients with malignant disease, the 5-year survival is 43% to 45%. In patients with high-grade, poorly differentiated tumors, however, the prognosis is similar to pancreatic adenocarcinoma, with 2-year survival of 19% to 25%.[43,84] In a series from M. D. Anderson of 163 patients with nonfunctioning islet cell carcinoma, patients with localized disease had a median survival of 7.1 years, whereas those with metastatic disease had a median survival of 2.1 years.[84] Given this poor prognosis, as well as the negative predictive factor of R1 or R2 resection, surgical resection without potential for complete resection is not warranted in patients with poorly differentiated and metastatic tumors.[43,84]

SOLID PSEUDOPAPILLARY TUMOR

Solid pseudopapillary tumor of the pancreas (SPT) was first described by Frantz[85] in 1959 and was given its current consistent terminology by the World Health Organization classification in 1996.[86] SPT is a rare entity, comprising 0.9% to 2.5% of solid pancreatic tumors.[87,88] SPT affects primarily women (82%–93% of cases) of young age (median age 26 to 39, range 12–79 years) and has a predilection for non-whites.[87–92]

Patients may present with an abdominal mass or vague abdominal pain, but are often asymptomatic.[87,90] Given the subtle nature of the associated symptomatology, tumors are typically quite large at presentation (median diameter 4.4–9.3 cm, range 0.5–25 cm).[87–89,91,92] SPT is fairly evenly distributed throughout the pancreas, with a slight propensity for the body and tail of the pancreas (46%–67%).[87,88,91,92]

SPT has characteristic radiographic features. On CT, it appears as a well-demarcated, large encapsulated mass arising from the parenchyma of the pancreas, often inflicting mass effect on surrounding structures (**Fig. 3**A). SPT typically has solid features of soft tissue density peripherally with cystic components (attenuation less than muscle but greater than water) centrally, and shows intravenous contrast enhancement on portal venous phase. Calcifications may be present. MRI may provide more morphologic details.[93]

The cell line of origin of SPT is unclear, but it may arise from pleuripotential cells of the pancreatic duct as there is evidence of features of both epithelial and neuroendocrine differentiation. Given its predilection for women, a role for both estrogen and progesterone in the pathogenesis of SPT has been investigated, although none has been supported.[94]

Histologic features of SPT include solid and cystic components, with pseudopapillae formation. The epithelioid cells are uniform (see **Fig. 3**B). Immunohistochemical studies can confirm diagnosis with positive staining for vimentin, synaptophysin, α-1-antitrypsin, CD10, and CD56, but absent staining for chromogranin, trypsin, and chymotrypsin. The genetic alterations involved in the pathogenesis of SPT appear to be related to the APC/β-catenin pathway.[90,94–96]

SPTs are neoplasms of low malignant potential, generally demonstrating benign or indolent behavior. Because of their typically large size on presentation, surgical resection can present a formidable challenge. Complete surgical resection, with preservation of surrounding structures when possible, is the primary treatment modality for SPT. All reasonable attempts at R0 resection should be made to prevent long-term recurrence in the typically young patient. The surgical approach depends on the location and size of the neoplasm. Laparoscopic resection is appropriate when feasible. Lymph node involvement is exceedingly rare and thus lymphadenectomy is not necessary. Local vascular invasion, particularly of the portosplenic confluence, or the presence of metastatic disease should not preclude resection, and metastatic disease should be resected at the time of surgery when possible.

Approximately 15% of SPTs are metastatic to the liver or peritoneum, either on presentation or as recurrent disease.[87,88,90,91,97] Potentially prognostic

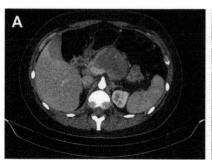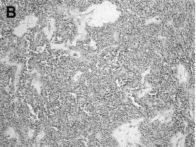

Fig. 3. (*A*) Axial contrasted dynamic CT image reveals a large solid pseudopapillary tumor of the body of the pancreas. (*B*) Histologic section at magnification ×10 demonstrating a solid pseudopapillary tumor of the pancreas.

clinicopathologic features of SPT have been evaluated by several groups and proposed as significant, including venous invasion, nuclear atypia, and mitotic activity[98]; diffuse growth pattern, extensive tumor necrosis, and high mitotic rate[90]; and microscopic margin positivity, local invasion, and size greater than 5 cm.[87] Also reported, however, are malignant-behaving tumors with benign-appearing pathology. Clearly, these are tumors of uncertain malignant potential.

Even in the event of metastasis, however, SPT is associated with excellent long-term survival. After surgical resection, long-term survival rates of greater than 92% are consistently reported.[87,88,90,91,99]

AUTOIMMUNE PANCREATITIS

In 1961, Sarles and colleagues[100] were the first to note pancreatitis with associated hypergammaglobulinemia and a potential autologous immunologic pathogenesis. In 1995, Yoshida and colleagues[101] described a patient with presumed unresectable pancreatic cancer who developed regression of her disease with steroid therapy. These investigators detailed a disease marked by an enlarged pancreas with diffuse and irregular narrowing of the main pancreatic duct, elevated serum IgG, and positive antinuclear antibody. Yoshida and colleagues proposed the term "autoimmune pancreatitis" (AIP) along with a definition based on common clinical criteria from 10 observed cases. The Japan Pancreas Society has since defined diagnostic criteria, most recently revised in 2006, as has the Mayo Clinic, to aid in the research and understanding of this enigmatic disease (**Boxes 1** and **2**).[102,103] Intrigue in this disease, whose importance lies in its differentiation from pancreatic adenocarcinoma, has stimulated much discussion and research over the past decade.

AIP is most commonly seen in men (2.8:1) older than 50 years. AIP accounts for approximately 2% of cases of chronic pancreatitis in Japan. On presentation, symptomatology is often vague, including jaundice, weight loss, fatigue, and mild abdominal pain, all more suggestive of malignancy than typical pancreatitis. Seventy percent of patients have endocrine or exocrine insufficiency of the pancreas either at diagnosis or developing shortly thereafter.[103–107]

Approximately half of patients have diffuse disease, with narrowing and irregularity of the entire main pancreatic duct. The remainder has segmental duct involvement, with approximately 10% showing short segment narrowing, less than one-third the length of the duct. The segmental and focal forms are most difficult to differentiate from adenocarcinoma.

Box 1
Clinical diagnostic criteria of AIP, Japan Pancreas Society 2006

I. Radiography: Diffuse or segmental narrowing of the main pancreatic duct with irregular wall and diffuse or localized enlargement of the pancreas by imaging studies

II. Immunology: High serum gammaglobulin, IgG, or IgG4, or the presence of autoantibodies, such as antinuclear antibodies and rheumatoid factor

III. Histology: Marked interlobular fibrosis and prominent infiltration of lymphocytes and plasma cells in the periductal area, occasionally with lymphoid follicles in the pancreas

Diagnosis requires I + II or III, along with the exclusion of pancreatobiliary malignancy

From Okazaki K, Kawa S, Kamisawa T, et al. Clinical diagnostic criteria of autoimmune pancreatitis: revised proposal. J Gastroenterol 2006;21:395–7; with permission.

Box 2
Clinical diagnostic criteria of AIP, "HISORt criteria", Mayo Clinic 2007

Histology: Periductal lymphoplasmacytic infiltrate with obliterative phlebitis and storiform fibrosis or lymphoplasmacytic infiltrate with storiform fibrosis and many IgG4 cells

Imaging: Diffusely enlarged gland with rim enhancement and diffusely narrow irregular pancreatic duct

Serology: Elevated serum IgG4 level

Other organ involvement: Proximal biliary strictures, sialadenitis, mediastinal lymphadenopathy, retroperitoneal fibrosis

Response to steroid therapy

From Chari ST. Diagnosis of autoimmune pancreatitis using its five cardinal features introducing the Mayo clinic's HISORTt criteria. J Gastroenterol 2007;42(S18):39–41; with permission.

AIP has some characteristic radiographic features. On contrasted CT, there is delayed enhancement of an enlarged and edematous pancreas. A low-density capsule-like rim may surround the pancreas and is highly suggestive of the diagnosis. Findings more typical of other causes of pancreatitis, such as pseudocysts, calcifications, and ductal dilation, are typically absent. Similar features are seen on MRI.[108,109] EUS may show distinguishing features of AIP, although this has not yet been validated in large studies.[110] Endoscopic retrograde cholangiopancreatography demonstrates the most characteristic features of AIP, with pancreatic ductal narrowing and irregularity. There is often associated distal biliary ductal narrowing secondary to associated fibrosis.[111]

Serum IgG4 as a valuable marker for AIP was recognized early by Hamano and colleagues,[112] who reported excellent sensitivity (90.2%) and specificity (97.5%) of this test for AIP, distinguishing it well from other benign and malignant entities. Experience with IgG4, however, has brought its uniform reliability as a disease-specific marker into question.[113,114] Ghazale and colleagues[115] reported that 10% of patients with pancreatic cancer have elevated serum IgG4 levels. These investigators note, however, that only 1% of patients with pancreatic cancer have serum IgG4 levels greater than 2 times normal, although this point of reference is then only 53% sensitive for AIP. They suggest that serum carbohydrate antigen 19-9 levels, which are more likely to be elevated in pancreatic cancer than AIP (71% vs 9%, $P<.001$), might be a useful adjunct to IgG4 level to help in disease distinction.

Histologically, AIP is marked by lymphoplasmacytic sclerosing pancreatitis (LPSP). There is fibrosis (storiform fibrosis) with infiltration of lymphocytes and plasma cells around medium-sized and large interlobular ducts (**Fig. 4**). Immunohistochemical staining of plasma cells is strongly positive for IgG4, although this finding is not entirely specific to AIP and may be seen in chronic pancreatitis and pancreatic cancer.[116–119]

An interesting feature of AIP is the potential for extrapancreatic manifestations of IgG4-related sclerosing disease, most commonly cholangitis and sialadenitis, but with a growing number of potentially involved organs.[107,120]

Treatment of AIP is with steroid therapy, most commonly oral prednisolone.[121] The current recommendation is initial high-dose therapy (30–40 mg per day) for 2 to 4 weeks, followed by a gradual taper over 3 months to a maintenance dose of 2.5 to 5 mg per day for 3 years.[107] Most patients respond to steroid therapy with improved pancreatic (and biliary) ductal changes, decreased pancreatic enlargement (in some

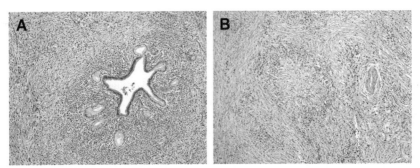

Fig. 4. (*A*) Histologic section at magnification ×10 demonstrating autoimmune pancreatitis affecting a pancreatic duct. (*B*) Classic storiform fibrosis is demonstrated on this histologic section of autoimmune pancreatitis.

cases pancreatic atrophy), and decreased serum IgG4 levels. There are reports of improvement in endocrine and exocrine insufficiency with steroid therapy, but these outcomes are inconsistent. Long-term follow-up is recommended as recurrence is described, and generally responds to steroid therapy.[111,122]

Despite the progress in understanding of this difficult disease, AIP often remains a diagnostic enigma. When the diagnosis is elucidated based on the proposed clinical criteria, steroid therapy should be instituted. Close follow-up should be obtained, with a measurable clinical response often within 2 weeks expected. In patients with atypical features and suboptimal response to therapy, surgical intervention may be warranted to exclude malignancy.[123]

METASTATIC TUMORS

Metastatic tumors to the pancreas are rare, representing less than 2% of all pancreatic malignancies. Isolated metastatic disease to the pancreas is unusual in that most patients present with diffuse metastatic disease without the option for operative therapy. Because of the relatively favorable biology and prognosis of many tumors that metastasize to the pancreas, for example, renal cell carcinoma and colorectal cancer, pancreatic resection of isolated pancreatic metastasis should be considered. Other tumors that metastasize to the pancreas with resection reported include melanoma, sarcoma, lung cancer, gastric cancer, gallbladder cancer, breast cancer, ovarian cancer, and gastrointestinal stromal tumors.[124]

According to a large retrospective analysis of 243 patients reported in the literature, the most common presentation for metastatic tumors to the pancreas is during a surveillance CT or incidentally on imaging performed for another reason. Forty-three percent of patients are asymptomatic. Other presentations include abdominal pain (24%), jaundice (22%), and gastrointestinal bleeding (10%).[125]

Metastases to the pancreas are typically hypervascular and enhance on contrast-enhanced imaging such as CT or MRI, in contrast to pancreatic adenocarcinoma.[124]

The largest single institution series of surgery for metastatic disease to the pancreas includes 49 patients. The median survival for all tumors is reported as 35.8 months, with a 36.2% 5-year survival.[124] Prognosis is related to the biology of the tumor of origin, with renal cell cancer having the best prognosis at median survival of 105 months after resection, with a 5-year survival of 66%.[124] In general, in patients with isolated pancreatic metastases with favorable tumor biology, resection is indicated.

SUMMARY

Solid lesions of the body and tail of the pancreas challenge all the diagnostic and technical skills of the modern gastrointestinal surgeon. The information available from modern CT, MR, and EUS imaging provide diagnostic and anatomic data that give the surgeon precise information with which to plan an operation and to discuss with the patient during the preoperative visit. Patients usually come to the surgeon with preliminary information they obtained from the Web, and expect to have clear answers about the risks, expected outcome, and alternatives to surgery. Because solid tumors of the body and tail of the pancreas carry a wide spectrum of potential pathology, with very different prognoses and in some cases, different therapies, a careful and complete preoperative evaluation is not only standard practice but necessary to answer all the questions the anxious, partially knowledgeable patient brings to the surgeon. A preoperative evaluation includes a thorough history and a pancreas protocol CT scan, supplemented by MRI and EUS when needed, to differentiate between the various potential diagnoses. These same modalities can be essential in proper staging in the case of malignant lesions, thus aiding in management decisions. Most lesions ultimately require operative resection, barring metastatic disease, with the notable exception of autoimmune pancreatitis. The laparoscopic approach to distal pancreatectomy and local resection of benign solid neoplasms of the tail and body of the pancreas has many champions who report notable success, with exciting prospects for continued advancement of laparoscopic techniques in managing tumors of the pancreas.

REFERENCES

1. Bipat S, Phoa SS, van Zeldan OM. Ultrasonography, computed tomography, and magnetic resonance imaging for diagnosis and determining respectability of pancreatic adenocarcinoma: a meta-analysis. J Comput Assist Tomogr 2005;29:438–45.
2. Anderson MA, Carpenter S, Thompson NW, et al. Endoscopic ultrasound is highly accurate and directs management in patients with neuroendocrine tumors of the pancreas. Am J Gastroenterol 2000;95:2271.
3. Omar S, Seewald S, Seitz U, et al. Reliability of EUS in exclusion of pancreatic cancer—results of the Hamburg-Eppendorf study. Endoscopy 2006;38S2:A35.
4. Maguchi H, Takahashi K, Osanai M, et al. Small pancreatic lesions is there need for EUS-FNA preoperatively? What to do with the incidental lesions? Endoscopy 2006;38S1:S53–6.
5. Chang KJ. Endoscopic ultrasound and FNA in pancreaticobiliary tumors. Endoscopy 2006;38S1:S56–60.
6. Papanikolaou IS, Adler A, Neumann U, et al. Endoscopic ultrasound in pancreatic disease—its influence on surgical decision making. Pancreatology 2009;9: 55–65.
7. Bournet B, Migueres I, Delacroix M, et al. Early morbidity of endoscopic ultrasound: 13 years experience at a referral center. Endoscopy 2006;38:349–54.
8. Gress FG, Hawes RH, Savides TH, et al. Role of EUS in the preoperative staging of pancreatic cancer: a large single center experience. Gastrointest Endosc 1999;50:786–91.
9. Yovino S, Darwin P, Daly B, et al. Predicting unresectability in pancreatic cancer patients: the additive effects of CT and endoscopic ultrasound. J Gastrointest Surg 2007;11:36–42.

10. Ferrone CR, Warshaw AL, Rattner DW, et al. Pancreatic fistula rates after 462 distal pancreatectomies: staplers do not decrease fistula rate. J Gastrointest Surg 2008;12:1691–7.
11. Warshaw AL. Conservation of the spleen with distal pancreatectomy. Arch Surg 1988;123:550–3.
12. Richardson DQ, Scott Connor LEH. Distal pancreatectomy with and without splenectomy, a comparison study. Am Surg 1989;55:21–5.
13. Fahy BN, Frey CF, Ho HS, et al. Morbidity, mortality, and technical factors of distal pancreatectomy. Am J Surg 2002;183:237–41.
14. Lillimoe KD, Kaushal S, Cameron JL, et al. Distal pancreatectomy: indications and outcomes in 235 patients. Ann Surg 1999;229:693–8.
15. Johnson CD, Flechtmacker J, Trede M. Resection for adenocarcinoma of the body and tail of the pancreas. Br J Surg 1993;80:1177–9.
16. Shoup M, Conlon KC, Klimstra D, et al. Is extended resection for adenocarcinoma of the body and tail of the pancreas justified? J Gastrointest Surg 2003;7:946–52.
17. Dalton RR, Sarr MG, van Heerden JA, et al. Cancer of the body and tail of the pancreas: is curative resection justified? Surgery 1992;111:489–94.
18. Nordback IH, Hruban R, Boitnot JK, et al. Cancer of the body and tail of the pancreas. Am J Surg 1992;164:26–31.
19. Brennan MF, Moccia RD, Klimstra D. Management of adenocarcinoma of the body and tail of the pancreas. Ann Surg 1996;223:506–12.
20. Christein JD, Kendrick ML, Iqbal CW, et al. Distal pancreatectomy for resectable adenocarcinoma of the body and tail of the pancreas. J Gastrointest Surg 2005; 9:922–7.
21. Bassi C, Dervenis C, Butturini G, et al. Postoperative pancreatic fistula: an international study group (ISGPF) definition. Surgery 2005;138:8–13.
22. Fingerhut A, Veyrie N, Ata T, et al. Use of sealants in pancreatic surgery: critical appraisal of the literature. Dig Surg 2009;26:7–14.
23. Nathan H, Cameron JL, Goodwin CR, et al. Risk factors for pancreatic leak after distal pancreatectomy. Ann Surg 2009;250:277–81.
24. Bernkeim BM. Organoscopy: cystoscopy of the abdominal cavity. Ann Surg 1911;53:764–7.
25. Cuschieri A, Hall AW, Clark J. Value of laparoscopy in the diagnosis and management of pancreatic carcinoma. Gut 1978;19:672–7.
26. Warshaw AL, Tepper JE, Shipley WU. Laparoscopy in the staging and planning of therapy for pancreatic cancer. Am J Surg 1986;151:76–80.
27. Shoup M, Winston C, Brennan MF, et al. Is there a role for staging laparoscopy in patients with locally advanced unresectable pancreatic adenocarcinoma. J Gastrointest Surg 2004;8:1068–71.
28. Liu RC, Traverso LW. Diagnostic laparoscopy improves staging of pancreatic cancer deemed locally unresectable by computed tomography. Surg Endosc 2005;19:638–42.
29. Soper NJ, Brunt LM, Dunnegan DL, et al. Laparoscopic distal pancreatectomy in the porcine model. Surg Endosc 1994;8:57–60.
30. Gagner M, Pomp A, Herrera MF. Early experience with laparoscopic resections of islet cell tumors. Surgery 1996;120:1051–4.
31. Melotti G, Butturini G, Piccoli M, et al. Laparoscopic distal pancreatectomy, results on a consecutive series of 58 patients. Ann Surg 2007;246:77–82.
32. Kooby D, Gillespie T, Bentrem D, et al. Left-sided pancreatectomy: a multicenter comparison of laparoscopic and open approaches. Ann Surg 2008;248: 438–46.

33. Sohn TA, Yeo CJ, Cameron JL, et al. Resected adenocarcinoma of the pancreas, 616 patients, results, outcomes and prognostic indicators. J Gastrointest Surg 2000;4:567–79.
34. Sasson AR, Hoffman JP, Ross EA, et al. En bloc resection for locally advanced cancer of the pancreas: is it worthwhile? J Gastrointest Surg 2002;6:147–58.
35. Watanabe I, Sasaki S, Konishi M. Onset, symptoms, and tumor location as prognostic factors of pancreatic cancers. Pancreas 2004;28:160–5.
36. Mansour JC, Chen H. Pancreatic endocrine tumors. J Surg Res 2004;120: 139–61.
37. Vagefi PA, Oswaldo R, Deshpande V, et al. Evolving patterns in the detection and outcomes of pancreatic neuroendocrine neoplasms. Arch Surg 2007;142: 347–54.
38. Gullo L, Migliori M, Falconi M, et al. Nonfunctioning pancreatic endocrine tumors: a multicenter study. Am J Gastroenterol 2003;98:2435–9.
39. Gomez-Rivera G, Stewart AE, Arnoletti JP, et al. Surgical treatment of pancreatic endocrine neoplasms. Am J Surg 2007;193:460–5.
40. Kazanjian KK, Rever HA, Hines OJ. Resection of pancreatic neuroendocrine tumors. Arch Surg 2006;141:765–70.
41. Kent RB III, van Heerden JA, Weiland LH. Nonfunctioning islet cell tumors. Ann Surg 1981;193:185–90.
42. Madeira I, Terris B, Voss M, et al. Prognostic factors in patients with endocrine tumours of the duodenopancreatic area. Gut 1998;43:422–7.
43. You DD, Lee HG, Paik KY, et al. The outcomes after surgical resection in pancreatic endocrine tumors: an institutional experience. Eur J Surg Oncol 2009;35: 728–33.
44. King AD, Ko GT, Yeung VT, et al. Dual phase spiral CT in the detection of small insulinomas of the pancreas. Br J Radiol 1998;71:20.
45. Chung MJ, Choi BI, Han JK, et al. Functioning islet cell tumor of the pancreas. Localization with dynamic spiral CT. Acta Radiol 1997;38:135.
46. Noone TC, Hosey J, Firat Z, et al. Imaging and localization of islet cell tumors of the pancreas on CT and MRI. Best Pract Clin Endocrinol Metab 2005;19:195–211.
47. Theoni RF, Mueller-Lisse UG, Chan R, et al. Detection of small, functional islet cell tumors in the pancreas: selection of MR imaging sequences for optimal sensitivity. Radiology 2000;214:483–8.
48. Modlin IM, Cornelius E, Lawton GP. Use of an isotopic somatostatin receptor probe to image gut endocrine tumors. Arch Surg 1995;130:367–71.
49. Gibril F, Jensen RT. Diagnostic uses of radiolabelled somatostatin receptor analogues in gastroenteropancreatic endocrine tumors. Dig Liver Dis 2004;36: S106–20.
50. Gibril F, Reynolds JC, Doppman JL, et al. Somatostatin receptor scintigraphy: its sensitivity compared with that of other imaging methods in detecting primary and metastatic gastrinomas: a prospective study. Ann Intern Med 1996;125: 26–34.
51. Rosch T, Lightdale CJ, Botet JF, et al. Localization of pancreatic endocrine tumors by endoscopic ultrasonography. N Engl J Med 1992;326:1721–6.
52. Proye C, Malvaux P, Pattou F, et al. Noninvasive imaging of insulinomas and gastrinomas with endoscopic ultrasonography and somatostatin receptor scintigraphy. Surgery 1998;124:1134–9.
53. Pais SA, McGreevy K, LeBlanc JK, et al. Utility of EUS-FNA in the diagnosis of pancreatic neuroendocrine tumors: correlation with histopathology in 76 patients. Gastrointest Endosc 2007;65:AB304.

54. Sundin A, Eriksson B, Bergstrom M, et al. PET in the diagnosis of NE tumors. Ann NY Acad Sci 2004;1014:246–57.
55. Wilder RM, Allan FN, Power MH, et al. Carcinoma of the islands of the pancreas. Hyperinsulinism and hypoglycemia. JAMA 1927;89:348–54.
56. Campbell WR, Graham RR, Robinson WL. Islet cell tumors of the pancreas. Am J Med Sci 1939;198:445–54.
57. Nilfarjan M, Warshaw AL, Axelrod L, et al. Improved contemporary surgical management of insulinomas: a 25 year experience at the Massachusetts General Hospital. Ann Surg 2008;247:165–72.
58. Service FJ, McMahon MM, O'Brien PC, et al. Functioning insulinoma: incidence, recurrence and longterm survival of patients: a 60 year study. Mayo Clin Proc 1991;66:711–6.
59. Whipple AO. Adenomas of the islet cells with hyperinsulinism: a review. Ann Surg 1935;101:1299.
60. Roland CL. Surgical approach and perioperative complications determine short term outcomes in patients with insulinoma: results of a bi-institutional study. Ann Surg Oncol 2008;15:3532.
61. Tseng LM, Chan JY, Won JG. The role of intraarterial calcium stimulated testing with hepatic venous sampling in the management of occult insulinoma. Ann Surg Oncol 2007;14:2121–7.
62. Hashimoto LA, Walsh RM. Preoperative localization of insulinoma is not necessary. J Am Coll Surg 1999;189:368–73.
63. Ravi K, Britton B. Surgical approach to insulinomas: are preoperative localization tests necessary? Ann R Coll Surg Engl 2007;89:212–7.
64. Patterson EJ, Gagner M, Salky B. Laparoscopic pancreatic resection: a single institution experience of 19 patients. J Am Coll Surg 2001;193:281–7.
65. SaCanha A, Beau C, Rault A, et al. Laparoscopic versus open approach for solitary insulinoma. Surg Endosc 2007;21:103–8.
66. Schindl M, Kadzirek K, Kaserer K, et al. Is the new classification of neuroendocrine pancreatic tumors of clinical help? World J Surg 2000;24:1312–7.
67. Zollinger RM, Ellison EH. Primary peptic ulcerations of the jejunum associated with islet cell tumors of the pancreas. Ann Surg 1955;142:709–23.
68. Gregory RA, Tracy HJ. The constitution and properties of two gastrins extracted from hog antral mucosa. Gut 1964;5:103–14.
69. Roy P, Venzon DJ, Shojamanesh H, et al. Zollinger-Ellison syndrome: clinical presentation in 261 patients. Medicine 2000;79:379–411.
70. Ectors N. Pancreatic endocrine tumors. Hepatogastroenterology 1999;46: 679–86.
71. Modlin IM, Lawton GP. Duodenal gastrinoma: the solution to the pancreatic paradox. J Clin Gastroenterol 1994;19:184–91.
72. Norton JA, Fraker DJ, Alexander HR, et al. Surgery to cure the Zollinger Ellison syndrome. N Engl J Med 1999;341:635–44.
73. Norton JA, Fraker DJ, Alexander HR, et al. Surgery increases survival in patients with gastrinoma. Ann Surg 2006;244:410–9.
74. Ellison EC, Sparks J, Verducci JS, et al. 50 year appraisal of gastrinoma: recommendations for staging and treatment. J Am Coll Surg 2006;202: 897–905.
75. Que FG, Nagorney DM, Batts KP, et al. Hepatic resection for metastatic neuroendocrine carcinomas. Am J Surg 1995;169:36–42.
76. Norton JA, Warren RS, Kelly MG, et al. Aggressive surgery for metastatic liver neuroendocrine tumors. Surgery 2003;134:1057–63.

77. Becker SW, Kahn D. Cutaneous manifestations of internal malignant tumors. Arch Dermatol Syph 1942;45:169.
78. Wermers RA, Fatourechi V, Kvols LK. Clinical spectrum of hyperglucagonemia associated with malignant neuroendocrine tumors. Mayo Clin Proc 1996;71: 1030.
79. Verner JV, Morrison AB. Islet cell tumor and a syndrome of refractory watery diarrhea and hypokalemia. Am J Med 1958;25:374–80.
80. Ghaferi AA, Chojnacki KA, Long WD, et al. Pancreatic VIPomas: subject review and one institutional experience. J Gastrointest Surg 2008;12:382–93.
81. Ganda OP, Weir GC, Soeldner JS, et al. Somatostatinoma: a somatostatin-containing tumor of the endocrine pancreas. N Engl J Med 1977;296:963–7.
82. Nesi G, Marcucci T, Rubio CA, et al. Somatostatinoma: clinicopathological features of three cases and literature reviewed. Gastroenterology 2007;23: 521–6.
83. Phan GQ, Yeo CJ, Hruban RH, et al. Surgical experience with pancreatic and peripancreatic neuroendocrine tumors: review of 125 patients. J Gastrointest Surg 1998;2:472–82.
84. Solarzano CC, Lee JE, Pisters PW, et al. Nonfunctioning islet cell carcinoma of the pancreas: survival results in a contemporary series of 163 patients. Surgery 2001;130:1078–85.
85. Frantz VK. Tumors of the pancreas. In: Blumberg CW, editor. Atlas of tumor pathology. 1st series. Washington, DC: US Armed Forces Institute of Pathology; 1959. p. 32–3.
86. Kloppel G, Socia E, Longnecker DS, et al. Histological typing of tumors of the exocrine pancreas, International histological classification of tumours. 2nd edition. New York: Springer Verlag, World Health Organization; 1996. p. 15–21.
87. Martin RC, Klimstra DS, Brennan MF, et al. Solid pseudopapillary tumor of the pancreas: a surgical enigma? Ann Surg Oncol 2002;9:35–40.
88. Lam KY, Lo CY, Fan ST. Pancreatic solid-cystic-papillary tumor: clinicopathologic features in eight patients from Hong Kong and review of the literature. World J Surg 1999;23:1045–50.
89. Chen SQ, Zou SQ, Dai QB, et al. Clinical analysis of solid-pseudopapillary tumor of the pancreas: report of 15 cases. Hepatobiliary Pancreat Dis Int 2008;7: 196–200.
90. Tang LH, Hakan A, Brennan MF, et al. Clinically aggressive solid pseudopapillary tumors of the pancreas. Am J Surg Pathol 2005;29:512–9.
91. Yang F, Jin C, Long J, et al. Solid pseudopapillary tumor of the pancreas: a case series of 26 consecutive patients. Am J Surg 2009;198:210–5.
92. Nakagohri T, Kinoshita T, Konishi M, et al. Surgical outcome of solid pseudopapillary tumor of the pancreas. J Hepatobiliary Pancreat Surg 2008;15:318–21.
93. Dong DJ, Zhang SZ. Solid-pseudopapillary tumor of the pancreas: CT and MRI features of 3 cases. Hepatobiliary Pancreat Dis Int 2006;5:300–4.
94. Adams AL, Siegal GP, Jhala NC. Solid pseudopapillary tumor of the pancreas: a review of salient clinical and pathologic features. Adv Anat Pathol 2008;15: 39–45.
95. Abraham SC, Klimstra DS, Wilentz RE, et al. Solid pseudopapillary tumors of the pancreas are genetically distinct from pancreatic ductal adenocarcinomas and almost always harbor beta-catenin mutations. Am J Pathol 2000;160:1361–9.
96. Tanaka Y, Kato K, Notohara K, et al. Frequent beta-catenin mutation and cytoplasmic/nuclear accumulation in pancreatic solid pseudopapillary neoplasm. Cancer Res 2001;61:8401–4.

97. Sclafani LM, Reuter VE, Coit DG, et al. The malignant nature of papillary and cystic neoplasm of the pancreas. Cancer 1991;68:153–8.

98. Nishihara K, Nagoshi M, Tsuneyoshi M, et al. Papillary cystic tumors of the pancreas, assessment of their malignant potential. Cancer 1993;71:82–92.

99. Salvia R, Bassi C, Festa L, et al. Clinical and biological behavior of pancreatic solid pseudopapillary tumors: report on 31 consecutive patients. J Surg Oncol 2007;95:304–10.

100. Sarles H, Sarles JC, Muratore R, et al. Chronic inflammatory sclerosis of the pancreas—an autonomous pancreatic disease? Am J Dig Dis 1961;6:688–98.

101. Yoshida K, Toki F, Takeuchi T, et al. Chronic pancreatitis caused by an autoimmune abnormality. Proposal of the concept of autoimmune pancreatitis. Dig Dis Sci 1995;40:1561–8.

102. Okazaki K, Kawa S, Kamisawa T, et al. Clinical diagnostic criteria of autoimmune pancreatitis: revised proposal. J Gastroenterol 2006;21:395–7.

103. Chari ST. Diagnosis of autoimmune pancreatitis using its five cardinal features introducing the Mayo clinic's HISORTt criteria. J Gastroenterol 2007;42(S18): 39–41.

104. Okazaki K, Chiba T. Autoimmune related pancreatitis. Gut 2002;51:1–4.

105. Okazaki K. Autoimmune pancreatitis: etiology, pathogenesis, clinical findings and treatment. The Japanese experience. JOP 2005;6S1:132–7.

106. Ectors N, Maillet B, Aerts R, et al. Non-alcoholic duct destructive chronic pancreatitis. Gut 1997;41:263–8.

107. Shimosegawa T, Kanno A. Autoimmune pancreatitis in Japan: overview and perspective. J Gastroenterol 2009;44:503–17.

108. Sahani DV, Kalva SP, Farrell J, et al. Autoimmune pancreatitis: imaging features. Radiology 2004;233:345–52.

109. Chang WI, Kim GB, Lee KJ, et al. The clinical and radiological characteristics of focal mass-forming autoimmune pancreatitis. Pancreas 2009;38:401–8.

110. Hoki N, Mizuno N, Sawaki A, et al. Diagnosis of autoimmune pancreatitis using endoscopic ultrasonography. J Gastroenterol 2009;44:154–9.

111. Horiuchi A, Kawa S, Hamano H, et al. ERCP features in 27 patients with autoimmune pancreatitis. Gastrointest Endosc 2002;55:494–9.

112. Hamano H, Kawa S, Horiuchi A, et al. High serum IgG4 concentrations in patients with sclerosing pancreatitis. N Engl J Med 2001;344:732–8.

113. Hochwald SN, Hemming AW, Draganov P, et al. Elevation of serum IgG4 in Western patients with autoimmune sclerosing pancreatocholangitis: a word of caution. Ann Surg Oncol 2008;15:1147–54.

114. Morselli-Labate AM, Pezzilli R. Usefulness of serum IgG4 in the diagnosis and follow up of autoimmune pancreatitis: a systematic literature review and meta-analysis. J Gastroenterol Hepatol 2009;24:15–36.

115. Ghazale A, Chari ST, Smyrk TC, et al. Value of serum IgG4 in the diagnosis of autoimmune pancreatitis and in distinguishing it from pancreatic cancer. Am J Gastroenterol 2007;102:1646–53.

116. Kawaguchi K, Koike M, Tsuruta K, et al. Lymphoplasmacytic sclerosing pancreatitis with cholangitis: variant of primary sclerosing cholangitis extensively involving pancreas. Hum Pathol 1991;22:387–95.

117. Deshpande V, Chicano S, Finkelberg D, et al. Autoimmune pancreatitis: a systemic immune complex mediated disease. Am J Surg Pathol 2007;30: 1537–45.

118. Zhang L, Notohara K, Levy MJ, et al. IgG4-positive plasma cell infiltration in the diagnosis of autoimmune pancreatitis. Mod Pathol 2007;20:23–8.

119. Kloppel G, Luttges J, Lohr M, et al. Autoimmune pancreatitis: pathological, clinical, and immunologic features. Pancreas 2003;27:14–9.
120. Kamisawa T, Okamoto A. Autoimmune pancreatitis; proposal of IgG4 related sclerosing disease. J Gastroenterol 2006;41:613–25.
121. Hirano K, Tada M, Isayama H, et al. Long-term prognosis of autoimmune pancreatitis with and without corticosteroid treatment. Gut 2007;56:1719–24.
122. Uchida K, Yazumi S, Nishio A, et al. Long-term outcome of autoimmune pancreatitis. J Gastroenterol 2009;44:726–32.
123. Gardner TB, Levy MJ, Takahashi N, et al. Misdiagnosis of autoimmune pancreatitis: a caution to clinicians. Am J Gastroenterol 2009;104:1620–3.
124. Reddy S, Wolfgang S. The role of surgery in the management of isolated metastases to the pancreas. Lancet Oncol 2009;10:287–93.
125. Reddy S, Edil BH, Cameron JL. Pancreatic resection of isolated metastases from nonpancreatic primary cancers. Ann Surg Oncol 2008;15:3199–206.

Portal Vein Resection

Kathleen K. Christians, MD*, Alysandra Lal, MD, Sam Pappas, MD,
Edward Quebbeman, PhD, MD, Douglas B. Evans, MD

KEYWORDS

- Pancreas cancer • Portal vein • Superior mesenteric vein
- Borderline resectable

Involvement of the superior mesenteric vein (SMV) or the portal vein (PV) by pancreatic cancer historically was a relative contraindication to pancreaticoduodenectomy (PD).[1] The Japanese,[2] and subsequently Fortner[3] in 1973, proposed the concept of "regional pancreatectomy," which involved deliberate and systematic resection of major peripancreatic vascular structures combined with wide soft tissue clearance. PV resection at the time of PD was originally performed in an attempt to improve survival,[1] but unfortunately this proved not to be true as this type of extended PD did not confer a survival advantage.[4,5] Confusion among treating physicians occurred when these regional pancreatectomy patients were equated to those patients having isolated tumor involvement of the SMV, PV, or SMV-PV confluence. The former had stage III disease with a median survival of 10 to 12 months, and the latter, survival of 2 years.[6–8] In contrast to regional pancreatectomy, contemporary vein resection (VR) is done when the operating surgeon cannot safely separate the SMV or the SMV-PV confluence from the tumor, but is not done for the purpose of achieving a greater extent of lymphatic clearance.[7] At present, resection and reconstruction of these veins at the time of PD to facilitate a complete (R0/R1) resection of a pancreatic tumor has been shown to be associated with a low rate of perioperative morbidity and similar rates of R0 resection and overall survival when compared with patients treated with standard PD without venous resection.[7,8]

The American Hepato-Pancreatico-Biliary Association and Society of Surgical Oncology (AHPBA/SSO) panel of experts joined forces to formulate a consensus statement published in 2009 on the subject of vein resection and reconstruction during PD. The investigators concluded that PD with vein resection and reconstruction is the standard of practice for pancreatic adenocarcinomas locally involving the SMV-PV confluence, provided that adequate inflow and outflow veins are present, that the tumor does not involve the superior mesenteric artery (SMA) or hepatic artery (HA), and that an R0/R1 resection is reasonably expected. The consensus statement went on to say that patients with nonmetastatic adenocarcinomas should be

Department of Surgery, Medical College of Wisconsin, 9200 West Wisconsin Avenue, Milwaukee, WI 53226, USA
* Corresponding author.
E-mail address: kchristi@mcw.edu

Surg Clin N Am 90 (2010) 309–322
doi:10.1016/j.suc.2009.12.001
0039-6109/10/$ – see front matter © 2010 Elsevier Inc. All rights reserved.

evaluated and resected at institutions capable of, and experienced in, resection and reconstruction of major mesenteric veins.[9]

PRINCIPLES OF MANAGEMENT

Accurately defining the extent of disease at the time of diagnosis (preoperative) and reserving surgery for those patients with localized, nonmetastatic pancreatic cancer who can undergo a complete gross resection of the primary tumor are critical elements to successful surgery for pancreatic adenocarcinoma.[10] To achieve results equivalent to those for patients with tumors that do not involve adjacent vascular structures, the following principles of management[11] must be adhered to when considering the performance of an extended PD to include vascular resection and reconstruction:

1. Appropriate patient selection based on high-quality computed tomography (CT) imaging and review of all cases at multidisciplinary disposition conferences[12] is key to avoiding operative intervention on patients with T4 (involving celiac axis or SMA) or M1 tumors.
2. Operative and pathologic attention to margins of resection. The technical aspects of the SMA dissection in large part will determine the likelihood of local recurrence. The final margin status is determined by the size and location of the tumor, the conduct of the operation itself (the removal of all soft tissue to the right of the SMA), and the effectiveness of adjuvant or neoadjuvant therapy.
3. Advances in surgical technique, surgeon experience, and improved understanding of the anatomy of the SMV allow vascular resection to become a routine part of PD.

PREOPERATIVE STAGING

Only patients characterized as resectable or borderline resectable are considered for PD. Staging should be established by a multidetector contrast-enhanced CT scan of the abdomen with 3-dimensional reconstruction,[13] and by review in a multidisciplinary conference.[12] The definitions of resectability are as follows:

1. **Resectable** pancreatic cancer, defined as:
    (a) The absence of extrapancreatic disease.
    (b) No evidence of tumor extension to the SMA, celiac axis, or HA; as defined by the presence of a normal tissue plane between the tumor and these arteries (**Fig. 1**).
    (c) Patent SMV-PV confluence assuming that resection and reconstruction of the SMV, PV, or SMV-PV confluence can be performed when necessary.[4]
    The AHPBA/SSO consensus statement further defined resectable tumors as those with no radiographic evidence of SMV and PV "abutment, distortion, tumor thrombus or venous encasement." In addition, "clear fat (soft tissue) planes" had to be present around the celiac axis, HA, and SMA.[13]
2. **Borderline resectable: Katz classification**[14]
    Type A
    (a) Tumor abutment (≤180°) of the SMA or celiac axis.
    (b) Tumor abutment or encasement (>180°) of a short segment of the HA (usually at the origin of the gastroduodenal artery [GDA]).
    (c) Short segment occlusion of the SMV, PV, or SMV-PV confluence with a suitable PV above and SMV below, for reconstruction (**Fig. 2**A,B and **Fig. 3**A,B).

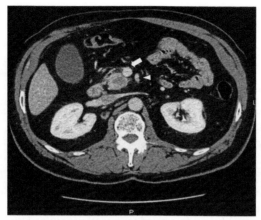

Fig. 1. Axial CT image of a resectable adenocarcinoma of the pancreatic head (low-density pancreatic head mass, *arrow* points to SMV and *arrowhead* indicates the SMA with normal surrounding tissue plane).

Type B

Patients with CT findings suspicious for, but not diagnostic of, metastatic disease as well as those with N1 disease from prereferral surgical biopsy or endoscopic ultrasound (EUS)-guided fine-needle aspiration (FNA) biopsy. These patients have primary tumors that may be technically resectable or borderline resectable by CT criteria.

Type C

Patients with borderline resectable disease due to a marginal performance status as well as those patients with severe preexisting comorbidities requiring protracted evaluation precluding immediate operation. This category does not include those with no potential for eventual operation.

Neoadjuvant therapy should be part of treatment sequencing for those patients with tumor-artery abutment. Patients with arterial encasement (tumor-vessel interface >180°) are considered to have locally advanced disease, and surgery is not a treatment option for those with this extent of local disease.[14]

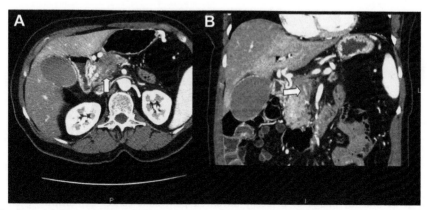

Fig. 2. Axial (*A*) and coronal (*B*) CT images of a borderline resectable pancreatic cancer. There is near complete occlusion of the SMV-PV confluence (*arrow*).

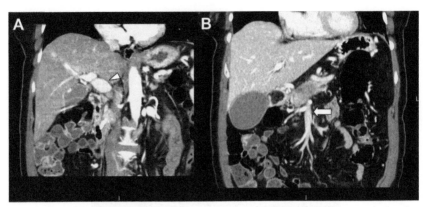

Fig. 3. Coronal CT images demonstrating (*A*) a normal portal vein above (*arrowhead*) and (*B*) a normal SMV (*arrow*) below an area of segmental venous occlusion. Of importance is that the tumor did not encase the celiac or SMA (not shown). Successful resection of this tumor required segmental venous resection and reconstruction with interposition grafting.

Locally advanced tumors have encasement (>180°) of adjacent arteries or an occluded SMV-PV with no technical option for resection and reconstruction (**Fig. 4**). Locally advanced, stage III tumors should not be considered for operation.[14] Current chemotherapy and radiation therapy will not convert a tumor with CT evidence of arterial encasement into a resectable situation. The goal of therapy for such patients is maximizing length and quality of life. Complete resection and cure should not be a realistic expectation.

It should be noted that the 2009 AHBPA/SSO consensus conference recommendations published in the *Annals of Surgical Oncology* (2009) differed with the definitions defined herein by including in the borderline category any radiographic evidence of involvement of the SMV-PV (abutment to short segment occlusion) if reconstruction was possible. In the absence of vein occlusion, such patients are considered resectable in these definitions.[9] The consensus statement arrived at a more conservative definition of resectable disease—one that required the tumor to be completely free

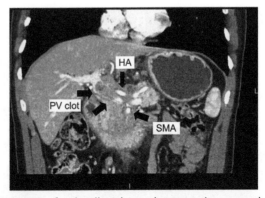

Fig. 4. Coronal CT image of a locally advanced pancreatic cancer demonstrating SMA encasement. This extensive tumor will never become resectable with currently available systemic therapies and radiation therapy techniques.

of the visceral veins and arteries. Any contact of the tumor with the SMA, HA, or SMV-PV was considered borderline resectable, and such tumors should not be considered for upfront surgery (neoadjuvant therapy strongly recommended).

RESECTION MARGINS
"R" Factor

Three categories are used to describe the presence or absence of residual tumor following surgical resection:

1. R0 is a grossly complete resection with microscopically negative margins.
2. R1 is a grossly complete resection with microscopically positive margins.
3. R2 is defined as a grossly incomplete resection.[15]

SMA Margin

The American Joint Committee on Cancer (AJCC) defined the soft tissue that contains autonomic nerves adjacent to the right lateral border of the proximal 3 to 4 cm of the SMA to be the retroperitoneal, mesenteric, or uncinate margin. The more anatomically precise term is the "SMA margin." The most critical resection margin in a PD is the SMA margin because whereas the bile duct and pancreatic margins can be reexcised, an SMA margin cannot (SMA not usually resected). Thus, the SMA margin is the margin most commonly positive following PD and is the most common site of local recurrence.[16,17] R2 resections are avoidable with proper preoperative imaging, patient selection, and surgical technique. In contrast, an R1 resection may occur despite the absence of gross tumor at the margin, as pancreatic adenocarcinoma may extend microscopically to the perineural autonomic plexus that surrounds the SMA beyond the extent of palpable or visible tumor.

The SMA margin should be evaluated according to the AJCC *Cancer Staging Manual* (sixth edition) guidelines,[18] and must be evaluated on permanent sections by inking the margin and sectioning the tumor perpendicular to the margin. It is critical that the surgeon and pathologist identify the margin at the time of resection because it cannot be assessed retrospectively.[11] The surgeon must also document the presence or absence of a complete gross resection at the time of PD. If the surgeon appreciates that the tumor extends to the left of (medial to) the SMA and is not completely removed at the time of surgery, a histologically positive margin should result in an R2 designation in the final operative report. If a gross complete resection has been performed but the SMA margin returns microscopically positive, the operative report should reflect the R1 designation.[7,11] It is important that the operative dictation not be finalized until the pathology report, to include the status of the SMA margin, is completed and reviewed by the surgeon.

TREATMENT SEQUENCING
Neoadjuvant Therapy

Patients with borderline resectable disease based on anatomic criteria are at higher risk for a margin-positive resection with a surgery-alone approach. These patients also may be at higher risk for perioperative complications based on the complexity of the surgery, and at higher risk for systemic failure because of the advanced nature of their primary tumor. For these reasons, a neoadjuvant approach has been advocated including systemic chemotherapy, chemoradiation, or both, rather than operation as the initial mode of therapy.

In this "surgery last" approach, those patients who have rapidly progressive disease in whom surgery would provide no clinical benefit may be identified at the time of posttreatment, preoperative restaging. These patients can therefore avoid major surgery with the attendant risk for morbidity and mortality. The "surgery last" approach ensures that patients receive chemotherapy or chemoradiation as opposed to a "surgery first" treatment sequence in which there may be treatment delays or complete failure to receive adjuvant therapy. Adjuvant therapy may not be received because of treatment-related problems (surgical complications, delayed recovery), disease-related problems (tumor progression), or patient-related problems (age, marginal performance status, medical comorbidities, patient refusal).[19,20] In addition, those who respond to neoadjuvant therapy, as evidenced by a decline in serum level of carbohydrate antigen 19-9 or a radiographic response, have a more favorable survival.[14] In 2009 Katz and colleagues[10] wrote, "when the magnitude of the operation and the risk for recurrence are both increased, neoadjuvant treatment sequencing becomes more attractive as a strategy to more precisely select patients who will benefit from pancreatectomy."

For borderline resectable patients, resectability rates are modest (41%) and perioperative death rates not inconsequential (3%), thus it is critically important to reserve this operation for patients most likely to benefit.[14] Katz and colleagues[14] reported that the borderline resectable patients who completed all intended therapy including surgical resection had a median survival of 40 months as opposed to those who had evidence of disease progression or poor performance status at posttreatment imaging (median survival 13 months). These 2 groups are indistinguishable at the time of diagnosis. However, they can be more accurately differentiated at the time of restaging 4 to 5 months into preoperative treatment. A neoadjuvant approach allows for early treatment of micrometastatic disease in all patients. The chemotherapy and chemoradiation is given to a well-vascularized primary tumor (potentially improving R0 resection rates). Neoadjuvant therapy also physiologically stresses the patient and may help identify those patients with poor physiologic reserve and less ability to tolerate a major operation.[19]

ADVANCES IN SURGICAL TECHNIQUE
Standard Anatomy

The SMV drains the mid gut, which extends from the duodenum to the transverse colon. The SMA supplies arterial flow to the mid gut including the pancreatic head, duodenum, small bowel, and proximal colon. The SMA arises from the aorta and courses caudally, posterior to the pancreas. Proximal branches of the SMA include the inferior pancreaticoduodenal arteries (usually 2) and very small unnamed tributaries to the uncinate process. Several centimeters distal to its origin, the SMA gives off the first jejunal branches. The SMA normally lies posteromedial to the SMV. The SMA is ensheathed by autonomic nerves and lymphatic tissue that extends to the celiac ganglia. This nerve plexus extends into the pancreatic parenchyma, and can allow microscopic extension of tumor back to the celiac ganglia (**Fig. 5**).[11]

Normally the PV arises posterior to the superior aspect of the pancreatic neck and is derived from the SMV and splenic vein (SV) confluence. The SMV lies anterior and to the right of the SMA and has 2 branches: the middle colic and the gastrocolic trunk of Henle. The gastrocolic trunk drains the right gastroepiploic, the right superior colic, and the anterosuperior pancreaticoduodenal veins. The main trunk of the SMV arises from the confluence of 2 first-order branches, the jejunal and ileal branches. The jejunal branch provides venous drainage from the proximal small bowel; after coursing transversely and posterior to the SMA the jejunal branch enters the right posterolateral

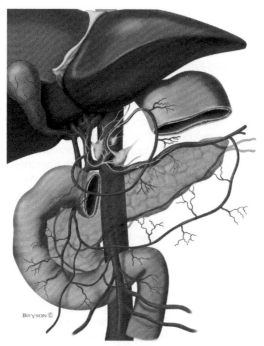

Fig. 5. Vascular arterial anatomy of the celiac axis and SMA with reference to surgery for pancreatic head neoplasms. (*Courtesy of* Mary K. Bryson; with permission. © 2009 Mary K. Bryson. Published by Elsevier Inc. All rights reserved.)

aspect of the main trunk of the SMV. In contrast, the ileal branch drains the distal small bowel and travels caudal to cranial in the root of the small bowel mesentery. The inferior mesenteric vein (IMV) usually drains into the SV (**Fig. 6**) but can also enter the SMV directly, usually inferior to the SV-SMV confluence.[21,22]

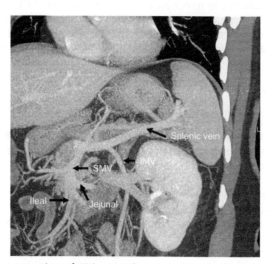

Fig. 6. Coronal reconstruction of CT images demonstrating the important venous anatomy with reference to surgery for pancreatic neoplasms.

Anatomic Variations

More than 90% of patients have a main trunk of the SMV; however, the ileal and jejunal branches occasionally may merge at the level of the SV without forming this common trunk. In these cases, the jejunal branch usually courses anterior to the SMA (20% of cases).[21,23,24] This variant is particularly important when performing PD with regard to medial mobilization of the SMV off of the uncinate process of the pancreas (which is necessary for visualization of the SMA). When the jejunal branch lies posterior to the SMA, the venous branches from the uncinate process to the jejunal branch must be divided to separate the jejunal branch from the uncinate and allow medial retraction of the SMV to fully expose the SMA. An anterior jejunal branch makes it easier to separate the uncinate from the SMV, and the small venous branches from the uncinate usually enter the ileal rather than jejunal branch. However, when an anterior jejunal branch exists, anatomic variations occur at a high rate, including the lack of a main SMV trunk and drainage of the IMV directly into the jejunal branch of the SMV.[23] The small bowel will have adequate venous return if either the ileal or the jejunal branch remains intact; if one of these first-order branches is resected, but not both, then venous reconstruction is usually not necessary.[11]

Surgical Approach

PD is performed as described by Evans and colleagues.[25] CT evidence of tumor involvement of the SMV or its first-order branches should prompt thorough scrutiny of the venous anatomy to determine the extent of vascular involvement and to develop an optimal strategy for vascular resection and reconstruction. High-quality preoperative CT imaging should prevent unexpected venous resections at the time of PD. The most important oncologic step of the PD is the division of the pancreas and completion of the mesenteric and retroperitoneal dissection, removing all soft tissue to the right of the adventitia of the SMA (SMA margin). Tangential or segmental resection of the SMV, PV, or SMV-PV confluence is performed when the surgeon cannot separate the pancreatic head or uncinate process from the SMV-PV confluence without leaving gross tumor on the vein or incurring a venotomy. Elective venous resection is not done in the absence of tumor adherence to the vessel.[11] Of note, tumor adherence to the SMV-PV is a judgment made at the time of surgery and does not always imply tumor infiltration of the vein wall; final pathologic assessment will demonstrate tumor infiltration of the vein wall in approximately 61% of PD specimens.[7]

TYPES OF VENOUS RESECTION

The different technical options for resection and reconstruction are illustrated in **Fig. 7**.

1. VR1: Tangential resection of the SMV-PV confluence for tumor adherence limited to a small part of the lateral or posterior wall of the SMV-PV confluence. Repair is by greater saphenous vein patch. If isolated tumor involvement of the lateral SMV-PV confluence occurs directly opposite the SV entrance and a pie-shaped defect can be repaired transversely, a vein patch is not used.[11]
2. VR2: Tumor involves the SMV-SV-PV confluence and requires SV ligation. The SMV and PV can be reapproximated without tension, and an end-to-end primary anastomosis is performed (**Fig. 8**).
3. VR3: Tumor involves the SMV-SV-PV and ligation of the SV is necessary, but there is inadequate length to allow a primary end-to-end anastomosis. An interposition graft is used and the internal jugular vein is the authors' preferred conduit.

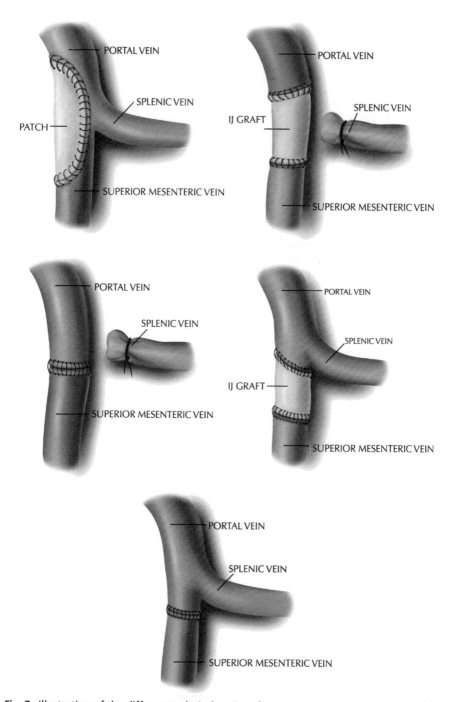

Fig. 7. Illustration of the different technical options for resection and reconstruction of the SMV, PV, or SMV-PV confluence. (*Courtesy of* Mary K. Bryson; with permission. © 2009 Mary K. Bryson. Published by Elsevier Inc. All rights reserved.)

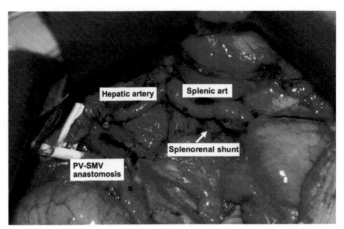

Fig. 8. Intraoperative photograph following pancreaticoduodenectomy with segmental resection of the SMV-PV confluence. In this patient, the area of SMV-PV encasement was at the SV confluence, which required division of the SV. Because the IMV entered the SMV (and not the SV), SV ligation carried the risk of left-sided venous hypertension (and gastroesophageal varices); for this reason, the SV was anastomosed into the left renal vein.

4. VR4: Tumor involves just the SMV or the PV such that the SV can be preserved and a primary end-to-end anastomosis is possible. This situation is limited to short segment resections as the intact SV tethers the PV and prevents a primary anastomosis of the SMV and PV in most cases.
5. VR5: Tumor involves just the SMV or the PV. The SV is preserved, and an interposition graft is needed to connect the SMV with the PV.[7]

MANAGEMENT OF THE SPLENIC VEIN

The standard technique for segmental venous resection historically included transection of the SV (to release the PV).[22] Division of the SV also allows complete exposure of the SMA medial to the SMV, and provides increased SMV and PV length to allow primary venous anastomosis. With the SV divided, the retroperitoneal dissection is then completed by dividing the tissues anterior to the aorta and to the right of the SMA, leaving the specimen only attached by the SMV-PV confluence. Vascular clamps are then placed 2 to 3 cm proximally on the PV and distally on the SMV. Systemic heparinization with 2500 to 5000 U is given and the SMA is occluded with a Rommel tourniquet. Inflow occlusion of the SMA prevents small bowel edema and makes the subsequent pancreatic and biliary reconstruction less difficult. The vein is then transected and the tumor is removed. The SMV-PV is then reapproximated using interrupted 6-0 prolene.[7]

SV preservation is possible when tumor invasion of the SMV or PV does not involve the SV confluence. Preservation of the SV-SMV-PV confluence, however, significantly limits mobilization of the PV and prevents primary anastomosis of the SMV to the PV unless the segmental resection is less than 2 cm. Thus, most patients with SV preservation require an interposition graft. The preferred conduit for the interposition graft is the internal jugular (IJ) vein.[26] The IJ vein is harvested when it becomes apparent to the surgeon that an interposition graft is necessary, before the venous dissection is complete and the specimen is removed. This graft should be ready to use once the vascular clamps are applied to the SMV, PV, and other vessels.[11] Preservation of the SV prevents direct access to the most proximal 3 to 4 cm of the SMA medial to the SMV and thus, in these cases, venous resection and reconstruction are done either before the specimen is separated from the right lateral wall of the SMA, or after complete mesenteric dissection by separating the specimen first from the SMA.[7,25,27]

MANAGEMENT OF JEJUNAL AND ILEAL BRANCHES

After transection of the pancreatic neck, the head and uncinate are separated from the SMV and PV when possible by dividing the small venous branches to the pancreas, including those from the jejunal branch to the uncinate. Isolated involvement of the jejunal branch of the SMV requires division of this branch and sometimes resection of a short segment. Reconstruction of the jejunal branch is not necessary if the ileal branch is intact and of reasonable diameter. The ileal branch is usually at least 1.5 times the diameter of the SMA as seen on axial CT imaging. The jejunal branch of the SMV is exposed by dissecting the root of mesentery to the right of the SMA and medial to, or to the left of, the SMA. The soft tissue between these vessels is carefully divided until the jejunal branch is identified coursing posterior to the SMA. This step is much simpler when the jejunal branch courses anterior to the SMA. In the rare situation whereby the tumor involves only the ileal branch, it too can be ligated and a short segment resected, often without reconstruction.[21]

When the ileal and jejunal branches as well as the proximal common trunk of the SMV is encased with tumor, the jejunal branch is ligated along with concurrent segmental resection and reconstruction of the main SMV and the proximal ileal branch, which may or may not require an interposition graft. If the SV is left intact, the PV remains relatively immobile, and an interposition graft is usually necessary to join the ileal branch to the main trunk of the SMV.[21]

Reconstruction of the ileal branch is always preferred over reconstruction of the jejunal branch because the jejunal branch is usually posteriorly located, thin-walled, and difficult to access for an anastomosis with the main trunk of the SMV. However, as a general rule, resection and reconstruction of the ileal branch (when the jejunal branch is ligated) is not done if the diameter of the ileal branch is not larger than the diameter of the SMA on axial CT images. This recommendation is based on the anecdotal clinical observation that long-term graft patency may be a concern the further out one travels in the small bowel mesentery and the smaller the diameter of the ileal branch. Acute thrombosis of the PV or SMV can lead to vascular congestion, bowel edema, hypotension, bowel ischemia, and necrosis, and is largely preventable with good surgical technique.[21]

OTHER VASCULAR RESECTIONS

Hepatic artery resection and reconstruction is performed when limited tumor involvement of the GDA necessitates short segment resection of the common or proper HA. If a replaced right HA is inseparable from tumor, it is resected. The need for revascularization in this setting is based on back bleeding from the distal artery. The anterior wall of the inferior vena cava (IVC) can also be resected with vein patch reconstruction, when the posterior aspect of the tumor cannot be separated from the IVC.[7]

RESULTS OF VASCULAR RESECTIONS

In 2004 Tseng and colleagues[7] reported on 572 patients who underwent PD for all histologic diagnoses, of whom 141 (25%) required major vascular resections. Resection of the SMV, PV, or SMV-PV confluence was performed in 126 (89%) of 141 patients. Venous resections included 36 VR1, 24 VR2, 15 VR3, 11 VR4, and 40 VR5. In addition, 17 (12%) of 141 required segmental resection of the HA with or without interposition grafting, and 7 of these also had concomitant venous resection and reconstruction. A part of the anterior wall of the IVC was resected in 6 (4%). The perioperative mortality rate was 2.1% (3 patients). Major perioperative complications occurred in 29 (21%) patients; 4 required reoperation including 3 for intra-abdominal hemorrhage, and one patient needed delayed biliopancreatic and gastrointestinal reconstruction due to bowel edema from prolonged venous occlusion at the time of resection/reconstruction. Median length of stay (LOS) was 13 days.

PD was performed for pancreatic ductal adenocarcinoma in 291 (51%) of the 572 patients; standard PD was performed in 181 (62%), and 110 (38%) required vascular resection and reconstruction. Venous resection was performed in 100 patients, 8 required isolated HA resection and reconstruction, and 2 required isolated resection of the anterior IVC. Of the 100 patients who required venous resection, 3 needed concomitant HA resection and 1 needed concomitant resection of the anterior surface of the IVC. The median overall survival was 24.9 months for all 291 patients. The only predictor of decreased survival on univariate analysis was N1 disease (21.1 months with node-positive disease versus 31.9 months for those who were node negative [$P = .005$]). The 110 patients who required vascular resection had a median survival of 23.4 months compared with 26.5 months for the 181 patients who underwent standard PD ($P = .18$). Multivariate analysis of those undergoing PD for pancreatic ductal adenocarcinoma demonstrated that the presence of N1 disease and the occurrence of one or more major perioperative complications were significant predictors of decreased survival (hazard ratio [HR] 1.50, $P = .01$ and HR 1.52, $P = .024$, respectively). Vascular resection was not associated with decreased survival (HR 1.1, $P = .499$). Of note, multimodality therapy was given to 88% of the vascular resection group and 91% of the standard PD group.[7]

SUMMARY

With proper patient selection, a detailed understanding of the anatomy of the root of mesentery, and adequate surgeon experience, vascular resection and reconstruction can be performed safely and does not impact survival duration. The median survival of patients with pancreatic ductal adenocarcinoma who underwent vascular resection was 23 months. This period was approximately 1 year longer than the expected survival of patients who did not have surgery because they were thought to have locally advanced pancreatic cancer (due to tumor extension to the SMV or PV), and only received chemotherapy or chemoradiation. Isolated venous involvement is not a contraindication to PD when performed by experienced surgeons at high-volume centers as part of a multidisciplinary and multimodal approach to localized pancreatic cancer.[9,11]

REFERENCES

1. Roder JD, Stein HJ, Siewert JR. Carcinoma of the periampullary region: who benefits from portal vein resection? Am J Surg 1996;171:170–4 [discussion: 174–5].
2. Asada S, Itaya H, Nakamura K, et al. Radical pancreatectomy and portal vein resection. Arch Surg 1963;87:608–13.
3. Fortner JG. Regional resection of cancer of the pancreas: a new surgical approach. Surgery 1973;73:307–20.

4. Yeo CJ, Cameron JL, Lillemoe KD, et al. Pancreaticoduodenectomy with or without distal gastrectomy for periampullary adenocarcinoma. Part 2: randomized controlled trial evaluating survival, morbidity, and mortality. Ann Surg 2002;236:355–68.

5. Pisters PW, Evans DB, Leung DH, et al. RE: surgery for ductal adenocarcinoma of the pancreatic head. World J Surg 2001;25:533–4.

6. Wolff R, Crane C, Li D, et al. Neoplasms of the exocrine pancreas. In: Kufe D, Bast R, Hait W, et al, editors. Holland-Frei cancer medicine. Ontario: B.C. Decker, Inc; 2006. p. 1331–59.

7. Tseng JF, Raut CP, Lee JE, et al. Pancreaticoduodenectomy with vascular resection: margin status and survival duration. J Gastrointest Surg 2004;8:935–49 [discussion: 49–50].

8. Raut CP, Tseng JF, Sun CC, et al. Impact of resection status on pattern of failure and survival after pancreaticoduodenectomy for pancreatic adenocarcinoma. Ann Surg 2007;246:52–60.

9. Evans DB, Farnell MB, Lillemoe KD, et al. Surgical treatment of resectable and borderline resectable pancreas cancer: expert consensus statement. Ann Surg Oncol 2009;16:1736–44.

10. Katz MH, Wang J, Fleming JB. Long-term survival after multidisciplinary management of resected pancreatic adenocarcinoma. Ann Surg Oncol 2009;16:836–47.

11. Tseng JE, Tamm EP, Lee JE, et al. Venous resection in pancreatic cancer surgery. Best Pract Res Clin Gastroenterol 2006;20(2):349–64.

12. Evans DB, Crane CH, Charnsangavej C, et al. The added value of multidisciplinary care for patients with pancreatic cancer. Ann Surg Oncol 2008;15(8):2078–80.

13. Callery MP, Chang KJ, Fishman EK, et al. Pretreatment assessment of resectable and borderline resectable pancreatic cancer: expert consensus statement. Ann Surg Oncol 2009;16:1727–33.

14. Katz MH, Pisters PW, Evans DB, et al. Borderline resectable pancreatic cancer: the importance of this emerging stage of disease. J Am Coll Surg 2008;206: 833–48.

15. General information on cancer staging and end-results reporting. In: Greene FL, Page DL, Fleming ID, et al, editors. AJCC cancer staging manual. Chicago: Springer; 2002. p. 1–16.

16. Yen TW, Abdalla EK, Pisters PW, et al. Pancreaticoduodenectomy. In: Von Hoff DD, Evans DB, Hruban RH, editors. Pancreatic cancer. Sudbury (MA): Jones and Bartlett; 2005. p. 256–86.

17. Scoggins CR, Lee JE, Evans DB. Pancreaticoduodenectomy with en bloc vascular resection and reconstruction for localized carcinoma of the pancreas. In: von Hoff DD, Evans DB, Hruban RH, editors. Pancreatic cancer. Sudbury (MA): Jones and Bartlett; 2005. p. 321–34.

18. Exocrine pancreas. In: Green FL, Page DL, Fleming ID, et al, editors. AJCC cancer staging manual. Chicago: Springer; 2002. p. 157–64.

19. Aloia TA, Lee JE, Vauthey JN, et al. Delayed recovery after pancreaticoduodenectomy: a major factor impairing the delivery of adjuvant therapy? J Am Coll Surg 2007;204(3):347–55.

20. Abrams RA, Lowy AM, O'Reilly EM, et al. Combined modality treatment of resectable and borderline resectable pancreas cancer: expert consensus statement. Ann Surg Oncol 2009;16:1751–6.

21. Katz MHG, Fleming JB, Pisters PW, et al. Anatomy of the superior mesenteric vein with special reference to the surgical management of first-order branch involvement at pancreaticoduodenectomy. Ann Surg 2008;248:1098–102.

22. Misuta K, Shimada H, Miura Y, et al. The role of splenomesenteric vein anastomosis after division of the splenic vein in pancreaticoduodenectomy. J Gastrointest Surg 2005;9:245–53.

23. Kim HJ, Jo YT, Kim JW, et al. Radiologic anatomy of the superior mesenteric vein and branching patterns of the first jejunal branch: evaluation using multi-detector row CT venography. Surg Radiol Anat 2007;29:67–75.

24. Graf O, Boland GW, Kaufman JA, et al. Anatomic variants of mesenteric veins: depiction with helical CT venography. AJR Am J Roentgenol 1997;168:1209–13.

25. Evans DB, Lee JE, Pisters PW. Pancreaticoduodenectomy (Whipple operation) and total pancreatectomy for cancer. In: Baker RJ, Fischer JE, editors. Mastery of surgery. Philadelphia: Lippincott/Williams & Wilkins; 2001. p. 1233–47.

26. Cusack JC Jr, Fuhrman GM, Lee JE, et al. Managing unsuspected tumor invasion of the superior-mesenteric-portal venous confluence during pancreaticoduodenectomy. Am J Surg 1994;168(4):352–4.

27. Leach SD, Davidson BS, Ames FC, et al. Alternative method for exposure of the retropancreatic mesenteric vasculature during total pancreatectomy. J Surg Oncol 1996;61(2):163–5.

Adjuvant and Neoadjuvant Therapy in Curable Pancreatic Cancer

F.W. Nugent, MD*, Keith Stuart, MD

KEYWORDS

• Pancreatic cancer • Adjuvant chemotherapy • Radiotherapy

Pancreatic cancer is the tenth most common cancer in the United States and the fourth leading cause of cancer death. Afflicting approximately 37,000 Americans yearly, more than 80% of patients are unresectable and, therefore, incurable at the time of their diagnosis.[1] Although surgical resection offers the only opportunity for cure, it remains largely unsuccessful; most patients who are candidates for surgical resection relapse and die in fewer than 5 years. This mortality leaves a 5-year overall survival (OS) of about 4% for patients diagnosed with pancreatic cancer.[2] Perhaps the most daunting realization for physicians involved in the management of this disease is the understanding that these numbers have not changed in more than 30 years. As surgery remains the foundation of curative therapy for pancreatic cancer, this article reviews the data on adjuvant chemotherapy and adjuvant chemotherapy with radiotherapy (CRT) as efforts to boost cure rates.

HISTORICAL PERSPECTIVE ON ADJUVANT THERAPY

Consideration for adjuvant therapy for resected pancreatic cancer first gained interest in the late 1960s. The rationale was twofold: first, data from other gastrointestinal malignancies such as rectal cancer proved the potential beneficial effects of postoperative chemotherapy and CRT in gastrointestinal malignancies; second, given the dismal prognosis for patients treated with surgical resection alone, attempts at additional therapy seemed warranted.[3] In 1974, the Gastrointestinal Tumor Study Group G19173 (GITSG) embarked on a randomized trial comparing adjuvant CRT to best supportive care for patients post surgical resection in pancreatic cancer.[4] Despite its small numbers, the GITSG trial established the beneficial effects of adjuvant pancreatic cancer treatment and established adjuvant therapy as a standard that

Department of Hematology/Oncology, Lahey Clinic Medical Center, 41 Mall Road, Burlington, MA 01805, USA
* Corresponding author.
E-mail address: Francis.w.nugent@lahey.org

Surg Clin N Am 90 (2010) 323–339
doi:10.1016/j.suc.2009.12.010
0039-6109/10/$ – see front matter © 2010 Published by Elsevier Inc.

surgical.theclinics.com

remains to this day. Exactly which treatment is the most beneficial, however, is hotly debated. The standard of care in the United States is still CRT, whereas in Europe adjuvant chemotherapy alone is the standard. This article provides a critical review of the data, evaluating chemotherapy alone and CRT in the adjuvant treatment of pancreatic cancer.

THE DEBATE: THE CASE FOR AND AGAINST ADJUVANT CRT
Randomized Trials

Much of the debate regarding CRT versus chemotherapy in adjuvant pancreatic cancer treatment arises from patterns of failure. For patients undergoing resection, there is a high rate of local and distant relapse (**Table 1**). Local failure rates following complete surgical resection vary widely and are reported as high as 86%, although many patients fail simultaneously with local and distant disease.[5–9] Given high local failure rates, combining locoregional therapy (radiation) with systemic treatment (chemotherapy) makes sense. Proponents of this combined modality approach dominate the discussion in North America.

GITSG G19173

Adjuvant CRT was adopted as standard in the United States shortly after the publication of the GITSG trial in 1985. Accruing 49 patients in 8 years, this is arguably the most influential trial of its size in oncologic history. GITSG ultimately randomized 43 patients (23 in the treatment arm) to observation versus CRT using split-course radiation in 10 20-Gray (Gy) fractions in a 2-week period, followed by a 2-week break, followed by 20 Gy for 2 additional weeks for a total of 40 Gy. Patients in the treatment arm received bolus 5-fluorouracil (5-FU) given on days 1 to 3 of each radiation cycle, followed by 2 years of maintenance 5-FU given weekly. Eligible patients were required to have pancreatic adenocarcinoma (no periampullary tumors) post R0 resection, although no standardized preoperative evaluation was required and no central pathologic review was attained. Also, no central review of designated radiation fields was obtained. In addition, no routine restaging or surveillance was performed postoperatively or following treatment completion. The trial was terminated early because of poor accrual and to the apparent benefit conferred from CRT in the treatment arm. After median follow-up of 56 months, median survival in the CRT arm was 20 months versus 11 months in the observation arm ($P = .04$).[4] Despite its small numbers and obvious flaws, and despite a methodology since abandoned for chemotherapy and for radiation, GITSG established a treatment standard that stood for 20 years.

Table 1
Patterns of failure following curative resection of pancreatic cancer

| Study | Patient Number | Pattern of Failure | | |
		Local, Number (%)	Extrapancreatic, Number (%)	Both ? Number (%)
Smeenk et al[5]	108	39 (36)	37 (34)	NA
Westerdahl et al[9]	74	64 (86)	68 (92)	NA
Tepper et al[7]	26	13 (50)	NA	NA
Griffin & Smalley[6]	35	19 (53)	27 (77)	NA
van den Broeck et al[8]	110	19 (17)	66 (60)	25 (23)

RTOG 9704

In 1996, gemcitabine was approved by the US Food and Drug Administration for the treatment of metastatic pancreatic cancer, the first newly approved chemotherapy for this disease in 35 years. Attempting to build on the successes of GITSG, an intergroup trial led by the Radiation Therapy Oncology Group (RTOG) embarked on a trial comparing 2 CRT strategies: the first using 5-FU and the second using gemcitabine. Accruing 538 patients, RTOG 9704 randomized 451 patients to 6 months of therapy: in the gemcitabine arm (arm A), patients received 1 month of gemcitabine followed by CRT with 5-FU (total radiation dose of 50.4 Gy given without interruption) followed by 3 additional months of gemcitabine. In arm B, patients received 1 cycle of 5-FU as a continuous infusion for 3 weeks followed by an identical radiation paradigm, followed by 3 additional months of infusional 5-FU.[10]

RTOG 9704 deserves credit for the rigor that it demanded of its participants: all patients were required to have a pre-enrollment computed tomography (CT) scan to rule out recurrent or metastatic disease; all patients were required to have an R0-R1 resection confirmed by central pathologic review; and radiation planning was subjected to prospective quality assurance. Surveillance following completion of therapy was mandatory. The arms were well balanced and approximately 85% to 90% of patients completed therapy on each arm. Results revealed a nonsignificant trend in survival favoring the gemcitabine arm: a median survival of 20.5 months and a 3-year OS of 31% in arm A versus a median survival of 16.9 months and a 3-year survival of 22% in arm B (hazard ratio [HR] 0.82, 95% confidence interval 0.65–1.03, $P = .09$).[10] Encouragingly for proponents of CRT, these data were consistent with GITSG. Further evidence supporting the benefit of radiation was the low rate of local recurrence in this trial, with only 23% of relapsing patients having a local recurrence as their initial site of failure, a low rate when compared with other trials. Given an R0 resection rate of only 42%, a locoregional benefit from radiation must be considered. Confounding this conclusion, however, is that the margin status of 25% of patients was listed as unknown.

Single-Institution Retrospective Analyses

Several large single-institutional experiences have been reported that suggest benefit for adjuvant CRT.

The Johns Hopkins experience

Swartz and colleagues[11] compared 162 patients post pancreatoduodenectomy (PD) treated with adjuvant CRT at their institution, comparing their outcome with 430 matched controls treated with PD alone. Collecting cases from 1993 to 2005, the investigators reported a median survival of 20.8 months for those receiving adjuvant CRT compared with 13 months for those treated with PD alone. Five-year survival was 25% versus 14.8% ($P = .001$).[12] These data have not been published in full form so any confounding variables remain unclear.

The Mayo Clinic experience

In 2008, Corsini and colleagues[13] published a retrospective review of 472 consecutive patients from 1975 to 2005 who underwent R0 resection of pancreatic cancer at their institution. Median follow-up was 32.4 months. Median survival for patients receiving adjuvant CRT was 25.2 months versus 19.2 months ($P = .001$) for no adjuvant therapy. An OS benefit was still seen at 10 years (20% vs 14%) when comparing the treatment arm with observation. These differences were noted despite significantly higher risk factors (node positivity, high histologic grade, disease extension outside the pancreas) in patients in the treatment arm compared with those in the observation arm ($P = .001$).

These data are compelling and mirror the apparent benefit and OS seen in the GITSG and RTOG 9704 trials. They do, however, suffer from the potential bias of all single-institutional retrospective analyses. In addition, CRT was the standard of care through much of the time during which these data were obtained. One must question why, given the near universal recommendation for adjuvant therapy, those in the observation arm were unable to receive it. Estimates of disease-specific survival may be a more useful indicator of benefit in such analyses.

Surveillance Epidemiology and End Results Data Analyses

At least 3 recent analyses of the Surveillance Epidemiology and End Results (SEER) database describe benefit for adjuvant radiation. Artinyan and colleagues[14] evaluated node-negative resected patients from 1988 to 2003. A cohort of 1930 patients was identified. The investigators found a median survival of 20 months for patients receiving adjuvant radiation versus 15 months for those who did not (P = .01). When accounting for early deaths as defined as death within 3 months of resection, a survival improvement was not found. Moody and colleagues[15] reviewed 3252 patients undergoing attempted curative resection of pancreatic cancer from 1988 to 2003, including node-positive patients. Just more than half of all patients received adjuvant radiation. Improved survival was seen (P = .005), but subsequent subgroup analyses revealed nearly all the benefit was derived by patients with stage IIb disease (HR 0.70, P = .0001). Greco and colleagues[16] evaluated data on 2636 patients with resected pancreatic cancer from 1973 to 2003. Median OS was 11 months for observation versus 18 months for irradiated patients.

These reports suffer from several important weaknesses. First, given that standard of care in the United States in the last 30 years has been CRT, it is unclear whether any potential benefit seen in the irradiated cohorts was as result of adjuvant chemotherapy rather than radiation, as many patients may have received both. Second, as CRT was standard, it is also unclear whether those who did not receive treatment suffered from surgical complications or comorbidities that could confound survival data. For example, Moody and colleagues[15] eliminated any patients from their analysis whose survival was less than 6 months from their diagnosis, surmising that they suffered significant morbidity associated with surgery. When these patients were eliminated, any benefit for adjuvant radiation was lost for those with less than IIb disease. The analysis of Artinyan and colleagues[14] showed a similar trend.

THE CASE AGAINST CRT

Despite high rates of local recurrence, pancreatic cancer that recurs following complete resection in most patients recurs as distant metastatic disease. Given that a radical local therapy has already been adopted (ie, resection), opponents of CRT argue that a second local therapy for a predominantly systemic process is unnecessary. The data against CRT compared with adjuvant chemotherapy in pancreatic cancer are now reviewed.

Randomized Trials

EORTC 40,891
In 1987, the European Organization for Research and Treatment of Cancer (EORTC) attempted to replicate the encouraging results of GITSG G19173. Randomizing 219 patients between CRT and observation, EORTC enrolled 110 patients on combined 5-FU and split-course radiation. Unlike GITSG, periampullary tumors were eligible and patients with T3-4 and T1-2N1a tumors were excluded. Chemotherapy was

continuous infusion 5-FU although schedules varied by patient and treatment site and no additional cycles of 5-FU were delivered following completion of radiation therapy, a major difference in the 2 study designs. All tumors and margins were reviewed by central pathology. Nonsignificant improvements were found in the treatment arm for median survival (24.5 months vs 19 months), 2-year survival (51% vs 41%), and 5-year survival (28% vs 22%).[17] The investigators concluded that EORTC 40,891 failed to confirm the benefit of CRT.

Since its publication, this trial has been heavily criticized. Some have argued that the statistical analysis was inappropriate, and if other, more valid statistical methods had been used the trial would have reached significance.[18] Others have pointed to the substandard radiation schedule as split-course radiation was no longer the standard of care (although the radiation schedule was in fact identical to GITSG G19173).[19] Still others felt that the addition of periampullary tumors, which have a more favorable prognosis, may have confounded any benefit.[20] The investigators, however, performed a separate analysis on patients with pancreatic head primaries and these data were also nonsignificant.

One can argue that the doses and duration of chemotherapy were substantially less than that delivered on GITSG and, hence, lessened any delay of recurrence and death in relapsed patients seen on GITSG. On all adjuvant pancreatic cancer trials most patients relapse and die of disease. It can be argued that adjuvant chemotherapy is actually palliative chemotherapy for most patients and, with less given, perhaps the time to disease progression was shortened, and with it, survival. Others point out that 5-FU has little benefit in the metastatic setting and therefore should not account for a substantial benefit in the adjuvant setting. Regardless, EORTC 40,891 did not confirm the benefit of CRT.

ESPAC-1

In 2004, Neoptolemos and colleagues[21] published the final results of the European Study Group for Pancreatic Cancer 1 (ESPAC-1) trial. Enrolling 541 patients from 1994 to 2000 in a 4-arm trial with a 2-by-2 factorial design, the investigators sought to answer 2 questions: does adjuvant CRT improve survival? and does adjuvant chemotherapy do the same? The 4 arms were: observation; chemotherapy alone; CRT; and CRT followed by maintenance chemotherapy. Radiation was given in a split-course fashion to 40 Gy (similar to GITSG), whereas chemotherapy was bolus 5-FU on day 1 to 3 during the 2 courses of radiation followed by 6 months of bolus 5-FU with leucovorin given 5 days a month. Chemotherapy was administered for a total of 6 months for those receiving maintenance. Patients receiving chemotherapy alone received 6 months of bolus 5-FU given 5 days a month. No central pathologic review was performed, no central radiology review was mandated, and no surgical quality control was arranged. No baseline imaging was obtained. Patients were followed every 3 months until death.

As noted, survival data were analyzed using a 2-by-2 factorial design (chemotherapy vs no chemotherapy and CRT vs no CRT). The investigators report a median survival of 15.9 months versus 17.9 months for CRT versus no CRT (HR 1.28; $P = .05$) with 2- and 5-year survivals of 29% and 10% versus 41% and 20%, suggesting a survival decrement for the addition of adjuvant radiation to chemotherapy. Conversely, the investigators describe a survival benefit with chemotherapy alone. Median survival for chemotherapy versus none was 20.1 months versus 15.5 months (HR 0.71; $P = .009$) with 2- and 5-year survivals of 40% and 21% for chemotherapy versus 30% and 8% for no chemotherapy.[21]

As with EORTC 40,891, ESPAC-1 has been heavily criticized. Once again, critics point to its outdated radiation schedule to explain the poor outcomes of radiated patients. No pre-enrollment imaging was obtained. Furthermore, the absence of central pathologic, radiologic, and surgical review is worrisome in the era of modern clinical trials. In addition, a troubling number of patients failed to receive their assigned therapy (31% in the chemotherapy group and 19% in the CRT group), perhaps mitigating any treatment effect.[21] Nonetheless, ESPAC-1 changed the standard of care for adjuvant treatment of pancreatic cancer in Europe, where radiation is no longer routinely given to patients who have undergone curative resection.

THE CASE FOR ADJUVANT CHEMOTHERAPY
Randomized Trials

CONKO-001
In 2007, the Charité Onkologie (CONKO) published the results of CONKO-001, a trial comparing adjuvant gemcitabine with observation. Randomizing 364 patients from 1998 to 2004 with resected T1-4 N0-1 pancreatic adenocarcinoma and a postoperative cancer antigen 19-9 less than 2.5 times normal limits, patients received weekly gemcitabine on a day 1, 8, 15, every 28 days schedule for 6 months total. A total of 186 patients were randomized to each arm with the primary end point being disease-free survival; OS was a secondary end point. No formal pathologic review was undertaken, no formal preoperative evaluation was mandated, and no surgical quality control was defined. CT scanning was performed at 6 months in both groups (ie, following completion of chemotherapy in the treatment arm) followed by abdominal ultrasonography (US) every 2 months to detect recurrence. Patients noted to have had recurrence were eligible for treatment with gemcitabine. After a median follow-up of 53 months, median disease-free survival was 13.4 versus 6.9 months (P<.001). OS showed a nonsignificant trend for improved survival favoring gemcitabine (P = .06, 22.1 months vs 20.2 months in the control arm).[22]

Proponents of adjuvant chemotherapy argue that CONKO-001 failed to show an improvement in OS for several reasons. First, patients in the observation arm were allowed to cross over to gemcitabine at the time of recurrence. Given that nearly all patients experienced recurrence and that no second-line chemotherapy has shown a survival benefit in the metastatic setting, this cross-over effect may have blunted any improvement in adjuvant treatment with gemcitabine as nearly all patients in both arms ended up receiving it. The only difference between the 2 groups was the timing of treatment. Second, in the intent-to-treat analysis, 32 (18.9%) patients in the treatment arm were excluded from the qualified survival analysis for a range of reasons, perhaps blunting any treatment effect.[22]

Final results of CONKO-001 were presented at the American Society of Clinical Oncology (ASCO) meeting in 2008. Longer follow-up revealed that improved disease-free survival was maintained (13.4 months vs 6.9 months; P<.001), and the data now showed a statistically significant improvement in OS (22.8 months vs 20.2 months; P = .05). Estimated survival at 3 and 5 years was 36.5% and 21% for the gemcitabine arm versus 19.5% and 9% for patients on observation.[23] These data are now consistent with a real but modest benefit to adjuvant gemcitabine chemotherapy.

ESPAC-3
Building on the results from ESPAC-1 and CONKO-001, Neoptolemos and colleagues presented the results of ESPAC-3 at the oral abstract session of ASCO 2009. This large, multicountry, open-labeled, randomized trial compared 6 months of adjuvant bolus

5-FU/folinic acid with 6 months of gemcitabine given on a day 1, 8, 15, every 28 days schedule. Enrolling patients in 17 countries from 2000 to 2007, nearly 1100 patients were first stratified by country and resection margin status (R0 vs R1) and then randomized to the 2 treatment arms. No mention was made regarding surgical quality control, central pathologic review, or prestudy imaging. Arms were balanced evenly for known prognostic factors such as resection margins status, node positivity, stage, and tumor grade. After 34 months' follow-up the data demonstrated no difference in OS or progression-free survival between treatment arms, suggesting that either chemotherapy was beneficial when given adjuvantly (median OS 23 months in both arms). Gemcitabine appeared to trend toward improved survival in patients with node-positive disease or positive resection margins and exhibiting a more favorable toxicity profile, and hence, was deemed the most appropriate choice for treatment.[24] As these data were presented in incomplete form, a formal assessment of the trial awaits. Nonetheless, this is the largest randomized trial ever organized in adjuvant pancreatic cancer treatment.

Ueno and colleagues
Recent data from Japan support the benefit of adjuvant gemcitabine. Enrolling 119 patients from 2002 to 2005, Ueno and colleagues[25] randomized patients to 3 months of postoperative gemcitabine versus observation, a design similar to CONKO-001, albeit of shorter duration. Patients were accrued from 10 centers across Japan and were required to have undergone an R0-R1 resection of pancreatic adenocarcinoma and begin treatment within 10 weeks of surgery. No pre-enrollment imaging was reported. Following completion of adjuvant treatment, patients were surveyed by CT or US scanning every 3 months until disease progression. The investigators reported a significantly longer disease-free survival (11.4 months vs 5.0 months; $P = .01$) but no improvement in OS (22.3 months vs 18.4 months; $P = .19$). These data mirror the benefit seen in CONKO-001, but may reflect the lack of power, given the small numbers (57 patients in the treatment arm).

THE CASE AGAINST ADJUVANT CHEMOTHERAPY
Randomized Trials

Bakkevold and colleagues
From 1984 to 1987, these investigators randomized 61 patients with pancreatic adenocarcinoma and carcinoma of the ampulla of Vater who had undergone R0 resections to adjuvant chemotherapy versus observation. Chemotherapy consisted of adriamycin, mitomycin C, and 5-FU administered on a day 1, every 21 days schedule. Again, no preoperative or postoperative staging was codified, no pathologic review was obtained, and no surgical quality control was described. Only 24 of 30 patients in the treatment arm actually received chemotherapy. Median survival was significantly prolonged in the treatment group (23 months vs 11 months; $P = .02$), but no improvement was noted in 5-year survival (4% for treatment vs 8% for observation).[26]

Takada and colleagues
From 1986 to 1992, the investigators randomized 508 patients with pancreatobiliary cancers (n = 173 with pancreatic cancer) to adjuvant chemotherapy or observation. Chemotherapy consisted of mitomycin C given perioperatively followed by continuous infusion 5-FU during the first and third week postoperatively. Patients were stratified by institution and by primary tumor site. Patients were then treated with oral 5-FU daily until disease progression. Although the investigators found a survival benefit for patients with gallbladder cancer, no such benefit was found for those with pancreatic

cancer (5-year survival of 11.5% in the chemotherapy arm vs 18.0% in the control arm).[27]

Both of the previous trials suffer from many of the same flaws as the trials described earlier. Neither controlled for confounding factors by implementing strict guidelines for preoperative assessment, central pathologic or radiologic review, or standardized surveillance. Both were underpowered and used chemotherapy regimens that were, at best, nonstandard in the modern treatment of pancreatic cancer. In addition, Bakkevold and colleagues[26] included patients with ampullary carcinoma, a disease that confers a better prognosis than adenocarcinoma of the pancreas. Including patients with a superior prognosis may have affected the investigators' ability to detect a difference in survival at 5 years.

FACTORS CONFOUNDING A CLEAR ASSESSMENT OF THE DATA

At this juncture, there is a clear consensus recommending some form of adjuvant therapy for patients undergoing curative resection of pancreatic cancer. Flaws in study design and treatment schedules, lack of rigor of preoperative evaluation and postoperative restaging, and variable means of surveillance allow for debate on which strategy is the most beneficial for patients. These flaws are reviewed next.

1. Flaws in study design

Many of the trials discussed earlier suffer from flaws in design that prevent any conclusions from being drawn regarding benefit. Many trials simply lack sufficient power to reveal the admittedly small benefit garnered from adjuvant chemotherapy or CRT. Initially, surgeons feared that their patients would suffer added harm from chemotherapy or CRT given after a complicated, morbid procedure such as PD. More recently, the larger European trials (CONKO-001, ESPAC-3) have omitted radiation altogether, arguing that ESPAC-1 was sufficient to rule out any benefit conferred by radiation despite using what was clearly outmoded, less intense radiation than is the standard today. Hence, many believe that modern CRT has never been truly compared with chemotherapy alone. Improvements in modern radiotherapy have been dramatic in the last 2 decades. Radiotherapists are able to deliver higher radiation doses more safely to more precise volumes than ever before. Modern radiotherapy for adjuvant pancreatic cancer treatment consists of approximately 50.4 Gy given in 28 fractions without interruption.[19] Split-course radiation given in 10 fractions with a 2-week interruption followed by 10 additional fractions to a total dose of 40 Gy is inferior in intensity to modern radiation and, as such, may not be a fair comparator with modern designs strategies. The only trial to use modern radiation techniques is RTOG 9704, which compared 2 CRT schedules rather than CRT versus chemotherapy.[10] A randomized trial comparing modern CRT with chemotherapy alone is necessary to end this debate.

2. Absence of standardized preoperative imaging

Trials studying the benefit of adjuvant therapy have rarely insisted on standardized preoperative imaging. Surgical resectability of localized pancreatic cancer is largely determined by the preoperative use of standardized radiological criteria using high-definition CT scanning regarding the relationship of the tumor to the superior mesenteric vessels and celiac axis.[28] These criteria are well defined but sometimes absent from preoperative assessments in the community. Such rigor is necessary for well-designed trials in adjuvant pancreatic cancer.

3. Absence of central pathologic review

Many trials have failed to adequately assess margin status in enrolled patients following curative resection. Involvement of lymph nodes and margins (most commonly the retroperitoneal margin adjacent to the superior mesenteric artery) portends poor prognoses in patients undergoing curative resection.[21] Pathologic quality control helps ensure appropriate surgical quality control and stratifies patients undergoing PD to different prognostic groups. In RTOG 9704 25% of enrolled patients had an unknown margin status, and another 33% to 35% of patients had an R1 resection.[10] Lack of clarity regarding postoperative resection margins contaminates many studies, leaving some to wonder if complete resections of all gross disease had been achieved and making comparisons between study populations more difficult. Such standardization is necessary to perform quality research in the future.

4. Absence of postoperative restaging

Nearly all patients with pancreatic cancer relapse following PD and some do quickly. In the absence of pre-enrollment restaging, as many as 20% of patients enrolled on adjuvant trials will have metastatic disease at the time of their enrollment.[29,30] These patients may obscure any beneficial effects of adjuvant therapy. All trials should incorporate standard reimaging before initiating treatment.

5. Absence of radiation oncology quality control
6. Absence of modern radiologic follow-up

Secondary end points on nearly all adjuvant pancreatic cancer trials include progression-free survival. Yet surveillance techniques vary widely between trials, making any comparison difficult. Patients found to have relapsed earlier may be candidates for palliative chemotherapy, stereotactic radiation, or other techniques that could potentially extend life and affect OS. Standardized follow-up for patients on adjuvant trials should be incorporated in trial design.

OTHER APPROACHES
Neoadjuvant Chemoradiotherapy

Moving adjuvant CRT to the preoperative setting has several theoretic advantages. As mentioned earlier, pancreatic cancer is a systemic disease at presentation for most patients, even if they seem resectable. Initiating chemotherapy earlier in the treatment paradigm means treating a systemic process with a systemic treatment at the earliest possible moment rather than waiting (often months) until patients heal from what is ultimately a local procedure. Given that more than 1 in 4 patients fail to recover sufficiently postoperatively to receive adjuvant chemotherapy, a neoadjuvant approach allows for all patients to receive first what may be the most important part of their treatment.[31] In addition, occult metastatic disease or aggressive biologies may declare themselves and patients may manifest identifiable metastatic disease before a morbid and unnecessary procedure is undertaken. Neoadjuvant therapy also allows for delivery of radiation and chemotherapy before the inflammatory insult of surgery occurs and issues such as tissue hypoxia and cytokine stimulation potentially affect the efficacy of adjuvant treatment.[32] Preoperative CRT may increase the likelihood of R0 resection also, a described risk factor following surgery.[21] Given the strong rationale, investigators have used a range of different neoadjuvant strategies in an effort to improve the chance of cure. Most reports describe single-institutional approaches aimed at refining preoperative treatment strategies. Whether these approaches are translatable to the general community is uncertain.

The Duke Experience

In 2004, researchers at Duke University related their experience with neoadjuvant CRT before PD in patients with pancreatic adenocarcinoma. The investigators[33] describe 96 resectable patients treated with CRT. Radiation schedules typically used daily fractionated doses of 180 cGy to a total dose of 50.4 Gy given concurrently with a range of chemotherapeutic agents, most commonly 5-FU-based treatment. Patients received a break of 3 to 4 weeks and were then restaged. Patients without metastatic progression were surgically explored. Of 96 original patients, 70% underwent surgical exploration and 55% were resected, rates that are consistent with series from other institutions. Negative resection margins were achieved in 75% of resected patients and operative mortality was 3.8%. Postoperative complications were similar to institutional experience in patients taken directly to the operating room. The incidence of pancreatic leak was lower (10% vs 43%) than rates for those who did not undergo preoperative therapy. OS for 67 patients surviving the postoperative period is 28% at 5 years, with a median survival of 23 months.[34]

The MD Anderson Experience

In a series of investigations begun in 1990 and culminating with 2 trials published in 2008, the MD Anderson Cancer Center explored the potential benefit of neoadjuvant CRT. The institution's most recently published analyses explored 2 treatment paradigms: first, neoadjuvant gemcitabine and radiation followed by surgical resection; and second, induction cisplatin and gemcitabine followed by neoadjuvant CRT with weekly gemcitabine and radiation followed by surgery. The investigators employed rigorous pretreatment and preoperative staging criteria coupled with standardized surgical approaches and pathologic evaluation. In the first trial, patients were treated with 7 doses of weekly gemcitabine given concurrently with radiation to a total dose of 30 Gy given in 10 fractions. Eighty-six patients were initially enrolled from 2004 to 2006, of whom 74 were resectable at radiologic restaging. On exploration, 64 of the original 86 (73%) patients were resectable at a mean of 5.6 weeks following completion of neoadjuvant therapy. Major perioperative complications occurred in 6 (9%) of patients, including 1 death. Surgical margins revealed microscopic disease in 7 (11%) patients, a low rate compared with most published series. The median survival of all 86 patients was 22.7 months and 5-year OS was 27%. For patients undergoing resection, 5-year OS was 36%.[30]

The MD Anderson Cancer Center sought to build on the potential benefit of this model with a second trial using combination chemotherapy followed by CRT followed by surgical resection. Enrolling 90 patients, Varadhachary and colleagues[31] treated patients with cisplatin and gemcitabine for 2 months followed by CRT using gemcitabine in a similar fashion to the prior trial. Again, strict quality control was maintained throughout. Seventy-nine patients (88%) completed neoadjuvant therapy with a mixture of treatment-related effects and progressive disease accounting for the dropout. Seventy-seven patients underwent restaging, with 15 patients (19%) unable to go on to resection. Sixty-two were deemed radiologically resectable and underwent exploratory surgery. A successful PD was completed in 52 (66%) patients. Positive margins were found in 1 patient (R1 resection rate 4%) and nodal disease found in 58% of patients undergoing successful resection. Median follow-up was 29.3 months. At that time, median survival was 17.4 months for all patients and 28.3 months for those undergoing resection for ductal adenocarcinoma. The investigators concluded that the addition of induction cisplatin and gemcitabine chemotherapy to neoadjuvant CRT did not add additional benefit.

The Fox Chase Experience

Hoffman and colleagues[35] enrolled 34 patients with localized pancreatic cancer in a 6-year period to preoperative CRT comprised of 5-FU and mitomycin given concurrently with radiation (to 50.4 Gy). One death from cholangitis was reported during preoperative treatment. Following CRT, patients were restaged for potential surgical resection. Nine patients were not operable and 25 underwent surgical exploration. Of this cohort, 11 had metastases and 3 underwent palliative pancreatectomies. Perioperative major morbidity and mortality involved 2 patients (9%). Of the remaining 11 patients (32% of the original cohort), median survival was 45 months, with a product limit estimate of 5-year survival of 40%.

Based on these favorable data, the Eastern Cooperative Oncology Group (ECOG) initiated a phase II trial (PD289) using the same design. Enrolling patients from 1991 to 1993, 64 patients (53 eligible patients) with resectable or locally advanced pancreatic cancer were treated with CRT. Chemotherapy consisted of infusional 5-FU with mitomycin C coupled with radiation to a total dose of 50.4 Gy over 28 fractions. Treatment-related toxicity included 2 deaths from cholangitis in endoscopically placed stents. Twenty-nine of 57 patients were hospitalized for complications (51%). Forty-one patients underwent surgical exploration, of whom 24 had resection with curative intent. One patient died postoperatively (mortality 4.2%). Three late deaths were noted, 2 secondary to liver abscesses and a third from pneumonia and superior mesenteric vein thrombosis. Median survival was 15.7 months for patients undergoing curative resection.[36]

ECOG PD289 provides a cautionary tale regarding extrapolating data from small single-institutional series to broader settings. The median survival of PD289 was one-third that of its pilot study. PD289 enrolled patients with adverse features and locally advanced disease; average tumor size was 3.5 cm for resected patients, a size that conferred an inferior prognosis on ESPAC-3.[24] In addition, 7 of 24 resected patients required extended resections involving either the superior mesenteric vein, adjacent colon, or both.[36] Neoadjuvant chemotherapy has not shown a consistent ability to convert unresectable or borderline resectable patients into better operative candidates and this was clearly a cohort with advanced disease. Better patient selection with an emphasis on patients with smaller, node-negative tumors may lead to proof of principle in neoadjuvant therapy. Regardless, this is a rational approach if solely to eliminate patients with aggressive biologies from candidacy for surgical resection. In this series, 15% or more of patients initially believed to be resectable never went to surgery. These patients were spared an operation from which they were unlikely to benefit. Ultimately, the biggest role of neoadjuvant therapy may be in determining who should not undergo attempted curative resection rather than improving patients' chances of operability or likelihood of cure. Efforts such as those of the MD Anderson Cancer Center, with strict quality control and paradigms building one on another, should be commended as we try to better understand the potential benefit of neoadjuvant therapy.

Chemoimmunotherapy

Several investigators have sought to enhance antineoplastic therapy in pancreatic cancer treatment by adding biologic modulators, the most common of which has been interferon. Interferon has reported capability to: enhance chemotherapeutic-induced cell kill; work synergistically with 5-FU and other chemotherapeutics; and sensitize cells to radiation.[37–39] Researchers at Virginia Mason Medical Center adopted a strategy using interferon with CRT with cisplatin and 5-FU, followed by additional cycles of 5-FU, and compared this approach to patients receiving a GITSG-type approach. Patients were given the choice between the 2 options. From 1993 to 1998, Nukui and colleagues[40] accrued 33 patients to the 2 arms: 16 to GITSG-type treatment and 17 patients to interferon-based therapy. As patients were not randomized, the arms were uneven, with 76% of patients in the interferon-based arm having stage III disease, whereas 56% of patients receiving the GITSG-type treatment were noted to have stage I disease. Despite a poorer prognosis, 2-year survival was superior for interferon-based therapy (84% vs 54%; $P = .04$). This superior 2-year survival came at a cost as toxicity was high. Seventy-six percent of patients on interferon-based treatment had interruptions in treatment caused by gastrointestinal toxicity. Still, there were no treatment-related fatalities and all patients completed the protocol.

Picozzi and colleagues[41] followed up that trial with a single-arm analysis evaluating a similar adjuvant treatment regimen. Once again evaluating patients postcurative resection at Virginia Mason Medical Center, the investigators accrued 43 patients to interferon-based therapy from 1995 to 2002. All patients received CRT with infusional 5-FU, weekly cisplatin, and interferon (this time daily rather than given every other day during radiation). Once again, all patients completed radiation, although 42% were hospitalized during treatment because of toxicity. With a mean follow-up of 31.9 months, actuarial 5-year survival was 55% despite a cohort with advanced disease (84% of patients had positive lymph nodes).

ACOSOG Z05031

Hoping to confirm the promising data from Virginia Mason Medical Center, the American College of Surgeons Oncology Group undertook a multicenter phase II trial of adjuvant cisplatin, 5-FU, and interferon, adopting a similar design to Picozzi and colleagues.[42] Opened in 2003, Z05031 planned enrollment of 93 patients but closed early because of toxicity after 89 patients were enrolled. Patients were treated with weekly cisplatin, infusional 5-FU during radiation, and 5-FU for 2 6-week cycles after radiation was completed. Interferon (3×10^6) was given 3 times a week during radiation. Radiation consisted of 50.4 Gy in 38 days. After a median 28 months' follow-up, 2-year and median OS was 55% and 27.1 months. respectively. Grade 3+ toxicity occurred in 81 of 84 (96%) of patients, although no long-term toxicity or deaths were noted. This trial has not been published in full form so a more thorough analysis awaits.

Linehan and Colleagues

In 2008, these investigators reported the results of a single-arm, single-institutional study attempting to build on the Virginia Mason Medical Center experience. Enrolling 53 patients from 2002 to 2005, the investigators treated patients following R0-R1 resection with adjuvant weekly cisplatin, infusional 5-FU, and interferon given concurrently with radiation. Cisplatin and 5-FU doses were slightly lower than in ACOSOG Z05031. Following CRT, patients were treated with 2 3-week cycles of gemcitabine (rather than infusional 5-FU). Restaging CT scanning was done before CRT and again before gemcitabine. Surveillance with CT scans began 2 months after completion of therapy and continued every 6 months for 2 years, then annually until disease progression. Sixty-eight percent of patients experienced grade 3 or 4 toxicity during CRT and the same number suffered grade 3 and 4 toxicity during postchemoradiation gemcitabine. No treatment-related deaths were noted, but 3 late deaths were described 1 from liver abscesses believed secondary to obliterative endarteritis, 1 from gastric outlet obstruction from an anastamotic stricture, and 1 from "a spectrum of radiation associated injuries." After a median follow-up of 38 months, 3-year OS was 41%, comparing favorably with other trials in adjuvant pancreatic cancer.[43]

CapRI

Investigators at the University of Heidelberg have sought to further expand on our understanding of interferon-based adjuvant therapy. The chemoimmunotherapy trials described earlier vary in the chemotherapy doses given with radiation and in the types and duration of postradiation chemotherapy. Dose schedules of interferon have varied from 3 days a week to daily. The ChemoRadioImmunotherapy of Pancreatic Cancer (CapRI) trial will attempt to clarify the relative benefit of chemotherapy, immuno-therapy, and radiation in the adjuvant setting. CapRI is an ongoing prospective randomized multicenter phase II trial comparing 3 variations of the Virginia Mason Medical Center regimen: in arm A, patients will receive a standard approach with weekly cisplatin, infusional 5-FU, and interferon, followed by more infusional 5-FU; in arm B, the cisplatin will be omitted and; in arm C, cisplatin and radiation will be omitted. Anticipated accrual is 135 patients. First clinical results (safety data) are expected at the end of 2009.[44]

The data supporting chemoimmunotherapy are compelling, although caution must be used when interpreting them. Aside from ACOSOG Z05031 (which reported inferior results compared with the other chemoimmunotherapy experiences described earlier), these data are single-institutional experiences and suffer from potential bias regarding patient selection. Little description is offered regarding how patients were enrolled on trial or how other patients treated at the same institutions fared following PD. The results of CapRI and larger randomized controlled trials comparing chemoim-munotherapy with more standard approaches are awaited as we try to determine if and how to incorporate biologic therapy into adjuvant pancreatic cancer treatment. These experiences may improve on chemotherapy and CRT, although proof of benefit awaits, as do treatment schema that better control for toxicity. Such changes will likely be needed before chemoimmunotherapies could be transferable to community-based practice.

CAN ANY CONCLUSION BE DRAWN?

Despite the absence of clear consensus and the methodological flaws listed in this article, several important conclusions can be drawn from the data regarding adjuvant pancreatic cancer treatment. First, adjuvant chemotherapy clearly confers a survival benefit for patients who have undergone curative resection. ESPAC-1 and CONKO-001, the largest and best-designed trials available for review, describe a 5-year survival of 20% or more for patients receiving adjuvant chemotherapy (**Table 2**). Recent data from Japan confirm the benefit derived from chemotherapy also. In comparison, most trials that randomized patients to observation report 5-year survival rates of approximately 10% in the untreated arm. Adjuvant chemotherapy seems to double the likelihood of cure for patients following complete surgical resection. These benefits are modest but equal to the modest benefit conferred from curative surgical resection alone. Second, the relative benefits of radiation added to chemotherapy have yet to be proven. Absent trials comparing CRT versus chemotherapy with stricter quality control and with modern radiation designs the debate regarding the relative benefits of radiation will continue. To be fair to our European counterparts, the present data opposing standard CRT for all patients following curative resection seem to outweigh the data favoring radiation although the rationale for incorporating

Table 2
5-year survival for patients receiving adjuvant chemotherapy versus surgery alone

Trial	Adjuvant Chemotherapy (%)	Observation (%)
ESPAC-1[21]	21	8
CONKO-001[23]	22	9
Ueno et al[25]	23.9	10.6[a]

[a] Estimated.

radiotherapy remains strong. Ongoing CRT trials using modern radiation designs should definitively answer this question in the next few years.

Few strides have been made in the fight against pancreatic cancer in the last 3 decades whether radiation is included or not. Surgeons, radiation oncologists, and medical oncologists must move beyond questions of the past decades and seek out newer better treatments rather than reliving the battles of the past. Greater rigor evaluating patients before either curative surgical resection or before enrollment on trials testing adjuvant strategies is a must. Novel approaches such as chemoimmunotherapy, vaccines, and targeted therapies, perhaps given neoadjuvantly, need a more thorough evaluation and must be combined with carefully considered surgery to raise the bar beyond the modest benefit we now offer to our patients with curable disease.

REFERENCES

1. American Cancer Society: 2008 Cancer facts and figures. Atlanta, GA; 2008.
2. Jemal A, Murray T, Samuels A, et al. Cancer statistics, 2003. CA Cancer J Clin 2003;53(1):5–26.
3. Prolongation of the disease-free interval in surgically treated rectal carcinoma. Gastrointestinal Tumor Study Group. N Engl J Med 1985;312(23):1465–72.
4. Kalser MH, Ellenberg SS. Pancreatic cancer adjuvant combined radiation and chemotherapy following curative resection. Arch Sug 1985;120:899–903.
5. Smeenk HG, van Eijck CH, Hop WC, et al. Long-term survival and metastatic pattern of pancreatic and periampullary cancer after adjuvant chemoradiation or observation long-term results of EORTC Trial 40891. Ann Surg 2007;246(5):734–40.
6. Griffin JF, Smalley SR. Patterns of failure after curative resection of pancreatic carcinoma. Cancer 1990;66(1):56–61.
7. Tepper J, Nardi G, Suit H. Carcinoma of the pancreas: review of MGH experience from 1963 to 1973 – analysis of surgical failure and implications for radiation therapy. Cancer 1976;37:1519–24.
8. Van den Broeck A, Sergeant G, Ectors N, et al. Patterns of recurrence after curative resection of pancreatic ductal adenocarcinoma. Eur J Surg Oncol 2009; 35(6):600–4.
9. Westerdahl J, Andren-Sandberg A, Ihse I. Recurrence of exocrine pancreatic cancer—local or hepatic? Hepatogastroenterology 1993;40(4):384–7.
10. Regine WF, Winter KW, Abrams R, et al. RTOG 9704 a phase III study of adjuvant pre and post chemoradiation (CRT) 5-FU vs. gemcitabine (G) for resected pancreatic adenocarcinoma. 2006 ASCO Annual Meeting Proceedings (Post Meeting Edition). J Clin Oncol 2006;24(18S):4007.

11. Swartz MJ, Abrams RA, Winter J, et al. Adjuvant chemoradiation for adenocarcinoma of the pancreas: the Johns Hopkins experience. Int J Radiat Oncol Biol Phys 2006;66(3 Suppl 1):S82.

12. Yeo CJ, Abrams RA, Grochow LB, et al. Pancreaticoduodenectomy for pancreatic adenocarcinoma: postoperative adjuvant chemoradiation improves survival. Ann Surg 1997;225(5):621–36.

13. Corsini MM, Miller RC, Haddock MG, et al. Adjuvant radiotherapy and chemotherapy for pancreatic carcinoma: the Mayo Clinic experience (1975–2005). J Clin Oncol 2008;26(21):3511–6.

14. Artinyan A, Hellan M, Mojica-Manosa P, et al. Improved survival with adjuvant external-beam radiation therapy in lymph node-negative pancreatic cancer. 2007 doi: 10.1002/cncr.23134 American Cancer Society Published online 13 November 2007 in Wiley InterScience. Available at: www.interscience.wiley.com. Accessed September 1, 2009.

15. Moody JS, Sawrie SM, Kozak KR, et al. Adjuvant radiotherapy for pancreatic cancer is associated with a survival benefit primarily in state IIB patients. J Gastroenterol 2009;44:84–91. DOI:10.1007/s00535-008-2280-8.

16. Greco JA, Castaldo ET, Feurer ID, et al. Survival benefit with adjuvant radiation in surgically resected pancreatic cancer [abstract 109]. ASCO Gastrointestinal Cancers Symposium Proceedings 2007.

17. Klinkenbijl JH, Jeekel J, Sahmoud T, et al. Adjuvant radiotherapy and 5-fluorouracil after curative resection of cancer of the pancreas and periampullary region: phase III trial of the EORTC gastrointestinal tract cancer cooperative group. Ann Surg 1999;230(6):776–84.

18. Garofalo MC, Regine WF, Tan MT. On statistical reanalysis, the EORTC trial is a positive trail for adjuvant chemoradiation in pancreatic cancer. Ann Surg 2006;244(2):332–3.

19. Gutt R, Liauw SL, Weichselbaum RR. Adjuvant radiotherapy for resected pancreatic cancer: a lack of benefit or a lack of adequate trials? Nat Clin Pract Gastroenterol Hepatol 2009;6(1):38–46. Available at: www.nature.com/clinicalpractice/gasthep Accessed September 1, 2009.

20. O'Connell JB, Maggard MA, Manunga J, et al. Survival after resection of ampullary carcinoma: a national population-based study. Ann Surg Oncol 2008;15(7):1820–7.

21. Neoptolemos JP, Stocken DD, Friess H, et al. A randomized trial of chemoradiotherapy and chemotherapy after resection of pancreatic cancer. N Engl J Med 350; 12. Available at: www.NEJM.Org. Accessed March 18, 2004.

22. Oettle H, Post S, Neuhaus P, et al. Adjuvant chemotherapy with gemcitabine vs observation in patients undergoing curative-intent resection of pancreatic cancer. A randomized controlled trial. JAMA 2007;297(3):267–77. Available at: http://www.jama.com. Accessed September 1, 2009.

23. Neuhaus P, Riess H, Post S, et al. Oettle Deutsche Krebsgesellschaft (CAO/AIO). CONKO-001: Final results of the randomized, prospective, multicenter phase III trial of adjuvant chemotherapy with gemcitabine versus observation in patients with resected pancreatic cancer (PC). J Clin Oncol 2008;26(15S (May 20 Supplement)):LBA4504. 2008 ASCO Annual Meeting Proceedings (Post-Meeting Edition).

24. Neoptolemos J, Buchler M, Stocken DD, et al. ESPAC-3(v2): a multicenter, international, open-label, randomized, controlled phase III trial of adjuvant 5-fluorouracil/folinic acid (5-FU/FA) versus gemcitabine (GEM) in patients with resected pancreatic ductal adenocarcinoma [abstract LBA4505]. J Clin Oncol 2009; 27(Suppl):18S.

25. Ueno H, Kosuge T, Matsuyama Y, et al. A randomized phase III trial comparing gemcitabine with surgery-only in patients with resected pancreatic cancer: Japanese Study Group of Adjuvant Therapy for Pancreatic Cancer. Br J Cancer 2009; 101:908–15.

26. Bakkevold KE, Arnesjo B, Dahl O, et al. Adjuvant combination chemotherapy (AMF) following radical resection of carcinoma of the pancreas and papilla of Vater – results of a controlled, prospective, randomised multicentre study. Eur J Cancer 1993;29(5):698–703.

27. Takada T, Amano H, Yasuda H, et al. Is postoperative adjuvant chemotherapy useful for gallbladder carcinoma? 2002 American Cancer Society Cancer 2002; 95(8):1685–95.

28. Fuhrman GM, Charnsangavej C, Abbruzzese JL, et al. Thin-section contrast-enhanced computed tomography accurately predicts resectability of malignant pancreatic neoplasms. Am J Surg 1994;167:104.

29. Evans DB, Varadhachary GR, Crane CH, et al. Preoperative gemcitabine-based chemoradiation for patients with resectable adenocarcinoma of the pancreatic head. J Clin Oncol 2008;26(21):3496–502.

30. Varadhachary GR, Wolff RA, Crane CH, et al. Preoperative gemcitabine and cisplatin followed by gemcitabine-based chemoradiation for resectable adenocarcinoma of the pancreatic head. J Clin Oncol 2008;26(21):3487–95. DOI:10.1200/JCO.2007.15.8642.

31. Sohn TA, Yeo CJ, Cameron JL, et al. Resected adenocarcinoma of the pancreas – 616 patients: results, outcomes, and prognostic indicators. From the Departments of Surgery, Pathology (RHH), and Oncology (RAA), The Johns Hopkins Medical Institutions, Baltimore, MD. Presented at the Forty-First Annual Meeting of The Society for Surgery of the Alimentary Tract, San Diego, CA, May 21–24, 2000.

32. Hirai T, Matsumoto H, Yamashita K, et al. Surgical oncotaxis—excessive surgical stress and postoperative complications contribute to enhancing tumor metastasis, resulting in a poor prognosis for cancer patients. Ann Thorac Cardiovasc Surg 2005;11(1):4–6.

33. Spitz FR, Abbruzzese JL, Lee JE, et al. Preoperative and postoperative chemoradiation strategies in patients treated with pancreaticoduodenectomy for adenocarcinoma of the pancreas. J Clin Oncol 1997;15(3):928–37.

34. White RR, Tyler DS. Neoadjuvant therapy for pancreatic cancer: the Duke experience. Surg Oncol Clin N Am 2004;13:675–84.

35. Hoffman JP, Weese JL, Solin LJ, et al. A pilot study of preoperative chemoradiation for patients with localized adenocarcinoma of the pancreas. Am J Surg 1995; 169(1):71–7 [discussion: 77–8].

36. Hoffman JP, Lipsitz S, Pisansky T, et al. Phase II trial of preoperative radiation therapy and chemotherapy for patients with localized, resectable adenocarcinoma of the pancreas: an Eastern Cooperative Oncology Group Study. J Clin Oncol 1998;16(1):317–23.

37. Wadler S, Schwartz EL. Antineoplastic activity of the combination of interferon and cytotoxic agents against experimental and human malignancies: a review. Cancer Res 1990;50(12):3473–86.

38. Vokes EE. The promise of biochemical modulation in combined modality therapy. Semin Oncol 1994;21(6 Suppl 14):29–33.

39. Holsti LR, Mattson K, Niiranen A, et al. Enhancement of radiation effects by alpha interferon in the treatment of small cell carcinoma of the lung. Int J Radiat Oncol Biol Phys 1987;13(8):1161–6.

40. Nukui Y, Picozzi VJ, Traverso LW. Interferon-based adjuvant chemoradiation therapy improves survival after pancreaticoduodenectomy for pancreatic adenocarcinoma. Am J Surg 2000;179:367–71.
41. Picozzi VJ, Kozarek RA, Traverso LW. Interferon-based adjuvant chemoradiation therapy after pancreaticoduodenectomy for pancreatic adenocarcinoma. Am J Surg 2003;185(5):476–80.
42. Picozzi VJ, Abrams RA, Traverso LW, et al. ACOSOG Z05031: Report on a multicenter, phase II trial for adjuvant therapy of resected pancreatic cancer using cisplatin, 5- FU, and alpha-interferon. 2008 ASCO Annual Meeting Proceedings (Post Meeting Edition). J Clin Oncol 2008;26(15S):4505.
43. Linehan DC, Tan MCB, Strasberg SM, et al. Adjuvant interferon-based chemoradiation followed by gemcitabine for resected pancreatic adenocarcinoma: a single-institution phase II study. Ann Surg 2008;248(2):145–51.
44. Marten A, Schmidt J, Ose J, et al. A randomized multicentre phase ii trial comparing adjuvant therapy in patients with interferon alpha-2b and 5-fu alone or in combination with either external radiation treatment and Cisplatin (CapRI) or radiation alone regarding event-free survival – CapRI-2. BMC Cancer 2009; 9:160. DOI:10.1186/1471-2407-9-160. Available at: http://www.biomedcentral. com/1471-2407/9/160. Accessed September 1, 2009.

Curative Radiation Therapy for Pancreatic Malignancies

Ellen W. Cooke, MD*, Lisa Hazard, MD

KEYWORDS

- Pancreatic cancer • Chemotherapy • Gemcitabine
- Radiotherapy

In the year 2009, the American Cancer Society estimates 42,470 new diagnoses of pancreatic cancer in the United States, with more than 80% dying of the disease.[1] The 5-year survival rate for individuals diagnosed between 1999 and 2005 is 5.7% as reported by the National Cancer Institute's Surveillance, Epidemiology, and End Results (SEER) database.[2]

The optimal management of pancreatic cancer remains unclear, specifically as to the role and sequencing of multimodality treatment. Surgery is the only curative modality, yet only 10% to 20% of patients present with resectable disease.[3] Furthermore, the long-term outcomes of surgery alone are poor, even in patients with resectable disease. In a randomized study by Oettle and colleagues,[4] out of 175 patients on the postoperative observation arm (80% R0 resection, 20% R1 resection), 92% had a recurrence, of which 41% were local with or without distant failures and 56% were distant failures alone. The most common distant site was the liver. These dismal results with curative resection alone highlight the need for adjunctive therapies to improve local and distant control. There are limited and conflicting data on the role of chemoradiation therapy (CRT) in the treatment of pancreatic cancer, and its use remains controversial. The use of CRT is more widely accepted in the setting of unresectable disease. This article reviews the evidence for definitive radiation therapy (RT) in both the adjuvant setting and the definitive treatment of unresectable pancreatic cancer.

ADJUVANT CRT

Several trials have investigated the use of CRT in the adjuvant setting (summarized in **Table 1**). The first trial to show a benefit to the addition of CRT after surgical resection

Department of Radiation Oncology, University of Utah, Huntsman Cancer Hospital, 1950 Circle of Hope, Salt Lake City, UT 84112, USA
* Corresponding author.
E-mail address: ellen.cooke@hci.utah.edu

Surg Clin N Am 90 (2010) 341–354
doi:10.1016/j.suc.2009.12.002
0039-6109/10/$ – see front matter © 2010 Elsevier Inc. All rights reserved.
surgical.theclinics.com

Table 1
Adjuvant therapy in pancreatic cancer: randomized phase 3 trials

Trial	Positive Margins (%)	Adjuvant Treatment	Number	Local Recurrence	Distant Metastasis	Disease-Free Survival	Overall Survival	Median Survival
GITSIG[5]	0	5-FU[b]/RT[a] → 5-FU[c]	21	33%	40% liver	48% (2 y)	14% (5 y)	20 mo
		Observation	22	47%	52% liver	14% (2 y)	4% (5 y)	11 mo; P<.05[n]
EORTC[7]	25	5-FU[d]/RT[a]	104	36%	49%	37% (2 y)	28% (5 y all)	24.5 mo (all)
							20% (5 y pancreas[e])	17.1 mo (pancreas[e])
		Observation	103	36%	49%	38% (2 y)	22% (5 y all)	19 mo (all)
							10% (5 y pancreas[e])	12.6 mo (pancreas[e])[o]
ESPAC-1[8,9]	18	5-FU[b]/RT[a]	73	For all patients	For all patients	Not reported	7% (5 y)	13.9
		5-FU[b]/RT[a] → 5-FU/leucovorin[f]	75	62%	61%		29% (5 y)	19.9
		5-FU/leucovorin[f]	72				13% (5 y)	21.6
		Observation	69				11% (5 y)	16.9[p]
RTOG 97-04[9]	>35	Gem[j] → 5-FU[k]/RT[l] → Gem[j]	221	23%	75%	Not reported	31% (3 y)	20.5
		5-FU[k] → 5-FU[k]/RT[l] → 5-FU[k]	230	28%	71%		22% (3 y)	16.9[q]
CONKO-001[4]	19	Gem[m]	179	34%	56%	23.5% (3 y)	34% (3 y)	22.1
		Observation	175	41%	49%	7.5% (3 y)[h]	20.5% (3 y)	20.5[i]

Abbreviations: CI, continuous infusion; CT, chemotherapy; 5-FU, 5-fluorouracil; Gem, gemcitabine; OS, overall survival.

a RT = 40-Gy split course, 2-week break after 20 Gy.

b 5-FU = bolus 500 mg/m² days 1 to 3 of each 20-Gy course of RT.

c Weekly 5-FU for 2 years or until progression.

d CI 5-FU 25 mg/kg/d first course RT and for 0, 3, or 5 days of second course depending on the toxicity.

e A subgroup analysis excluding patients with periampullary tumors revealed that the survival difference with the addition of CRT approached but did not reach statistical significance (P = .09).

f Intravenous 5-FU, 425 mg/m², and folinic acid, 20 mg/m², daily for 5 days, monthly for 6 months.

g The trial did not have enough statistical power to compare all 4 arms. When patients were grouped into CT (arms 2 and 3) versus no CT (arms 1 and 4), CT showed a survival benefit (20.1 vs 15.5 months, P = .009). Patients grouped into RT (arms 1 and 2) versus no RT (arms 3 and 4) and a survival detriment was shown (15.9 months vs 17.9 months, P<.05).

h P<.001.

i P=.06.

j Gem, 1000 mg/m², once per week for a 30-minute infusion 3 weeks before CRT and 12 weeks after.

k CI 5-FU 250 mg/m²/d.

l RT 5 daily fractions for 28 total to a dose of 50.4 Gy.

m Gem, 1000 mg/m², 30-minute infusion every 4 weeks for 6 cycles.

n P = .035.

o P = .09.

p P = not significant.

q P = .09.

was performed by the Gastrointestinal Tumor Study Group (GITSG).[5] Patients had undergone initial resection with negative margins, and periampullary tumors were excluded. Twenty-eight percent of patients had node-positive disease. The trial randomized patients between postoperative CRT and observation. CRT included a 40-gray (Gy) split course of radiation with a 2-week break after 20 Gy, given with concurrent bolus 5-fluorouracil (FU) (500 mg/m^2 on days 1–3 of each 20-Gy course of RT), followed by additional weekly 5-FU for 2 years or until progression. The trial closed early because of poor accrual (43 patients during 8 years) and the detection of a survival benefit on the interim analysis. After the closure of the trial, 30 additional patients were enrolled on the combined modality therapy arm and had a 2-year actu-arial survival of 46%.[6]

Another trial by the European Organization for Research and Treatment of Cancer (EORTC) did not show a benefit to adjuvant CRT.[7] Patients were allowed in the trial if they had periampullary tumors, positive margins (25%), or positive nodes (47%). One hundred and fourteen patients were randomized between CRT and 40-Gy split course given identically to the GITSG trial, with continuous infusion 5-FU (25 mg/kg/d during the first course of RT and for 0, 3, or 5 days of second course depending on the toxicity). No maintenance chemotherapy was given. Twenty percent of randomized patients did not receive the intended therapy. Although no significant survival benefit was reported for the whole group, when patients with periampullary cancers (which have a better prognosis than cancers of the pancreatic head) were excluded, the difference in overall survival approached but did not reach significance (overall survival at 5 years, 20% with CRT vs 10% with observation; $P = .07$). Potential explanations for the lack of a benefit to adjuvant CRT include the omission of maintenance chemotherapy, higher percentage of patients with node-positive disease than included in the initial GITSG trial, and the inclusion of patients with positive surgical margins.

After the report of the GITSG and the EORTC randomized trials, the role of adjuvant CRT in pancreatic cancer remained controversial, given their conflicting results. Specifically, a conclusion could not be drawn as to whether the benefit seen in the GITSG trial could be attributed to the combination of CRT with maintenance chemo-therapy or if the benefit could be attributed solely to one of these treatments. The European Study Group for Pancreatic Cancer 1 (ESPAC-1) trial was designed to answer this question.[8] Enrollment criteria included patients with adenocarcinoma of the pancreas having undergone prior surgical resection. As in the EORTC study, posi-tive margins were allowed (18%) in this trial. The study used a 2-by-2 factorial design in which patients were randomized to 1 of the 4 arms: RT and bolus 5-FU, RT and bolus 5-FU followed by 6 months of maintenance 5-FU, 5-FU alone for 6 months, and observation. As an alternative, physicians could choose to randomize patients between no treatment versus chemotherapy and no treatment versus CRT. RT was a 40-Gy split course. Bolus 5-FU was given as 500 mg/m^2 on days 1 to 3 of each course of RT in the combined modality arm. Intravenous 5-FU was given at a dosage of 425 mg/m^2 along with folinic acid, 20 mg/m^2, daily for 5 days on a monthly basis for 6 months in the chemotherapy arm. In the final analysis, only those patients who have undergone a randomization to any 1 of the 4 arms were reported (n = 289) because of concerns about potential biases introduced by physician-directed enrollment. Median survival was 16.9 months for observation (95% confidence interval [CI], 12.3–24.8), 13.9 months for CRT (95% CI, 12.2–17.3), 21.6 months for chemotherapy (95% CI, 13.5–27.3), and 19.9 months for CRT with maintenance chemotherapy (95% CI, 14.2–22.5). There was not enough statistical power to compare the 4 groups directly. Additional analysis was performed grouping patients who received chemotherapy (defined as chemotherapy alone and CRT with maintenance chemotherapy) versus no chemotherapy (defined as observation and CRT alone). Patients who received chemotherapy had a survival benefit when compared with those who did not receive chemotherapy ($P = .009$). A subsequent analysis was performed grouping patients who received radiotherapy (defined as CRT and CRT with maintenance chemotherapy) versus no radiotherapy (defined as observation and chemotherapy). Patients who received radiotherapy had a survival detriment ($P = .05$), thus resulting in the conclusion that CRT had a deleterious effect on survival.

Despite the results of the ESPAC-1 trial, a consensus as to the role of RT in the adjuvant setting has not yet been reached. The major criticism of this trial is the lack of quality assurance in multiple areas of the trial, including surgical, pathologic, and RT planning. RT field size and technique were not specified in the protocol, and no central review of RT plans was performed. RT technique has been shown to affect survival outcomes in other trials. In Radiation Therapy Oncology Group (RTOG) 97-04, patients received 5-FU and RT and were randomized between 5-FU before and after CRT and gemcitabine before and after CRT. All radiation plans were centrally reviewed. In the 5-FU arm 51% were treated per protocol, 35% had acceptable variation, and 5% had unacceptable variation in RT plans, resulting in corresponding median survivals of 1.47 years, 1.34 years, and 1.18 years, respectively ($P = .055$). In the gemcitabine arm 45% of patients were treated per protocol, 43% had acceptable variation, and 5% had unacceptable variation in RT plans, resulting in median survivals of 1.89 years, 1.41 years, and 1.37 years, respectively ($P = .023$). These results highlight the importance of RT technique and quality review, and give evidence for the effect of these issues on survival outcomes.

Additional criticisms of the GITSG, EORTC, and ESPAC-1 trials are the use of split-course RT and the fairly low total dose of 40 Gy. Split-course RT theoretically allows for accelerated repopulation of malignant cells during the treatment break and has been shown to be detrimental to tumor control in other disease sites, such as head and neck cancer, cervical cancer, and anal cancer.[9–12] Furthermore, typically doses of at least 45 to 50 Gy are required to control microscopic disease.[13] Many other tumor sites show evidence of a dose response in that improved control is obtained with increasing radiation dose. One particular challenge in pancreatic cancer is the low tolerance of the nearby small bowel, which limits the ability to deliver high doses of radiation. Intraoperative radiation therapy (IORT) has been investigated by single institutions to try to overcome this challenge. IORT allows the delivery of higher dose to the tumor bed at the time of surgery, as the bowel can be manually retracted out of the radiation field. IORT is usually combined with a course of external beam irradiation. Although not confirmed in randomized trials, data from single institution series suggest that a dose response exists for pancreatic cancer.[14–17] The GITSG performed a randomized trial examining the issue of radiation dose escalation and was unable to show improvement in survival outcomes. Patients with unresectable pancreatic cancer were randomized to 1 of the 3 arms: external beam radiation alone to 40 Gy, external beam radiation alone to 60 Gy, and CRT to 40 Gy.[18] A split course and 2-dimensional anterior/posterior:posterior/anterior fields were used. No improvement in the survival was shown with higher doses of radiation. There were no response rates or local control data reported. Older radiation technique; split-course RT; and the inclusion of only those patients with gross, unresectable disease call into question whether this trial can be considered applicable in the adjuvant setting and the modern era. Further studies are needed to investigate in a randomized fashion the question of whether a dose response exists in pancreatic cancer.

An additional consideration when analyzing these 3 trials is the lack of surgical and pathologic quality control. In these trials, preenrollment computed tomography (CT) scans were not required to exclude obvious gross residual disease or the interval development of metastatic disease after surgery. Although the reported rates of margin positivity are low (none in GITSG, 25% in EORTC, and 18% in ESPAC-1), local tumor recurrence was reported as a component of failure in 39% of patients from GITSG, 53% from EORTC, and 62% from ESPAC-1. The high rates of local recurrence suggest that the incidence of microscopic or gross residual disease was underreported in these studies. Patients with positive surgical margins have a median survival of less than 12 months, similar to patients with unresectable disease, regardless of whether they undergo adjuvant therapy.[19] Therefore, meticulous evaluation and reporting of margin status is essential to interpret the results of clinical trials. This criticism, and many other previously discussed criticisms of the available randomized data, makes interpretation of these trials challenging.

Adjuvant gemcitabine has been evaluated in 2 recently published trials. In the Charité Onkologie (CONKO)-001 trial, 368 patients with resected pancreatic cancer were randomized between gemcitabine (1000 mg/m^2 intravenously for 30 minutes on days 1, 8, and 15 every 28 days) versus observation. The disease-free survival was improved in the gemcitabine arm, 13.9 months (95% CI, 11.4–15.3) versus 6.9 months (95% CI, 6.1–7.8; $P<.001$). There was no statistically significant difference in the overall survival, but most of the patients received gemcitabine at relapse (median survival 22.1 months vs 20.2 months, $P = .06$). In the RTOG trial 97-04, 451 patients were randomized between chemotherapy with 5-FU for 3 weeks before CRT and 5-FU for 12 weeks after CRT versus gemcitabine before and after CRT. 5-FU was given as continuous infusion, 250 mg/m^2/d, and gemcitabine as 30-minute infusion, 1000 mg/m^2, once per week. CRT was 5-FU (250 mg/m^2 continuous infusion per day) and 28 fractions of radiotherapy to 50.4 Gy in both arms. There was no survival difference between the 2 arms; however, in patients with resected pancreatic head lesions, the median survival was 20.5 months for gemcitabine versus 16.9 months for 5-FU (hazard ratio [HR] for death 0.82; 95% CI, 0.65–1.03; $P = .09$). Although it is tempting to compare the outcomes of the gemcitabine arms of CONKO-001 and RTOG 97-04 to elucidate the role of RT, such comparisons are not valid given the differing patient populations in the 2 trials. The CONKO-001 trial defined an inclusion criterion of a carbohydrate antigen (CA) 19-9 serum value of less than 2.5 times the normal, whereas RTOG did not define an upper limit for CA19-9. Furthermore, the RTOG trial had a higher rate of margin-positive disease than the CONKO-001 trial (34% vs 19%). The CONKO-001 trial suggests a role for gemcitabine in the adjuvant setting but does not prove or disprove the role of RT.

A recently published analysis of the SEER database investigated the use of adjuvant RT in resected pancreatic carcinoma.[20] Patients with nonmetastatic, completely resected adenocarcinoma treated between 1988 and 2003 were included, totaling 3252 patients. Disease stage affected survival, and patients with more advanced disease stage were more frequently treated with RT, but despite this, the use of adjuvant RT was associated with increased survival (HR 0.87; 95% CI, 0.80–0.96). The investigators concluded that most benefit was seen in patients with T1-3N1, stage IIB disease (HR 0.70; 95% CI, 0.62–0.79).

Attempts at improving the survival outcomes at individual institutions are continually being reported. The University of Michigan recently published their data on an adjuvant program consisting of combination chemotherapy for 4 cycles (gemcitabine at 1000 mg/m^2 on days 1 and 8 with either cisplatin, 35 mg/m^2, on days 1 and 8 or capecitabine, 1500 mg/m^2, on days 1–14) followed by radiotherapy to 54 Gy with concurrent capecitabine (1330 mg/m^2/d).[21] The treatment was well tolerated, with a median progression-free survival of 21.7 months and median overall survival of 45.9 months.

These promising results may lead to further testing in a phase 3 setting. Investigators from Virginia Mason Medical Center reported impressive results with a regimen consisting of 5-FU, cisplatin, and subcutaneous alpha interferon concurrent with 45 to 50 Gy of external beam radiotherapy (known as the CapRI scheme).[22] With this regimen, they achieved a 55% 5-year overall survival rate, significantly improved over historical controls. Considerable acute gastrointestinal (GI) toxicity was observed, with more than 40% of patients requiring hospitalization during treatment. A phase 3 multicenter randomized trial was then performed in Germany to evaluate this regimen.[3] Clinical results have not yet been reported, but preliminary findings noted significantly less acute toxicity, presumably because of dose reduction in most patients as a result of hematologic toxicity.[22] Currently underway in Germany is a phase 2, three-armed trial investigating dose reduction with this regimen in which patients are randomized among CapRI in its standard form, CapRI with omission of cisplatin, and CapRI with omission of both cisplatin and RT.

Other areas of investigation include the role of novel molecular-targeted approaches in combination with CRT, including bevacizumab, epidermal growth factor receptor (EGFR) inhibitors (gefitinib, erlotinib, and cetuximab), and TNFerade (GenVec Inc, MD, USA).[23–26] EGFR inhibitors in preliminary data have shown the most promise.

DEFINITIVE CRT FOR UNRESECTABLE DISEASE

The role of RT in unresectable pancreatic cancer remains controversial. Patients with unresectable disease are generally considered incurable; however, RT may slow the progression of local disease and offer palliation of symptoms, such as pain, biliary obstruction, bleeding, or bowel obstruction. Long-term (>5 years) survivors have been reported with CRT. In a series out of Massachusetts General Hospital, 5-year survival was 4% for patients treated with intraoperative electron beam radiotherapy followed by 5-FU–based external beam CRT.[27] Patients with small tumor size had better long-term control as evidenced by the surrogate maker of intraoperative radiation field size. The intraoperative field size is typically the size of the tumor plus a 2-cm margin. There were no patients who had an intraoperative field size of greater than 9 cm who lived beyond 18 months. The highest 3-year survival of 17% was seen in patients with a 5- to 6-cm intraoperative field size. These findings suggest that patients with smaller tumors may have better outcome with CRT, and that not all patients with locally advanced disease harbor micrometastasis at the time of diagnosis.

A randomized study by the GITSG revealed that the addition of 5-FU to radiotherapy in unresectable disease improved overall survival.[18] Several subsequent trials have compared chemotherapy alone with CRT in the unresectable setting in a randomized fashion, including 2 Eastern Cooperative Oncology Group (ECOG) trials (1989, 2008),[28] 1 GITSG trial (1988), and 1 trial by the *Fondation Francophone de Cancerologie Digestive* and *Societe Francaise de Radiotherapie Oncologique* (FFCD/SFRO) (summarized in **Table 2**). The results of these trials are contradictory, and they make it difficult to draw conclusions as to the role of RT, with 2 trials showing a survival benefit in the combined modality arm (GITSG 1988 and ECOG 4201) and 2 trials showing no benefit to CRT (ECOG 1985 and FFCD/SFRO). The GITSG (1988) study and the initial ECOG study (1985) did not incorporate gemcitabine chemotherapy, which has been shown to have a significantly higher response rate than 5-FU.[29] In addition, these trials used a split-course RT technique, which is subject to the concerns discussed previously, and therefore their application in the modern setting is questionable. The SMF regimen (streptozocin, mitomycin, and 5-FU) used in the GITSG trial (1988) has higher toxicity in comparison with that of gemcitabine and therefore may have altered the survival rate. Similarly, the FFCD/SFRO study, which was closed early after an interim analysis, failed to show a benefit of RT, and used a toxic regimen (cisplatin, 5-FU, and high-dose radiation to 60 Gy) that may have masked the benefit of RT. The reported median survival of 8.4 months on the CRT arm was unusually low compared with other series in which median survivals are typically 10 to 12 months. This result may be explained by the high rates of acute toxicity with the prescribed regimen, leading to poor compliance. The current National Cancer Care Network standard is 5-FU monotherapy concurrent with 50.4 Gy of external beam radiotherapy.

Thus far, the most applicable trial to modern practice is the ECOG 4201 trial published in abstract form in 2008.[28] This trial randomized patients between CRT (50.4 Gy using 3-dimensional [3D] conformal technique with concurrent gemcitabine, 600 mg/m^2, weekly × 6, followed by gemcitabine, 1000 mg/m^2, weekly × 3 every 4 weeks for 5 cycles) and chemotherapy alone (gemcitabine 1000 mg/m^2 weekly for 3 days every 4 weeks for 7 cycles). The accrual goal was 316 patients; however, the trial was able to accrue only 74 total patients. Despite the small numbers, the results show a small but significant 2-month improvement in median survival with the addition of RT (11.0 months vs 9.2 months, $P<.05$). The median time to progression was also improved with RT, although minimally (6.3 months vs 6.1 months). These results suggest that there may be a role for RT in patients with locally advanced disease, in conjunction with gemcitabine chemotherapy.

Most of the published trials have looked at survival as the primary end point, but in this disease, which is generally considered incurable, evaluation of quality of life, palliation, and control of cancer-related symptoms is also important. Published literature on the evaluation of these end points is lacking. In the ECOG 4201 trial, grade 3 or greater GI toxicity was worse in the combined modality arm (38% vs 14%, $P = .03$), but the investigators comment that these toxicities were "generally manageable." Higher acute toxicity may be acceptable if the treatment results in improved quality of life after recovery from the treatment. Data regarding long-term quality of life have not yet been reported.

Given that the likelihood of micrometastatic distant disease is high in patients who present with locally advanced disease, many centers have adopted an approach in which chemotherapy is given for 3 months up front, followed by reevaluation for combined modality treatment. If after several cycles of gemcitabine the patient has no evidence of progression of disease and acceptable performance status, CRT is delivered. This approach theoretically gives time for the highly aggressive disease that is resistant to therapy to become evident, therefore sparing the patient from the morbidity of RT; it has been evaluated in a randomized phase 2 and a phase 3 trial by the *Groupe Cooperateur Multidisciplinaire en Oncologie*, examining various chemotherapy regimens.[30] Patients who had been enrolled in these trials were restrospectively evaluated. Out of a total 181 patients who received 3 months of gemcitabine-based chemotherapy, 53 (29.3%) had progression of disease during chemotherapy and were ineligible for CRT. Of the remaining 128 patients, 72 received CRT, whereas 56 received further chemotherapy alone at the discretion of the treating physician. The 2 groups were balanced in regard to performance status, sex, age, type of neoadjuvant chemotherapy, and response to neoadjuvant chemotherapy. The progression-free survival times were 10.8 months for CRT versus 7.4 months for chemotherapy alone ($P = .005$), and the median overall survival times were 15 months versus 11.7 months ($P = .0009$). Patients who progressed during chemotherapy had

Table 2
Definitive CRT in locally advanced pancreatic cancer: randomized phase 3 trials

Trial	Treatment	Number	Median Survival (mo)	Overall Survival	Median Time to Progression (mo)	RT Technique
GITSG (1981)	(1) 40-Gy RT (2-wk break between each 20 Gy course) and CT (bolus 5-FU 500 mg/m² days 1–3 of each 20-Gy course of radiation and then every 4 wk for 2 y)	83	10	40% (1 y)	6	AP:PA
	(2) 60-Gy RT (2-wk break between each 20-Gy course) and CT (bolus 5-FU 500 mg/m² days 1–3 of each 20-Gy course of RT and then every 4 wk for 2 y)	86	10	40% (1 y)	8	
	(3) 60-Gy RT (2 wk break between each 20-Gy course)	25	6[a]	10% (1 y)	3[a]	
ECOG (1985)	(1) 40-Gy RT (2-wk break between each 20-Gy course) and 5-FU (600 mg/m² IV bolus days 1–3 of each course RT and weekly after the completion of RT)	34	8.3	28% (1 y)[b]	4.4	AP:PA
	(2) 5-FU (600 mg/m² weekly)	37	8.2	28% (1 y)[b]	4.2	
GITSG (1988)	(1) RT (2-wk break between each 20-Gy course) and CT (bolus 5-FU 350 mg/m² days 1–3 of each course of radiation, then SMF for 2 y starting d 64)	24	10	41% (1 y)	Not reported	CT plan
	(2) SMF chemotherapy for 2 y or until progression	24	8[a]	19% (1 y)[a]		3–4 fields

Study	Treatment	n				RT technique
FFCD/SFRO (2008)	(1) RT (60 Gy) and CT (5-FU 300 mg/m²/d days 1–5 for 6 wk and cisplatin 20 mg/m²/d wk 1 and 5 during radiation and Gem after radiation 1000 mg/m² weekly for 3–4 wk)	59	8.6	32% (1 y)	6[b]	Conformal RT recommended
	(2) Gem 1000 mg/m² weekly for 7 wk	60	13[a]	53% (1 y)	7[b]	
ECOG 4201 (2008)	(1) 50.4 Gy RT with concurrent Gem 600 mg/m² weekly × 6, then Gem 1000 mg/m² weekly × 3 every 4 wk for 5 cycles	34	11.0	45% (1 y)[b]	6.3	3D conformal RT
	(2) Gem 1000 mg/m² weekly × 3 every 4 wk for 7 cycles	35	9.2[a]	30% (1 y)[b]	6.1	

Abbreviations: AP:PA, anterior/posterior:posterior/anterior; CI, continuous infusion; CT, chemotherapy; 5-FU, 5-fluorouracil; Gem, gemcitabine; OS, overall survival; RT, radiation therapy; SMF, streptozocin, mitomycin, 5-FU.

[a] $P<.05$.
[b] Extrapolated from curve.

a median survival of only 4.5 months. Phase 3 trials are ongoing evaluating this promising approach in patients with unresectable disease.

In summary, patients with locally advanced, unresectable pancreatic cancer likely benefit modestly from chemotherapy and radiotherapy in improving survival and palliation. These treatments should be considered complementary, and a focus on improving the quality of life is essential.

RADIATION THERAPY TECHNIQUE

Conventional RT, as was used in the trials published before the early 1990s, consisted of 2 opposed anterior and posterior fields encompassing the pancreas or pancreatic bed and regional nodes with margin. Currently, 3D conformal therapy is standard, which uses acquired CT images to allow delineation of target volumes and precise localization of normal structures. A radiation plan is then generated that provides optimum coverage of the target and maximal sparing of normal tissues. Multiple custom-shaped fields are used, and beam angles are varied according to individual patient anatomy. Treatments are typically given in 5 daily fractions per week during the course of 5 to 6 weeks. Split-course radiotherapy is no longer used given the concerns regarding accelerated repopulation during the break. Smaller treatment volumes and better normal tissue sparing have been achieved with 3D conformal techniques; however, given the proximity of the pancreas to the duodenum, the small bowel is not completely excluded from the field and remains the major dose-limiting structure.

Intensity modulation radiation therapy (IMRT) is a more recent advance in the delivery of RT. Unlike 3D conformal therapy whereby the intensity of each treatment beam is constant throughout, the intensity of the radiation beam in IMRT is nonuniform, allowing dose distribution across each treatment field to vary, therefore minimizing dose to normal tissues. Dose escalation to the target volume can be achieved if normal tissue dose can be optimally minimized. The challenges of IMRT delivery in pancreatic cancer are related to the variation in target position with respiration and bowel filling. A precise knowledge of target position is essential for an accurate delivery of an IMRT plan. The use of daily pretreatment cone beam CT scans, implanted fiducial markers, and respiratory gating are all being explored as ways to improve target localization. Preliminary studies have shown improved dosimetry when comparing IMRT plans with 3D conformal plans, including reduction in dose to the liver, kidneys, stomach, and small intestines.[31,32] Small clinical trials showing the feasibility of IMRT have been performed.[31–34] It is yet to be seen whether the dosimetric advantages of IMRT will translate into the clinical benefit of decreased toxicity. Further investigation is ongoing.

Several other methods for precise targeting and dose escalation have been studied, including stereotactic body radiation therapy (SBRT) and IORT. SBRT delivers 1 to 5 high-dose fractions of radiation, as opposed to conventional fractionation of 25 to 28 lower-dose fractions. The rationale for conventional fractionation is that by using low dose per fraction, large amounts of normal tissue can be included in the radiation field, as they will have time between fractions to recover. Injury to normal tissues is therefore minimized by relying on the body's ability to repair radiation damage. With SBRT, ablative doses of radiation are used, and tissues within the field are expected to have significant radiation damage. Fields, therefore, include only areas of gross disease and not areas at risk for micrometastatic disease, such as lymph node regions. As discussed previously, the close proximity of the pancreas to the duodenum is challenging with regard to the aim of dose escalation. Small bowel is particularly intolerant to high doses of radiation, which can result in ulceration, obstruction, or perforation. In a phase 2 trial, SBRT was used to deliver 30 Gy in 3 fractions to unresectable pancreatic carcinoma.[35] The local control rate was 57%; however, small-bowel toxicity was high with 18% of patients experiencing severe GI mucositis/ulceration and 4.5% experiencing perforation. A trial from Stanford investigated 25 Gy given as a single fraction with a small radiation field and reported 84% local control at 12 months, with 4% grade 2 late toxicity and 9% grade 3 or 4 late GI toxicity.[36,37] Alternatively, Stanford investigated the use of SBRT as a method of boost delivery after 45 Gy of conventionally fractionated therapy. Using this approach, they were able to achieve 94% local control, with 12.5% incidence of late duodenal ulcers.[38] Median survival times have not been improved compared with historical controls in these trials, ranging from 6 to 11 months, with most patients developing distant metastatic disease. Although the local control rates have been impressive, given the GI toxicities observed and that improved local control has not translated into a survival benefit in these trials, caution should be exercised in future studies. Careful patient selection to include those patients at the lowest risk of developing metastatic disease may play a key role.

IORT has also been studied as a method for safely increasing the radiation dose. IORT allows high-dose delivery to the tumor bed, with a minimization of normal tissue dose by direct shielding or mobilization from the treatment volume. The National Cancer Institute performed a study in which patients were randomized between IORT and standard therapy (defined as observation if disease limited to the pancreas or external beam radiation if the disease was extrapancreatic or if lymph nodes were involved).[39] IORT resulted in improved local control. Data from Massachusetts General Hospital suggest that the combination of IORT with 5-FU–based CRT can result in long-term survival for a small number of patients.[27] In their series, 150 patients with unresectable, nonmetastatic pancreatic cancer were treated with this approach. Five patients lived longer than 5 years, and an additional 3 patients lived between 3 and 4 years. RTOG 85-05 investigated the use of 20 Gy IORT in addition to CRT (50.4 Gy with concurrent 5-FU 500 mg/m^2/d on days 1–3 of RT).[40] IORT was generally well tolerated. Median survival was 9 months and actuarial 18-month survival was 9%, not different from historical controls. Overall, the data suggest that IORT results in improved local control.[39] This, however, has not translated into a survival benefit and so has not been adopted as a standard treatment.

RADIATION THERAPY FIELD SIZE

RT field size is a current topic of interest and research, especially given the increasing interest in dose escalation. Historically, radiation fields have been large, encompassing the pancreas or pancreatic bed with a 2- to 3-cm margin and including lymph node regions, which may be harboring microscopic disease. Fields of this size are generally well tolerated when using doses on the order of 45 to 50 Gy with concurrent 5-FU–based chemotherapy. Recent interest in the use of concurrent gemcitabine has resulted in the investigation of smaller RT field size. When large RT fields are used, full-dose concurrent gemcitabine is not well tolerated.[41] With field reduction to gross disease plus margin, full-dose gemcitabine can be used, in an effort to deliver effective chemotherapy more efficiently with the aim of preventing metastatic disease.[42] In a phase 1 trial of full-dose concurrent gemcitabine and localized radiotherapy for unresected pancreatic cancer, only 1 of 23 patients developed regional nodal recurrence, suggesting that smaller RT field size may be reasonable.[42] Although these data are encouraging, no prospective randomized data exist to guide RT field size.

SUMMARY

Although surgery is generally considered the only curative modality in the treatment of pancreatic cancer, the dismal outcome with surgery alone highlights the need for continued study of adjuvant therapies. Therapeutic strategies are yet to result in significant improvements in survival for these patients, and the application of chemotherapy and particularly radiotherapy is controversial because of difficulties interpreting the available randomized data. In the adjuvant setting, the role of radiation remains unclear, as existing data do not clearly define its role. Prospective, randomized data are needed using modern radiation techniques, dose/fractionation, and gemcitabine-based chemotherapy regimens. In the setting of unresectable, nonmetastatic disease, radiation in conjunction with chemotherapy seems to play a role in improving local control, survival, and cancer-related symptoms in select groups of patients. A reasonable therapeutic strategy in the adjuvant and the definitive settings includes an initial 2 to 4 months of gemcitabine-based chemotherapy, followed by restaging and delivery of 5-FU–based CRT, typically to 50.4 Gy in 28 fractions, in those patients who have not developed metastatic disease. Further study is needed to define more clearly the optimal timing of radiotherapy, dose, field size, and technique, and to study the effect of treatment on quality of life and palliation of cancer-related symptoms.

REFERENCES

1. American Cancer Society. Cancer facts and figures 2009. Atlanta (GA): American Cancer Society; 2009.
2. SEER database. Cancer statistics, section: pancreas, Table 22.7. Available at: http://seer.cancer.gov/csr/1975_2006/browse_csr.php?section=22&page=sect_22_table.07.html. Accessed September 9, 2009.
3. Knaebel HP, Marten A, Schmidt J, et al. Phase III trial of postoperative cisplatin, interferon alpha-2b, and 5-FU combined with external radiation treatment versus 5-FU alone for patients with resected pancreatic adenocarcinoma—CapRI: study protocol [ISRCTN62866759]. BMC Cancer 2005;5:37.
4. Oettle H, Post S, Neuhaus P, et al. Adjuvant chemotherapy with gemcitabine vs observation in patients undergoing curative-intent resection of pancreatic cancer: a randomized controlled trial. JAMA 2007;297:267.
5. Kalser MH, Ellenberg SS. Pancreatic cancer. Adjuvant combined radiation and chemotherapy following curative resection. Arch Surg 1985;120:899.
6. Further evidence of effective adjuvant combined radiation and chemotherapy following curative resection of pancreatic cancer. Gastrointestinal Tumor Study Group. Cancer 1987;59:2006.
7. Klinkenbijl JH, Jeekel J, Sahmoud T, et al. Adjuvant radiotherapy and 5-fluorouracil after curative resection of cancer of the pancreas and periampullary region: phase III trial of the EORTC gastrointestinal tract cancer cooperative group. Ann Surg 1999;230:776.
8. Neoptolemos JP, Dunn JA, Stocken DD, et al. Adjuvant chemoradiotherapy and chemotherapy in resectable pancreatic cancer: a randomised controlled trial. Lancet 2001;358:1576.
9. Regine WF, Winter KA, Abrams RA, et al. Fluorouracil vs gemcitabine chemotherapy before and after fluorouracil-based chemoradiation following resection of pancreatic adenocarcinoma: a randomized controlled trial. JAMA 2008;299:1019.
10. John M, Pajak T, Flam M, et al. Dose escalation in chemoradiation for anal cancer: preliminary results of RTOG 92-08. Cancer J Sci Am 1996;2:205.

11. Overgaard J, Hjelm-Hansen M, Johansen LV, et al. Comparison of conventional and split-course radiotherapy as primary treatment in carcinoma of the larynx. Acta Oncol 1988;27:147.
12. Withers HR, Taylor JM, Maciejewski B. The hazard of accelerated tumor clonogen repopulation during radiotherapy. Acta Oncol 1988;27:131.
13. Withers HR, Peters LJ, Taylor JM. Dose-response relationship for radiation therapy of subclinical disease. Int J Radiat Oncol Biol Phys 1995;31:353.
14. Garton GR, Gunderson LL, Nagorney DM, et al. High-dose preoperative external beam and intraoperative irradiation for locally advanced pancreatic cancer. Int J Radiat Oncol Biol Phys 1993;27:1153.
15. Mohiuddin M, Cantor RJ, Biermann W, et al. Combined modality treatment of localized unresectable adenocarcinoma of the pancreas. Int J Radiat Oncol Biol Phys 1988;14:79.
16. Mohiuddin M, Regine WF, Stevens J, et al. Combined intraoperative radiation and perioperative chemotherapy for unresectable cancers of the pancreas. J Clin Oncol 1995;13:2764.
17. Roldan GE, Gunderson LL, Nagorney DM, et al. External beam versus intraoperative and external beam irradiation for locally advanced pancreatic cancer. Cancer 1988;61:1110.
18. Moertel CG, Frytak S, Hahn RG, et al. Therapy of locally unresectable pancreatic carcinoma: a randomized comparison of high dose (6000 rads) radiation alone, moderate dose radiation (4000 rads + 5-fluorouracil), and high dose radiation + 5-fluorouracil: the Gastrointestinal Tumor Study Group. Cancer 1981;48:1705.
19. Small W Jr, Berlin J, Freedman GM, et al. Full-dose gemcitabine with concurrent radiation therapy in patients with nonmetastatic pancreatic cancer: a multicenter phase II trial. J Clin Oncol 2008;26:942.
20. Moody JS, Sawrie SM, Kozak KR, et al. Adjuvant radiotherapy for pancreatic cancer is associated with a survival benefit primarily in stage IIB patients. J Gastroenterol 2009;44:84.
21. Desai S, Ben-Josef E, Griffith KA, et al. Gemcitabine-based combination chemotherapy followed by radiation with capecitabine as adjuvant therapy for resected pancreas cancer. Int J Radiat Oncol Biol Phys 2009;75:1450–5.
22. Marten A, Schmidt J, Ose J, et al. A randomized multicentre phase II trial comparing adjuvant therapy in patients with interferon alpha-2b and 5-FU alone or in combination with either external radiation treatment and cisplatin (CapRI) or radiation alone regarding event-free survival—CapRI-2. BMC Cancer 2009;9:160.
23. Crane CH, Ellis LM, Abbruzzese JL, et al. Phase I trial evaluating the safety of bevacizumab with concurrent radiotherapy and capecitabine in locally advanced pancreatic cancer. J Clin Oncol 2006;24:1145.
24. Crane CH, Winter K, Regine WF, et al. Phase II study of bevacizumab with concurrent capecitabine and radiation followed by maintenance gemcitabine and bevacizumab for locally advanced pancreatic cancer: Radiation Therapy Oncology Group RTOG 0411. J Clin Oncol 2009;27:4096.
25. Duffy A, Kortmansky J, Schwartz GK, et al. A phase I study of erlotinib in combination with gemcitabine and radiation in locally advanced, non-operable pancreatic adenocarcinoma. Ann Oncol 2008;19:86.
26. Iannitti D, Dipetrillo T, Akerman P, et al. Erlotinib and chemoradiation followed by maintenance erlotinib for locally advanced pancreatic cancer: a phase I study. Am J Clin Oncol 2005;28:570.

27. Willett CG, Del Castillo CF, Shih HA, et al. Long-term results of intraoperative elec-tron beam irradiation (IOERT) for patients with unresectable pancreatic cancer. Ann Surg 2005;241:295.
28. Loehrer P, Cardenes H, wagner L, et al. A randomized phase III study of gemci-tabine in combination with radiation therapy versus gemcitabine alone in patients with localized, unresectable pancreatic cancer: E4201 [abstract 4506]. J Clin On-col 2008;26(Suppl).
29. Burris HA 3rd, Moore MJ, Andersen J, et al. Improvements in survival and clinical benefit with gemcitabine as first-line therapy for patients with advanced pancreas cancer: a randomized trial. J Clin Oncol 1997;15:2403.
30. Huguet F, Andre T, Hammel P, et al. Impact of chemoradiotherapy after disease control with chemotherapy in locally advanced pancreatic adenocarcinoma in GERCOR phase II and III studies. J Clin Oncol 2007;25:326.
31. Brown MW, Ning H, Arora B, et al. A dosimetric analysis of dose escalation using two intensity-modulated radiation therapy techniques in locally advanced pancreatic carcinoma. Int J Radiat Oncol Biol Phys 2006;65:274.
32. Milano MT, Chmura SJ, Garofalo MC, et al. Intensity-modulated radiotherapy in treatment of pancreatic and bile duct malignancies: toxicity and clinical outcome. Int J Radiat Oncol Biol Phys 2004;59:445.
33. Ben-David MA, Griffith KA, Abu-Isa E, et al. External-beam radiotherapy for local-ized extrahepatic cholangiocarcinoma. Int J Radiat Oncol Biol Phys 2006;66:772.
34. Crane CH, Antolak JA, Rosen II, et al. Phase I study of concomitant gemcitabine and IMRT for patients with unresectable adenocarcinoma of the pancreatic head. Int J Gastrointest Cancer 2001;30:123.
35. Hoyer M, Roed H, Traberg Hansen A, et al. Phase II study on stereotactic body radiotherapy of colorectal metastases. Acta Oncol 2006;45:823.
36. Chang DT, Schellenberg D, Shen J, et al. Stereotactic radiotherapy for unresect-able adenocarcinoma of the pancreas. Cancer 2009;115:665.
37. Koong AC, Le QT, Ho A, et al. Phase I study of stereotactic radiosurgery in patients with locally advanced pancreatic cancer. Int J Radiat Oncol Biol Phys 2004;58:1017.
38. Koong AC, Christofferson E, Le QT, et al. Phase II study to assess the efficacy of conventionally fractionated radiotherapy followed by a stereotactic radiosurgery boost in patients with locally advanced pancreatic cancer. Int J Radiat Oncol Biol Phys 2005;63:320.
39. Sindelar WF, Kinsella TJ. Studies of intraoperative radiotherapy in carcinoma of the pancreas. Ann Oncol 1999;10(Suppl 4):226.
40. Tepper JE, Noyes D, Krall JM, et al. Intraoperative radiation therapy of pancreatic carcinoma: a report of RTOG-8505. Radiation Therapy Oncology Group. Int J Radiat Oncol Biol Phys 1991;21:1145.
41. Crane CH, Abbruzzese JL, Evans DB, et al. Is the therapeutic index better with gemcitabine-based chemoradiation than with 5-fluorouracil-based chemoradia-tion in locally advanced pancreatic cancer? Int J Radiat Oncol Biol Phys 2002; 52:1293.
42. McGinn CJ, Zalupski MM, Shureiqi I, et al. Phase I trial of radiation dose escala-tion with concurrent weekly full-dose gemcitabine in patients with advanced pancreatic cancer. J Clin Oncol 2001;19:4202.

Palliation in Pancreatic Cancer

E. James Kruse, DO

KEYWORDS

- Palliative care/methods • Pancreas neoplasms
- Cholestasis/etiology/therapy
- Duodenal Obstruction/etiology/therapy • Humans
- Pain/etiology/therapy • Stents

Most patients with newly diagnosed pancreatic cancer will not be cured and will need palliative treatment. The American Cancer Society estimates that in 2009 there will be 42,470 new cases of pancreatic adenocarcinoma and 35,240 deaths. These statistics reflect the aggressive nature of this malignancy and the vague symptom presentation. Most patients present these symptoms at an advanced stage. In most series, the possibility of resection for cure is approximately 20%. Despite undergoing a "curative" resection, the 5 year survival rate remains at 5% due to recurrence. Because most of the pancreatic cancer patients will have disease progression or recurrence, palliation of symptomatology is a necessity. The common symptoms specifically associated with pancreatic cancer are biliary obstruction, duodenal obstruction, and pain. Historically, a patient undergoing an exploratory operation for painless jaundice was frequently discovered to have an unresectable pancreatic head cancer. There were limited options for palliating biliary obstruction and gastric outlet obstruction, which occur secondary to locally advanced tumors. A double bypass is performed in anticipation of the ensuing symptoms. This double-bypass surgery consists of a gastrojejunostomy combined with either a cholecystojejunostomy or choledochojejunostomy. At present, better selection of patients is possible for surgical exploration with the intent of resection because of better preoperative radiologic and endoscopic evaluation. Most of the patients deemed unresectable are evaluated on the basis of preoperative staging studies, and they do not undergo exploratory operations. Eighty percent of the patients explored for an apparently resectable pancreatic head mass are able to undergo the operation with a curative intent. The improvement in patient selection results in a discussion regarding palliation in 2 discrete situations. The first situation involves patients discovered intraoperatively to have an unresectable malignancy. In this case the question becomes whether to perform an intervention to alleviate symptoms or a prophylaxis against possible future symptoms. The second

---

Department of Surgery, Surgical Oncology Section, Medical College of Georgia, 1120 15th Street, BB 4518, Augusta, GA 30912, USA
E-mail address: ekruse@mcg.edu

Surg Clin N Am 90 (2010) 355–364
doi:10.1016/j.suc.2009.12.004
0039-6109/10/$ – see front matter

surgical.theclinics.com

situation is the palliative procedure, which is an option in patients known to be unresectable at the time of diagnosis or who later have recurrence. The surgical intervention, particularly in the latter circumstance, carries a morbidity that has decreased in recent years but is not insignificant. This article aims to address the options for palliating symptomatic patients in each scenario, and discusses the alternatives for prophylactic intervention in asymptomatic patients.

PALLIATION OF BILIARY OBSTRUCTION

Approximately 80% of pancreatic cancers arise in the pancreatic head. Lillemoe and Pitt[1] point out that obstructive jaundice is the most common presenting symptom of pancreatic cancer, occurring in 70% of patients at the time of diagnosis. Untreated biliary obstruction leads to jaundice, pruritis, coagulopathy, and eventually to death due to liver failure. An extensive review of the literature that included more than 8000 patients by Sarr and Cameron[2] in 1982 found that patients who underwent an operative biliary bypass lived a longer and a more comfortable life than patients undergoing only exploratory laparotomy. The current palliative options to relieve biliary obstruction are endoscopic stenting, operative bypass through a laparotomy or laparoscopically, or external drainage via radiologic guidance. Each of these methodologies is briefly reviewed in this section.

Endoscopic Palliation

Advancements in endoscopic treatment have replaced the need for operative treatment of this condition in most unresectable patients, with excellent results. In 1994, a prospective randomized controlled trial of endoscopic versus surgical biliary bypass in 200 patients found equal initial success rates but lower complication, procedure-related mortality, and length of hospitalization in the endoscopically treated group.[3] In the endoscopically treated group, however, recurrent jaundice occurred in 38% of the patients and gastric outlet obstruction in 18% compared with only 7% and 2%, respectively, of the surgical group. Advancements in endoscopic self-expanding stents and the replacement of plastic stents with metal and covered stents have improved the performance of this methodology. Stents are still prone to occlusion and subsequent cholangitis with time; metal stents have more longevity than plastic stents, which are replaced every 3 months approximately. A French study looked at the experience with each type of stent and calculated the actuarial survival of endoscopically placed stents.[4] The median patency for plastic stents was 2.5 months compared with 7 months for metal stents. Another study looked at the cost effectiveness of the stent placement and reinterventions. The investigators found plastic stents to be the best modality for palliating patients surviving less than 6 months, but metallic stents seemed to be better for palliating patients surviving longer.[5] Another study from the Netherlands concluded that for this reason, endoscopic bypass was the best treatment for patients surviving less than 6 months, whereas surgical bypass was optimal for those surviving longer.[6,7]

Surgical Palliation

The common surgical options involve direct anastomosis of the biliary tree to the intestine via a choledochoduodenostomy, choledochojejunostomy, or cholecystojejunostomy. Because most of the malignancies arise in the pancreatic head, the choledochoduodenostomy is not typically an option but has been practiced at the Cleveland Clinic with good results.[8,9] The proximity of the primary malignancies to the new anastomosis could potentially give rise to a subsequent obstruction as the malignancy grows. A choledochojejunostomy is typically performed with a side-to-side or end-to-side anastomosis between the common bile duct and a Roux-en-Y loop of the jejunum. This technique has been described in detail elsewhere.[10] This option is associated with a better long-term patency rate but can be applied only when access to the common bile duct is feasible. Large malignancies or bulky portal lymphadenopathy may make this difficult to perform safely. Cholecystectomy may improve access to the common bile duct when present and distended. Another option is the cholecystojejunostomy: the anastomosis of the gallbladder to the jejunum to allow retrograde decompression of the biliary tract. This procedure has been described as either a direct connection to a functional loop of jejunum or as a Roux-en-Y loop.[2,8,9,11–15] Cholecystojejunostomy is technically easier to perform but limited to patients with a gallbladder that retains patency with the common bile duct. The procedure has been performed laparoscopically in many centers, and a stapled anastomosis is possible.[12–14,16–19] However, Lillemoe and Pitt[1] point out that recurrent jaundice is more frequent with a cholecystojejunostomy than with a choledochojejunostomy (hepaticojejunostomy).

Radiologic Palliation

Percutaneous biliary drainage is typically reserved for patients with unresectable disease on initial imaging, and who are unable to undergo endoscopic drainage. Due to the marked biliary dilation, percutaneous drainage is successful in 96% to 100% of cases when endoscopic retrograde cholangiopancreatography fails. Endoscopic drainage is often not possible when patients have previously undergone a pancreaticoduodenectomy or when they have locally very advanced lesions.[20,21] Radiology-guided procedures may involve placement of internal stents similar to those placed endoscopically, or may involve external drainage when placement of a stent is not possible. External drains have the possibility of cholangitis, dislodgment, occlusion, leaking ascites, and pain at the catheter site, and are an encumbrance to the patient. After establishment of external drainage, the drainage catheter may sometimes be converted to an internal drain by the interventional radiologist or as a simultaneous combined effort with the endoscopists.

PALLIATION OF DUODENAL OBSTRUCTION

Retrospective data show that duodenal obstruction occurs in 11% to 20% of patients with pancreatic head carcinomas, but less than 5% initially present with these symptoms.[22–24] When total obstruction occurs late in the disease process, alleviating this with a palliative surgical bypass is associated with a significant mortality, but endoscopic stenting may not be an option. There is some controversy over when to perform a prophylactic gastroenterostomy when a patient is discovered to be unresectable at the time of surgical exploration. Few would argue against a bypass in a patient with obstructive symptoms if they were found to be unresectable at the time of operation. The argument of prophylactic bypass hinges on the additional 10% to 15% of patients who will later develop duodenal obstruction, and they are briefly covered in this section. The options for symptomatic patients known to be unresectable are also discussed.

Endoscopic Palliation

Endoscopic stenting of the duodenum with self-expanding metal endoprostheses has been reported in numerous small series with success rates of 90% to 100%.[25,26] Technical failures are usually the result of a complete obstruction that cannot be traversed by a guidewire.[27] Endoscopic stenting was effective in a Mayo Clinic series of 36 patients, in which only 1 was unable to tolerate anything by mouth after stenting.[28] Another article reviewed 600 published reports and found a success rate of stent placement at 97%, with all of these patients subsequently tolerating oral intake.[29] The rate of severe complications in these series was 1.2%. Late stent obstruction occurred in 18% due to tumor ingrowth. Compared with surgical bypass, endoscopic treatment is approximately one-third of the cost, can be performed as an outpatient procedure, and has a lower mortality rate.[26,30] Complications such as stent migration or tumor ingrowth necessitating reintervention are uncommon problems in these series. Stenting may be unsuccessful in distal obstructing lesions or in patients with multiple levels of obstruction.[31] Fluoroscopic guidance is often used to guide final stent placement, but total fluoroscopic placement is possible only by a skilled interventional radiologists, and produces similar results.[32,33] In patients known to be unresectable or who later recur, endoscopic treatment seems to be an efficacious, cost effective, and less invasive option to offer patients. If patients are not candidates and their life expectancy is short, then decompressive percutaneous endoscopic gastrostomies may be an option.

Surgical Palliation

There is some controversy over whether to perform a prophylactic gastric bypass (ie, gastroenterostomy) in asymptomatic patients found to be unresectable at the time of operation. The debate lies between the risk of subsequent gastric outlet obstruction and the risk of additional morbidity to the patient. Morbidity and mortality are still significant in patients undergoing surgical exploration when they are found to be unresectable. A prospective study from Johns Hopkins randomized 87 patients found to be unresectable at the time of operation due to either a prophylactic retrocolic gastroenterostomy or no enteric bypass.[23] All of these patients were considered not to have an impending duodenal obstruction based on the surgeon's assessment of symptoms and tumor location. The 2 groups had similar hospitalization lengths and complication rates. It is significant that 19% of those not undergoing prophylactic bypass subsequently developed gastric outlet obstruction at a median 2 months after the exploratory operation. In the investigator's hands, prophylactic bypass was safe, and averted future problems in many patients. Another multicenter randomized trial from the Netherlands randomized patients discovered intraoperatively to be unresectable to a single (hepaticojejunostomy) or double (hepaticojejunostomy and gastrojejunostomy) bypass.[24] In the single bypass group, 20% subsequently developed symptoms of gastric outlet obstruction requiring reoperation. Postoperative morbidity was 30% in both groups. The trial was terminated midway because of the superiority of double over single bypass. Another study agreed that palliation of gastric outlet obstruction does not increase the morbidity when added to a palliative biliary bypass.[34] A significant cause of morbidity relates to delayed gastric emptying, a persistent problem for this operation. In Denmark, Poulsen and colleagues[35] performed a retrospective review of 165 patients undergoing gastroenterostomy for all causes of gastric outlet obstruction (42% pancreatic cancer). In this review, patients had complication rate of 39% and a 30-day mortality rate of 30%. Preoperative hypoalbuminemia, comorbidity, advanced age, emergency operations, and hyponatremia were predictors of morbidity and mortality. Fujino and colleagues[36] found that gastroenteric bypass only improved dietary intake in the subset of asymptomatic patients with high oral intake preoperatively. There are several reported small series of patients who have successfully undergone laparoscopic palliative enteric bypass, at times in conjunction with laparoscopic biliary bypass. These procedures require a high level of laparoscopic skill not available in most institutions, but offer promise in expert hands. These procedures may be offered to patients who undergo laparoscopic staging or as an intended therapeutic intervention. The outcomes of laparoscopic therapy in comparison to open techniques are yet to be determined by randomized studies.

PALLIATION OF PAIN

The pain associated with retroperitoneal malignancies can be difficult to control with oral or transcutaneous narcotic administration. Opioid dosage varies widely in patients with cancer-related pain and requires continual reassessment.[37] Additional modalities need to be considered in patients not receiving adequate relief with narcotic administration. The celiac plexus is a nerve cluster in proximity to the celiac artery adjacent to the aorta. Sympathetic and parasympathetic nerves to the viscera are in this region along with nociceptive fibers from the pancreas.[38] Celiac plexus ablation is a technique first described in 1914, and has been used since then to attempt to alleviate pain of pancreatic origin. Current ablative techniques involve injection of a neurolytic agent, but cryotherapy or excision has also been described; alcohol is used in most series. Despite multiple reports of the efficacy of celiac plexus neurolysis (CPN) in relieving pain, few patients are offered this intervention. Most reports, however, are poorly controlled and do not effectively compare side effects or the other purported benefits of CPN such as relief from nausea or appetite enhancement.[39] A splanchnic neurolysis can achieve good control of deep pain associated with advanced pancreatic cancers, and can be performed via surgical, endoscopic, or radiologic approaches. Minor adverse events that are common to splanchnic neurolysis include transient hypotension, local injection site pain, and diarrhea.[40] For the patient known to have unresectable disease, less invasive approaches are the preferred route.

Surgical Palliation

CPN at the time of operation is easy, quick, and effective.[41] Operative neurolysis is usually described concurrent with aborted resection in the face of unresectable tumors. Neurolysis is achieved by injecting approximately 40 cc of 50% alcohol solution directly into the celiac plexus. Half of the volume is injected adjacent to the aorta at the level of the celiac artery on each side; this is safe and associated with minimal morbidity. The first prospective randomized trial looking at chemical splanchnicectomy was performed at Johns Hopkins and subsequently published in 1993.[7] All patients (137 in total) over a 5 year period found to be unresectable at the time of operation were randomized to saline injection or chemical ablation of the celiac plexus as described earlier. There were no significant differences in postoperative courses, complications, or hospital readmissions for pain. Short- and long-term follow-up found that all patients receiving the alcohol ablation reported a significant improvement in pain scores, longer pain-free interval, and less narcotic use compared with the placebo group. Although 10% of the ethanol-injected patients subsequently required a second percutaneous ablation for pain, it took place a mean of 12 months later. The alcohol ablation group also had a significant improvement in survival.

Less invasive thoracoscopic splanchnicectomy or laparoscopic approaches have been reported.[42,43] The laparoscopic injections may be performed in conjunction with palliative bypass as described previously, or when used for staging purposes.

Nonsurgical Palliation

Neurolysis traditionally has been performed using fluoroscopic or computed tomography (CT) guidance via a posterior approach. There are rare serious complications associated with this approach, which may be reduced with greater levels of experience. CPN may be provided by an anterior approach using ultrasound guidance, or via a posterior approach using fluoroscopic or CT guidance. Rare serious complications to the posterior approach include paraplegia due to spinal cord injury.[44] Advancements in endoscopic ultrasound have allowed therapeutic endoscopists to perform neurolysis via a transgastric injection. A prospective study of 50 consecutive Swedish patients found CPN to be effective in 74% of the patients, with the best results in those with tumors originating in the pancreatic head.[45] This efficacy is consistent across a multitude of studies. A recent meta-analysis of endoscopic ultrasound-guided celiac plexus neurolysis (EUS-CPN) found that 80% of patients had pain relief from pancreatic cancer pain.[46] A small randomized controlled trial comparing EUS-CPN with CT-guided CPN in patients with chronic pancreatitis, found the EUS approach to be less costly and preferable to patients who had undergone both methodologies.[47] Despite its efficacy, EUS-CPN is probably underutilized. The majority of oncologists have never referred a patient with unresectable pancreatic cancers for EUS-guided CPN.[48] Potential but rare serious complications to EUS-CPN include enteric ischemia, gastroparesis, and retroperitoneal abscesses.[38,49,50]

PALLIATIVE PANCREATICODUODENECTOMY

This topic is more controversial and deserves special mention. The goal of radical resection of locally advanced or metastatic pancreatic cancers is palliation of one or more of the aforementioned problems. Although not widely practiced, this can be achieved with good results and involves acceptable morbidity in very high volume centers. An article from Johns Hopkins published in 1996 described a retrospective review of 64 patients with grossly or microscopically positive margins who underwent pancreaticoduodenectomy compared with a cohort that underwent biliary and gastric bypass.[51] The 2 groups had no significant differences in postoperative mortality or complications. The pancreaticoduodenectomy group had a 3.4-day longer hospitalization, but significantly improved survival. Some studies have shown a correlation between survival and margin status,[52–58] but others have not found that correlation.[59–61] A recent meta-analysis of randomized controlled trials concluded that resection margins did not influence survival.[62] In fact, after a rigorous pathologic assessment, resection margins were changed from negative to positive in up to 62% of patients.[63] These results and high recurrence rates suggest that palliative pancreaticoduodenectomies may actually be performed commonly, although not as intended procedures but as a consequence of an aggressive disease process. The key issue is patient selection, and margin-positive patients have been shown to have an improved survival over patients undergoing a palliative bypass.[64] However, a planned palliative resection cannot be recommended as a common practice for metastatic lesions or as a debulking procedure outside a clinical trial in a very high volume center.

SUMMARY

Pancreatic cancer is a devastating disease, with few patients cured or even offered surgical resection. The morbidity of the disease progression is considerable, but many palliative options are possible that can alleviate symptoms, improve quality of life, and prolong survival. The pancreatic surgeon should be familiar with the options available when a patient is found intraoperatively to be unresectable. Most patients will benefit from a palliative biliary and enteric bypass and chemical splanchnicectomy in the appropriate setting. Morbidity and mortality of these operations can be considerable, but are significantly better in high volume centers. For the patient found to have unresectable disease at the time of diagnosis, palliation may be provided by operative, radiologic, or endoscopic methods. The best option to offer patients will depend on local expertise and experience. These decisions should be made in a multidisciplinary fashion.

REFERENCES

1. Lillemoe KD, Pitt HA. Palliation. Surgical and otherwise. Cancer 1996;78(Suppl 3):605–14.
2. Sarr MG, Cameron JL. Surgical management of unresectable carcinoma of the pancreas. Surgery 1982;91(2):123–33.
3. Smith AC, Dowsett JF, Russell RC, et al. Randomised trial of endoscopic stenting versus surgical bypass in malignant low bile duct obstruction. Lancet 1994; 344(8938):1655–60.
4. Maire F, Hammel P, Ponsot P, et al. Long-term outcome of biliary and duodenal stents in palliative treatment of patients with unresectable adenocarcinoma of the head of pancreas. Am J Gastroenterol 2006;101(4):735–42.
5. Prat F, Chapat O, Ducot B, et al. Predictive factors for survival of patients with inoperable malignant distal biliary strictures: a practical management guideline. Gut 1998;42(1):76–80.
6. van den Bosch RP, van der Schelling GP, Klinkenbijl JH, et al. Guidelines for the application of surgery and endoprostheses in the palliation of obstructive jaundice in advanced cancer of the pancreas. Ann Surg 1994;219(1):18–24.
7. Lillemoe KD, Cameron JL, Kaufman HS, et al. Chemical splanchnicectomy in patients with unresectable pancreatic cancer. A prospective randomized trial. Ann Surg 1993;217(5):447–55 [discussion: 456–7].
8. Potts JR 3rd, Broughan TA, Hermann RE. Palliative operations for pancreatic carcinoma. Am J Surg 1990;159(1):72–7 [discussion: 77–8].
9. Singh SM, Longmire WP Jr, Reber HA. Surgical palliation for pancreatic cancer. The UCLA experience. Ann Surg 1990;212(2):132–9.
10. Watanapa P, Williamson RC. Single-loop biliary and gastric bypass for irresectable pancreatic carcinoma. Br J Surg 1993;80(2):237–9.
11. Casaccia M, Diviacco P, Molinello P, et al. Laparoscopic gastrojejunostomy in the palliation of pancreatic cancer: reflections on the preliminary results. Surg Laparosc Endosc 1998;8(5):331–4.
12. Mullin TJ, Damazo F, Dawe EJ. Cholecystoenteric anastomosis with the EEA stapler for cancer of the pancreas. Am J Surg 1983;145(3):338–42.
13. Thompson E, Nagorney DM. Stapled cholecystojejunostomy and gastrojejunostomy for the palliation of unresectable pancreatic carcinoma. Am J Surg 1986; 151(4):509–11.
14. Scudamore CH, Chow Y, Shackleton CR, et al. Choledochocholecystojejunostomy: a quick, effective method of biliary decompression for carcinoma of the pancreas. Can J Surg 1991;34(6):543–6.
15. Deziel DJ, Wilhelmi B, Staren ED, et al. Surgical palliation for ductal adenocarcinoma of the pancreas. Am Surg 1996;62(7):582–8.
16. Tang CN, Siu WT, Ha JP, et al. Endo-laparoscopic approach in the management of obstructive jaundice and malignant gastric outflow obstruction. Hepatogastroenterology 2005;52(61):128–34.
17. Tang CN, Siu WT, Ha JP, et al. Laparoscopic biliary bypass—a single centre experience. Hepatogastroenterology 2007;54(74):503–7.

18. Fletcher DR, Jones RM. Laparoscopic cholecystojejunostomy as palliation for obstructive jaundice in inoperable carcinoma of pancreas. Surg Endosc 1992; 6(3):147–9.

19. Shimi S, Banting S, Cuschieri A. Laparoscopy in the management of pancreatic cancer: endoscopic cholecystojejunostomy for advanced disease. Br J Surg 1992;79(4):317–9.

20. McGrath PC, McNeill PM, Neifeld JP, et al. Management of biliary obstruction in patients with unresectable carcinoma of the pancreas. Ann Surg 1989;209(3): 284–8.

21. Kaufman SL. Percutaneous palliation of unresectable pancreatic cancer. Surg Clin North Am 1995;75(5):989–99.

22. Schantz SP, Schickler W, Evans TK, et al. Palliative gastroenterostomy for pancreatic cancer. Am J Surg 1984;147(6):793–6.

23. Lillemoe KD, Cameron JL, Hardacre JM, et al. Is prophylactic gastrojejunostomy indicated for unresectable periampullary cancer? A prospective randomized trial. Ann Surg 1999;230(3):322–8 [discussion: 328–30].

24. Van Heek NT, De Castro SM, van Eijck CH, et al. The need for a prophylactic gastrojejunostomy for unresectable periampullary cancer: a prospective randomized multicenter trial with special focus on assessment of quality of life. Ann Surg 2003;238(6):894–902 [discussion: 902–95].

25. Feretis C, Benakis P, Dimopoulos C, et al. Duodenal obstruction caused by pancreatic head carcinoma: palliation with self-expandable endoprostheses. Gastrointest Endosc 1997;46(2):161–5.

26. Yim HB, Jacobson BC, Saltzman JR, et al. Clinical outcome of the use of enteral stents for palliation of patients with malignant upper GI obstruction. Gastrointest Endosc 2001;53(3):329–32.

27. Lopera JE, Brazzini A, Gonzales A, et al. Gastroduodenal stent placement: current status. Radiographics 2004;24(6):1561–73.

28. Adler DG, Baron TH. Endoscopic palliation of malignant gastric outlet obstruction using self-expanding metal stents: experience in 36 patients. Am J Gastroenterol 2002;97(1):72–8.

29. Dormann A, Meisner S, Verin N, et al. Self-expanding metal stents for gastroduodenal malignancies: systematic review of their clinical effectiveness. Endoscopy 2004;36(6):543–50.

30. Wong YT, Brams DM, Munson L, et al. Gastric outlet obstruction secondary to pancreatic cancer: surgical vs endoscopic palliation. Surg Endosc 2002;16(2): 310–2.

31. Carr-Locke DL. Role of endoscopic stenting in the duodenum. Ann Oncol 1999; 10(Suppl 4):261–4.

32. Akinci D, Akhan O, Ozkan F, et al. Palliation of malignant biliary and duodenal obstruction with combined metallic stenting. Cardiovasc Intervent Radiol 2007; 30(6):1173–7.

33. Aviv RI, Shyamalan G, Khan FH, et al. Use of stents in the palliative treatment of malignant gastric outlet and duodenal obstruction. Clin Radiol 2002;57(7): 587–92.

34. Potts JR 3rd, Vogt DP, Broughan T, et al. Indications for gastric bypass in palliative operations for pancreatic carcinoma. Am J Surg 1991;57(1):24–8.

35. Poulsen M, Trezza M, Atimash GH, et al. Risk factors for morbidity and mortality following gastroenterostomy. J Gastrointest Surg 2009;13(7):1238–44.

36. Fujino Y, Suzuki Y, Kamigaki T, et al. Evaluation of gastroenteric bypass for unresectable pancreatic cancer. Hepatogastroenterology 2001;48(38):563–8.

37. Brescia FJ, Portenoy RK, Ryan M, et al. Pain, opioid use, and survival in hospitalized patients with advanced cancer. J Clin Oncol 1992;10(1):149–55.
38. Moore JC, Adler DG. Celiac plexus neurolysis for pain relief in pancreatic cancer. J Support Oncol 2009;7(3):83–7, 90.
39. Sharfman WH, Walsh TD. Has the analgesic efficacy of neurolytic celiac plexus block been demonstrated in pancreatic cancer pain? Pain 1990;41(3):267–71.
40. Eisenberg E, Carr DB, Chalmers TC. Neurolytic celiac plexus block for treatment of cancer pain: a meta-analysis. Anesth Analg 1995;80(2):290–5.
41. Sharp KW, Stevens EJ. Improving palliation in pancreatic cancer: intraoperative celiac plexus block for pain relief. Southampt Med J 1991;84(4):469–71.
42. Ihse I, Zoucas E, Gyllstedt E, et al. Bilateral thoracoscopic splanchnicectomy: effects on pancreatic pain and function. Ann Surg 1999;230(6):785–90 [discussion: 790–1].
43. Andren-Sandberg A, Zoucas E, Lillo-Gil R, et al. Thoracoscopic splanchnicectomy for chronic, severe pancreatic pain. Semin Laparosc Surg 1996;3(1):29–33.
44. Kumar A, Tripathi SS, Dhar D, et al. A case of reversible paraparesis following celiac plexus block. Reg Anesth Pain Med 2001;26(1):75–8.
45. Rykowski JJ, Hilgier M. Efficacy of neurolytic celiac plexus block in varying locations of pancreatic cancer: influence on pain relief. Anesthesiology 2000;92(2):347–54.
46. Puli SR, Reddy JB, Bechtold ML, et al. EUS-guided celiac plexus neurolysis for pain due to chronic pancreatitis or pancreatic cancer pain: a meta-analysis and systematic review. Dig Dis Sci 2009;54(11):2330–7.
47. Gress F, Schmitt C, Sherman S, et al. A prospective randomized comparison of endoscopic ultrasound- and computed tomography-guided celiac plexus block for managing chronic pancreatitis pain. Am J Gastroenterol 1999;94(4):900–5.
48. Reddy NK, Markowitz AB, Abbruzzese JL, et al. Knowledge of indications and utilization of EUS: a survey of oncologists in the United States. J Clin Gastroenterol 2008;42(8):892–6.
49. Ahmed HM, Friedman SE, Henriques HF, et al. End-organ ischemia as an unforeseen complication of endoscopic-ultrasound-guided celiac plexus neurolysis. Endoscopy 2009;41(Suppl 2):E218–9.
50. O'Toole TM, Schmulewitz N. Complication rates of EUS-guided celiac plexus blockade and neurolysis: results of a large case series. Endoscopy 2009;41(7):593–7.
51. Lillemoe KD, Cameron JL, Yeo CJ, et al. Pancreaticoduodenectomy. Does it have a role in the palliation of pancreatic cancer? Ann Surg 1996;223(6):718–25 [discussion: 725–8].
52. Murakami Y, Uemura K, Hayashidani Y, et al. Prognostic significance of lymph node metastasis and surgical margin status for distal cholangiocarcinoma. J Surg Oncol 2007;95(3):207–12.
53. Winter JM, Cameron JL, Campbell KA, et al. 1423 pancreaticoduodenectomies for pancreatic cancer: a single-institution experience. J Gastrointest Surg 2006;10(9):1199–210 [discussion: 1210–1].
54. Verbeke CS, Leitch D, Menon KV, et al. Redefining the R1 resection in pancreatic cancer. Br J Surg 2006;93(10):1232–7.
55. Pingpank JF, Hoffman JP, Ross EA, et al. Effect of preoperative chemoradiotherapy on surgical margin status of resected adenocarcinoma of the head of the pancreas. J Gastrointest Surg 2001;5(2):121–30.
56. Benassai G, Mastrorilli M, Quarto G, et al. Factors influencing survival after resection for ductal adenocarcinoma of the head of the pancreas. J Surg Oncol 2000;73(4):212–8.

57. Benassai G, Mastrorilli M, Mosella F, et al. Significance of lymph node metastases in the surgical management of pancreatic head carcinoma. J Exp Clin Cancer Res 1999;18(1):23–8.

58. Riediger H, Keck T, Wellner U, et al. The lymph node ratio is the strongest prognostic factor after resection of pancreatic cancer. J Gastrointest Surg 2009;13(7): 1337–44.

59. Dillhoff M, Yates R, Wall K, et al. Intraoperative assessment of pancreatic neck margin at the time of pancreaticoduodenectomy increases likelihood of margin-negative resection in patients with pancreatic cancer. J Gastrointest Surg 2009; 13(5):825–30.

60. Schnelldorfer T, Ware AL, Sarr MG, et al. Long-term survival after pancreatoduo-denectomy for pancreatic adenocarcinoma: is cure possible? Ann Surg 2008; 247(3):456–62.

61. Hernandez J, Mullinax J, Clark W, et al. Survival after pancreaticoduodenectomy is not improved by extending resections to achieve negative margins. Ann Surg 2009;250(1):76–80.

62. Butturini G, Stocken DD, Wente MN, et al. Influence of resection margins and treatment on survival in patients with pancreatic cancer: meta-analysis of randomized controlled trials. Arch Surg 2008;143(1):75–83 [discussion: 83].

63. Esposito I, Kleeff J, Bergmann F, et al. Most pancreatic cancer resections are R1 resections. Ann Surg Oncol 2008;15(6):1651–60.

64. Lavu H, Mascaro AA, Grenda DR, et al. Margin positive pancreaticoduodenec-tomy is superior to palliative bypass in locally advanced pancreatic ductal adenocarcinoma. J Gastrointest Surg 2009. [Epub ahead of print].

Palliative Chemotherapy for Pancreatic Malignancies

Sharmila P. Mehta, MD

KEYWORDS

- Pancreatic cancer • Chemotherapy
- Management • Palliative

Metastatic pancreatic cancer is often one of the most challenging malignancies a medical oncologist faces. The management includes more than simply chemotherapy, and the response rates in the past and present have been dismal at best. Multimodality treatments with supportive and palliative measures are a crucial part of the treatment algorithm. The author first outlines the most common chemotherapeutic modalities, such as single agent chemotherapy, combination therapy, and targeted therapy, and finally briefly discusses second line treatment.

INCIDENCE

Pancreatic adenocarcinoma is the fourth most common cancer in the United States. It was estimated that more than 40,000 people would develop pancreatic cancer in 2009 and that more than 35,000 would die from the disease in that year.[1] Surgery is rarely an option for patients with pancreatic cancer and therefore, less than 20% are curative on diagnosis. The only curative surgery for these patients involves complete resection of the primary tumor and surrounding pancreatic tissue. Therefore, the primary treatment for most of these patients is chemotherapy. Overall survival (OS) for patients with localized and metastatic pancreatic cancer is usually less than a year for localized disease and less than 6 months for metastatic disease.[2–4]

When discussing chemotherapy, it is important to remember that although in most studies the primary endpoint remains OS, palliation and quality of life are now more commonly being addressed in these trials because they are also of primary importance in the treatment of the disease.

Palmetto Hematology/Oncology Internal Medicine, Marsha and Jimmy Gibbs Regional Cancer Center, Spartanburg Regional Health Systems, 380 Serpentine Drive, Suite 200, Spartanburg, SC 29303, USA
E-mail address: smehta@srhs.com

Surg Clin N Am 90 (2010) 365–375
doi:10.1016/j.suc.2009.12.005
0039-6109/10/$ – see front matter © 2010 Elsevier Inc. All rights reserved.

surgical.theclinics.com

SINGLE AGENT CHEMOTHERAPY
Fluorouracil

5-FU has been extensively studied in the treatment of pancreatic cancer since the 1950s. 5-FU is a pyrimidine analogue that is cell specific for the S phase of cell division. After it is converted into its active metabolite in the surrounding tissue, it inhibits RNA and DNA synthesis.[5]

In the past, several agents have been combined with 5-FU but the results have never been promising. Single agent 5-FU in the metastatic setting has an OS usually in the range of 10 to 24 weeks at best.[6] In 2 larger meta-analyses of chemotherapy in advanced pancreatic cancer, use of 5-FU alone was not found to be superior to combination regimens.[7,8]

Taxanes

The benefit of taxanes in the treatment of metastatic pancreatic cancer has not been overtly successful. Most clinical trials performed in the past have been with docetaxel and with or without gemcitabine. Some of these early trials have shown a significant improvement in OS with the addition of docetaxel to gemcitabine compared with gemcitabine alone. Initially, several phase 2 trials showed a small benefit with a tolerable side effect profile while using a combination of these drugs.[9] Most trials reported an OS in the range of 7 to 10.5 months.[10,11] However, to date no phase 3 trials have been done to support this.

Gemcitabine

Gemcitabine is a deoxycytidine analogue that is cell-cycle specific with activity in the S phase. It requires activation into the active diphosphonate and triphosphonate nucleotides, which then inhibit ribonucleotide reductase.[12] It competes with deoxycytidine triphosphonate for incorporation into DNA. It primarily works by resulting in chain termination and inhibition of DNA synthesis and function.[12]

In 1997, Burris and colleagues[13] initially conducted the trial that led to the approval of the use of gemcitabine for the treatment of pancreatic cancer. A total of 126 patients with untreated pancreatic cancer were randomized to receive either 5-FU 600 mg/m^2 once weekly or gemcitabine 1000 mg/m^2 weekly $\times$ 7 with 1 week off, followed by weekly $\times$ 3 weeks every fourth week. Median survival was 5.63 months and 4.41 months after treatment with gemcitabine and 5-FU, respectively. The survival rate at 12 months was 18% for the gemcitabine arm and 2% for the 5-FU arm. In addition to measuring response rates, progressive disease, and OS, there is a clinical benefit response (CBR) measurement as well. The primary efficacy measurement was the CBR, which is a composite measurement of pain, Karnofsky performance status and weight. CBR required a sustained improvement in at least 1 of these 3 parameters. The CBR rate was 23.8% in the gemcitabine arm versus 4.8% in the 5-FU arm.[13]

The measurement of CBR, as mentioned earlier, is an important measurement and endpoint to define symptom control in malignancies. Pancreatic cancer is a disease that frequently has more quality of life issues than most solid tumor malignancies; so much so that there are separate guidelines and recommendations for managing many of these complications included in most standard texts and even in National Comprehensive Cancer Network (NCCN) guidelines.[2]

The major toxicity associated with gemcitabine is myelosuppression, although kidney and renal function should also be monitored closely in patients on treatment with gemcitabine in a fixed dose rate (FDR) infusion.

FDR GEMCITABINE

Some evidence suggests that, although increasing doses of gemcitabine, greater than 1000 mg/m^2, does not improve response rate, increasing the dose intensification may improve outcomes. Dose intensification is achieved by increasing infusion time for gemcitabine while holding the dose rate constant. Initial trials were done by Tempero and colleagues[14] to test this hypothesis, in which patients were administered gemcitabine in FDR of 10 mg/m^2/min or gemcitabine given at standard doses in a 30-minute bolus technique. Patients treated with FDR had a trend toward improved survival when compared with conventional dose gemcitabine, 8 months versus 5 months respectively. This provocative result led to further studies of fixed dose gemcitabine. After this trial, a phase 2 trial was conducted by Louvet and colleagues[15] that included the use of oxaliplatin in combination with gemcitabine. Once again this trial showed improved survival with gemcitabine/oxaliplatin given at FDR, which led to a larger Eastern Cooperative Oncology Group (ECOG) trial.

In the ECOG trial, 833 patients were assigned to treatment with gemcitabine (1000 mg/m^2 every week, 7 out of 8 weeks then 3 out of 4 weeks) and FDR gemcitabine 1500 mg/m^2 over 150 minutes weekly for 3 out of 4 weeks. A third arm used the combination of FDR gemcitabine and oxaliplatin. There was no significant difference in relative response between FDR gemcitabine and gemcitabine/oxaliplatin in terms of OS.[16]

Therefore, based on these most recent data, currently most institutions have continued using standard methods of gemcitabine administration over FDR to minimize toxicities. However, NCCN guidelines do continue to recommend FDR as a reasonable alternative and as a category 2B recommendation.[2]

Capecitabine

Capecitabine is an orally administered fluoropyrimidine carbamate prodrug that is converted to 5-FU intracellularly.[17] It is converted to 5′-deoxy-5-fluorocytidine in the liver and then to 5′-deoxy-5-fluorouridine by cytidine deaminase.[17] This drug is incorporated into the RNA as a false nucleotide and causes cell damage by causing alterations in RNA processing and translation.[17] It also results in inhibition of DNA synthesis and function.

Capecitabine has been studied independently and in combination in patients with metastatic pancreatic cancer, and early results suggested that follow-up studies may be useful.

A landmark phase 2 trial enrolled 42 patients treated with oral capecitabine at 1250 mg/m^2 administered twice daily for 14 days, followed by a 1-week treatment holiday. Median OS duration was 6 months with a CBR of approximately 24%, which compared favorably to gemcitabine.[6] This study included patients with locally advanced disease and metastatic pancreatic cancer. This is a potential option in patients who may have failed first line treatment with gemcitabine, although NCCN guidelines recommend a reduced dose of 1000 mg/m^2 in their most recent guidelines.[2]

COMBINATION REGIMENS
Gemcitabine and Irinotecan

Two phase 3 trials have compared gemcitabine with a combination therapy of gemcitabine and irinotecan in patients with advanced pancreatic cancer. One of these trials published by Stathopoulos and colleagues[18] randomized patients to receive gemcitabine monotherapy (900 mg/m^2) on weeks 1, 8, and 15 every 4 weeks or gemcitabine same doses given on days 1 and 8 plus irinotecan administered 300 mg/m^2 day 8 every 3 weeks. The overall response rate was 15% in the irinotecan/gemcitabine arm and 10% in the gemcitabine arm. The median survival time was 6.4 months for the irinotecan/gemcitabine arm and 6.5 months for the gemcitabine arm. There was no statistically significant benefit in the addition of irinotecan for the treatment of advanced pancreatic cancer.

Gemcitabine and Oxaliplatin

Two phase 3 randomized trials compared the addition of oxaliplatin to gemcitabine. The largest trial, the ECOG 6201 trial, compared the standard dose gemcitabine (1000 mg/m^2/30 min) with FDR gemcitabine (1500 mg/m^2/150min) or GemOx (1000 mg/m^2 gemcitabine on day 1 plus oxaliplatin 100 mg/m^2 on day 2 every 14 days). Eight hundred thirty-two patients were enrolled and the median survival was 4.9 months for the standard gemcitabine arm, 6.2 months for the FDR arm, and 5.7 months for the GemOx arm. None of these were statistically significant differences, and GemOx caused higher rates of neuropathy, nausea, and vomiting.[16]

The results of the French Multidisciplinary Clinical Research Group (GERCOR) and Italian Group for the Study of Gastrointestinal Tract Cancer (GISCAD) trials were a comparison of gemcitabine and GemOx in the patient with metastatic pancreatic cancer. One hundred fifty-seven patients were allocated to the GemOx arm (gemcitabine 1 g/m^2 in day 1 and oxaliplatin 100 mg/m^2 on day 2 every 14 days), and 156 patients received gemcitabine alone (1 g/m^2 weekly as a 30-minute infusion). Median OS was 9.0 months for the GemOX arm and 7.1 months for the gemcitabine arm.

Once again, although these numbers showed a trend toward improvement in the combination arm the median OS did not reach statistical significance and the combination arm did have higher grade 3 and 4 toxicity.

Although the results of the trials reported earlier are promising, the GemOX combination used in these trials should not be considered the standard of care for the treatment of metastatic pancreatic cancer because neither trial showed a statistically significant improvement.

Gemcitabine and Cisplatin

Gemcitabine and cisplatin are promising in much the same way that oxaliplatin is in the treatment of metastatic pancreatic cancer. They show benefits in median OS and progression-free survival (PFS), although the benefits are not statistically significant. In a phase 3 trial that compared the use of gemcitabine and cisplatin, patients were randomized to receive GemCis (gemcitabine 1000 mg/m^2 and cisplatin 50 mg/m^2 on days 1 and 15 of a 28-day cycle) and gemcitabine (1000 mg/m^2 days 1, 8, and 15 of a 28-day cycle). Median OS was superior in the GemCis arm than the gemcitabine arm (7.5 vs 6 months). The rate of stable disease was greater in the combination arm (60.2% vs 40.2%; $P<.001$).[19]

Once again this study supported that there may be some benefit achieved with the use of platinum agents in the setting of metastatic pancreatic cancer. There is clearly synergy between the 2 agents and recent meta-analysis suggested a survival benefit when compared with gemcitabine alone.[20] A pooled analysis of the GERCOR/GISCAD study came to similar conclusions and the benefit was clearly superior in patients with a good performance status.[21]

Gemcitabine and Capecitabine

There are conflicting data regarding the efficacy of gemcitabine and capecitabine used together in the treatment of metastatic pancreatic cancer.

In a phase 3 trial that randomized patients to receive capecitabine 650 mg/m^2 twice daily, days 1 to 14, plus gemcitabine 1000 mg/m^2 in 30-minute infusions on days 1 and

8 every 3 weeks and gemcitabine alone at 1000 mg/m^2 weekly for 7 weeks, followed by a 1-week break and then weekly for 3 weeks out of 4 weeks; patients with increased performance status fared better (Karnofsky performance status>90%). CBR criteria and quality of life indicators were assessed over this period. Of the 319 patients, 19% treated with gemcitabine/capecitabine and 20% treated with gemcitabine alone experienced a quality-of-life benefit, based on CBR criteria. There was an improvement for patients in terms of median OS (10.4 vs 7.4 months) but only for patients with a Karnofsky performance status score of 90 to 100. There was no indication of a difference in both CBR and quality of life between the gemcitabine/capecitabine and the gemcitabine arms in other patients.[22] Median OS was 8.4 months for patients treated with gemcitabine/capecitabine and 7.3 months for patients treated with gemcitabine alone. This was not statistically significant and the overall frequency of grade 3 and grade 4 toxicities was similar in both arms.[22]

An abstract published in 2005 compared the effects of gemcitabine with those of gemcitabine/capecitabine. In this study, gemcitabine in combination with capecitabine did show a specifically significant longer median OS time of 7.4 months versus 6.0 months for gemcitabine alone.[23] This was considered to be a statistically significant survival benefit; however, this has appeared only in the abstract form presented at the 13th Annual European Cancer Conference in 2005. No follow-up article was published. One reason suggested for these conflicting data was that in the latter trial capecitabine was given on a more prolonged schedule of 1660 mg/m^2 for 21 out of 28 days.[24,25]

Targeted Therapy

An important part of treating metastatic pancreatic cancer is the issue of quality of life palliation and performance status. One of the greatest challenges for medical oncologists in treating these patients is maintaining a good performance status by palliating symptoms—primarily pain, nausea, diarrhea, obstructive jaundice, and anorexia on treatment. For this reason and because standard chemotherapeutic agents have made little dent in the treatment of this disease, it has made sense to investigate targeted therapy. Several pathways have been targeted in an attempt to treat pancreatic cancer but most of them have been disappointing or have failed to improve outcomes. The failure of targeted agents in treatment is multifactorial. It probably is secondary to the loss of molecular heterogeneity found in pancreatic cancer including downregulation of tumor suppressor genes, loss or gain of function in the form of upregulation of oncogenes, and epigenetic changes, and dysregulation of apoptotic and survival pathways.[26]

Epidermal Growth Factor Receptor Inhibitors

Overexpression of EGFR has been reported in pancreatic cancers and the idea behind developing EGFR inhibitors is that halting the growth activity in this pathway would be rational for a therapeutic approach in pancreatic cancer. EGFR can be inhibited by small molecular tyrosine kinase inhibitors such as erlotinib and gefitinib that block the intrinsic tyrosine kinase activity pathway. This pathway is usually required to transmit survival signals downstream of EGFR and inhibit EGFR signaling. Inhibition of EGFR tyrosine kinase inhibits mitogenic and antiapoptotic signals involved in growth, metastasis, and angiogenesis. Phase 3 studies have shown a small but modest improvement with the use of erlotinib and gemcitabine, which was not seen with the use of gefitinib despite similar mechanisms of action.[24]

Erlotinib is an orally administered molecule that interrupts the HER-1/EGFR signal by inhibiting the tyrosine kinase that is integrated in the intracellular receptor domain.[27] The original approval for erlotinib to be used in the treatment of pancreatic cancer was obtained in 2005 after a total of 569 patients were randomly assigned to receive standard gemcitabine plus erlotinib at 100 mg or 150 mg daily or gemcitabine alone plus placebo in a double-blind international stage 3 trial. The primary endpoint of OS was achieved statistically with a hazard ratio of 0.82 and median survival duration of 6.2 months versus 5.91 months.[28] One-year survival was also greater with erlotinib plus gemcitabine, 23% versus 17%. PFS was significantly longer with erlotinib plus gemcitabine with an estimated hazard ratio of 0.77.[28] However, objective response rates were not significantly different and most patients had disease stabilization. Although this study was statistically significant, major concerns still remain about using erlotinib with the minimal median survival duration benefit and cost effective benefit. Patients receiving erlotinib did have higher frequencies of rash, diarrhea, infection, and stomatitis, although generally they were well tolerated and were notably of grade 1 or 2.[28] It should also be noted that despite the difference in doses of erlotinib between 100 mg and 150 mg, in the initial trial most centers outside Canada used the 100 mg dose of erlotinib, which is the Food and Drug Administration–approved dose.[29]

Recent analysis has also shown that patients with pancreatic cancer treated with erlotinib/gemcitabine who had rashes of grade 2 or higher may have a higher OS than patients who had rashes of less than grade 2 or no rash. These results should be interpreted with caution.[29] There has been no clinical benefit from erlotinib alone as a single agent in the treatment of metastatic pancreatic cancer. There was an abstract presented in 2007 at GI ASCO conference that suggested that there may be some small benefit; however, this small phase 2 trial of 13 patients did not show any statistically significant data suggesting that erlotinib alone would be beneficial in the treatment of metastatic pancreatic cancer.[30]

Bevacizumab

The role of vascular endothelial growth factor (VEGF) inhibitors is a recent field of exploration in the treatment of pancreatic cancer with the idea that this new and unexplored class of drugs may have improved response over traditional chemotherapy drugs discussed earlier. VEGF inhibitors are a class of drugs that play an important role in angiogenesis. VEGF is known to stimulate cell growth, survival, and proliferation. VEGF inhibitors effectively reduce neovascularization. They inhibit new and recurrent tumor vessel growth and improve the tumor vasculatures' capacity for effective delivery of antitumor growth compounds.[31] Currently one of the most commonly used VEGF inhibitors is bevacizumab (Avastin), a recombinant humanized monoclonal antibody.

Studies to date on bevacizumab in the treatment of metastatic pancreatic cancer were not successful. There are 2 main phase 3 trials that evaluated the use of bevacizumab with and without gemcitabine,[32,33] and a more recent phase 3 trial evaluating gemcitabine plus erlotinib with or without bevacizumab.[34,35]

A recent phase 3 trial from Belgium randomized 306 patients to treatment with gemcitabine (1000 mg/m^2) weekly plus erlotinib (100 mg by mouth daily) and bevacizumab at 5 mg/kg every 2 weeks and compared them with 301 patients who were treated with gemcitabine plus erlotinib and placebo at the same doses. Median survival was not statistically significant with 7.1 months in the bevacizumab plus gemcitabine plus erlotinib arm versus 6.0 months in the gemcitabine plus erlotinib arm.[34,35] Although the drugs were well tolerated (toxicity was similar in both arms) and PFS was improved (4.6 vs 3.6 months), these results were not statistically significant to suggest a change in the current management.[34,35]

The Cancer and Leukemia Group B (CALGB) 80303 trial enrolled 590 patients with advanced pancreatic cancer to treatment with gemcitabine plus bevacizumab versus gemcitabine plus placebo. Gemcitabine was given at a standard dose (1000 mg/m^2 weekly) and bevacizumab was given at a dose of 10 mg/m^2 on days 1 and 15 of a 28-day cycle.[32] This was done after encouraging data from a phase 2 trial by Kindler and colleagues[33] suggested a 1-year survival rate of 29%. But the data from a phase 3 trial demonstrated that the combination of the 2 drugs was not superior to gemcitabine alone, with a median OS of 5.8 months and 6.1 months in the bevacizumab plus gemcitabine arm and gemcitabine arm, respectively.[32]

Two other trials have been performed with the VEGF inhibitors sorafenib and sunitinib, both in phase 2 and 1, respectively[36,37] and are still need to be studied in larger phase 3 trials to suggest any clinical benefit. Another randomized phase 2 trial with bevacizumab and gemcitabine plus cetuximab or erlotinib in preliminary analysis suggest potential activity by dual inhibition of VEGF and EGFR pathways synergistically.[38,39]

Although evidence from clinical and experimental data has potentially suggested a benefit from antiangiogenic drugs, clinical trials have failed to support this association. Potential reasons for this may include that not all proteins have simultaneously been blocked with current agents and pancreatic cancers are more hypovascular than originally thought, owing to the inability of these VEGF inhibitors to significantly impair growth in these tumors.[24]

Targeting the P13K-Akt mTOR Pathways Using Mammalian Target of Rapamycin Inhibitors

mTOR is a drug that inhibits downstream signaling of the P13K/Akt/mTOR pathway that has shown increased activation in about half of the pancreatic cancers.[40,41]

In a novel attempt to use mTOR inhibitors in metastatic pancreatic cancer a phase 2 trial was done by Wolpin and colleagues[40] to test the oral mTOR inhibitor, everolimus. Thirty-three patients who were considered to have gemcitabine refractory metastatic pancreatic cancer were enrolled in this initial trial. Patients were given everolimus (RAD100) 10 mg daily. Although it was well tolerated, single agent everolimus did not show any significant statistical activity in this patient population. There was no objective response with a median PFS of 1.8 months and median OS of 4.5 months.[40] These results were most disappointing because theoretically targeting these pathways should lead to inhibition of cell growth, reproduction, survival, and neoangiogenesis.[26]

In fact, dual blocking of both EGFR and mTOR pathways should theoretically be even more successful than mTOR inhibition alone, but this was also a failure in phase 2 trials. A study evaluating everolimus (30 mg/wk) with erlotinib (150 mg/d) showed a median PFS of only 49 days with significant increased toxicity in terms of fatigue, hyponatremia, cholangitis, and so on.[42]

These 2 trials reinforce the true frustration most researchers feel when trying these novel biologic agents with complex molecular signaling pathways alone and in conjunction with chemotherapy. Although they sound promising on paper, the trials have failed to show a significant combination of agents that have changed outcomes.

Cetuximab

Cetuximab is a recombinant chimeric monoclonal antibody directed against EGFR. It is overexpressed in a broad range of human solid tumors, which led to it being tested in pancreatic malignancy. The precise mechanism of action is not clearly known; however, it is known that cetuximab binds with a 10-fold higher affinity to EGFR than normal ligands do to EGF and transforming growth factor α, which then results in inhibition of EGFR. This prevents both homodimerization and heterodimerization of EGFR, which leads to inhibition of autophosphorylation in EGFR signaling.[43] Inhibition of this pathway leads to inhibition of mitogenic and antiapoptotic signals involved in proliferation, growth invasion, metastases, and angiogenesis. Other proposed mechanisms of action include immunologic mechanisms, which may be involved in antitumor activity, including commencement of antibody-dependent cell-mediated cytotoxicity and/or complement-mediated cell lysis.[43]

In a large phase 3 study, comparing gemcitabine plus cetuximab with gemcitabine alone, patients in the gemcitabine plus cetuximab arm showed a median survival of 6.5 months compared with patients in the gemcitabine arm who showed a median survival of 6.0 months. There was no clinically significant advantage of adding cetuximab to gemcitabine in terms of OS, PFS, and response rate.[42]

SECOND LINE THERAPY

A larger problem is what to give the patients after first line therapy with gemcitabine fails. Should multiple agents be added to gemcitabine knowing that response rates will be minimal? There are few second line agents that show benefit after treatment with gemcitabine. Most or any of these regimens usually use 2 or more agents, and in patients with dwindling performance statuses, tolerability may be difficult. There is a desperate need for further investigation of new regimens for second line treatment in phase 3 trials. The data on best supportive care compared with second line treatment is lacking. The trial mentioned later is the only small randomized controlled trial that has shown marginal benefit.[44]

A study in Germany[45] investigated the use of OFF (oxaliplatin, 5-FU, and folinic acid) as a second line agent after failure of first line gemcitabine. Thirty-seven patients were treated with this regimen with oxaliplatin (85 mg/m^2 on days 8 and 22) administered along with folinic acid (500 mg/m^2) and 5-FU (2600 mg/m^2) on days 1, 8, 15, and 22 every 6 weeks. Median time to progression was 12 weeks and OS was 22 weeks. Forty-three percent of the patients were found to have stable disease for more than 12 weeks. Primary toxicities associated with this regimen were hematologic and neurologic toxicities.[45]

Other therapies and drug combinations have been tried with little success and usually higher amounts of toxicity. Single agent docetaxel given weekly had a median PFS of only 1.5 months.[46] A combination of irinotecan and docetaxel did not have any objective response criteria but was associated with increased toxicity, with only half of the patients able to tolerate more than 1 cycle.[47]

Most combination regimens or single agents have shown little benefit over supportive care alone. Many questions still need to be answered about second line treatment including amount of palliation, cost effectiveness, and efficacy of further treatment.[44]

SUMMARY

In more than 20 years of research into chemotherapy trials in the treatment of metastatic pancreatic cancer, there is no clear benefit in survival outcomes. This is truly a painful, frustrating and difficult malignancy to manage on several levels. The importance of other palliative measures should not be forgotten when managing these patients. In fact, quality-of-life parameters and performance status are large predictors of response and play an important role in determining how long these patients should be treated. Gemcitabine remains the clear choice of first line chemotherapy in patients with metastatic pancreatic cancer; the choice for second line therapy is not clear, but an OFF regimen is a candidate. Ideally, the future will bring the medical breakthrough that is so desperately needed in the treatment of this very complicated, painful, debilitating, and frustrating disease process.

REFERENCES

1. Jemal A, Siegel R, Ward E, et al. Cancer statistics, 2009. CA Cancer J Clin 2009; 59:225–49.
2. National Comprehensive Cancer Network (NCCN). Available at: http://www.nccn. org/professionals/physcian_gls/f_guidelines.asp. Accessed November 3, 2009.
3. Heinemann V, Boeck S, Hinke A, et al. Meta-analysis of randomized trials: evaluation of benefit form gemcitabine-based combination chemotherapy applied in advanced pancreatic cancer. BMC Cancer 2008;8:82.
4. Wolff R. Chemotherapy for pancreatic cancer: from metastatic disease to adjuvant therapy. Cancer J 2007;13(3):175–81.
5. Chu E, DeVita V. 5-fluorouracil: cancer chemotherapy drug manual 2009. Sudbury (MA): Jones and Bartlett; 2009. p. 179–84.
6. Cartwright TH, Cohn A, Varkey J, et al. Phase II study of oral capecitabine on patients with advanced or metastatic pancreatic cancer. J Clin Oncol 2002; 20(1):160–4.
7. Sultana A, Smith CT, Cunningham D, et al. Meta-analyses of chemotherapy for locally advanced and metastatic pancreatic cancer. J Clin Oncol 2007;25(18): 2607–15.
8. Yip D, Karapetis C, Strickland A, et al. Chemotherapy and radiotherapy for inoperable advanced pancreatic cancer. Cochrane Database Syst Rev 2006;(3): CD002093.
9. Ridwelski K, Fahlke J, Kuhn R, et al. Multicenter phase I/II study using combination of gemcitabine and docetaxel in metastasized and unresectable, locally advanced pancreatic carcinoma. Eur J Surg Oncol 2006;32(3):297–302.
10. Jacobs AD, Otero H, Picozzi VJ, et al. Gemcitabine combined with docetaxel for the treatment of unresectable pancreatic carcinoma. Cancer Invest 2004;22(4): 505–14.
11. Schneider BP, Ganjoo KN, Seitz DE, et al. Phase II study of gemcitabine plus docetaxel in advanced pancreatic cancer: a Hoosier Oncology Group study. Oncology 2003;65(3):218–23.
12. Skeel R. Gemcitabine: handbook of cancer chemotherapy. 6th edition. Philadelphia: Lippincott, Williams, and Wilkins; 2003. p. 116–7.
13. Burris HA, Moore MJ, Andersen J, et al. Improvements in survival and clinical benefit with gemcitabine as first-line therapy for patients with advanced pancreas cancer: a randomized trial. J Clin Oncol 1997;15(6):2403–13.
14. Tempero M, Plunkett W, Van Haperen Ruiz, et al. Randomized phase II comparison of dose intense gemcitabine: thirty minute infusion and fixed dose rate infusion in patients with pancreatic adenocarcinoma. J Clin Oncol 2003;21(18): 3402–8.
15. Louvet C, Labianca R, Hammel P, et al. Gemcitabine in combination with oxaliplatin compared with gemcitabine alone in locally advanced or metastatic pancreatic cancer; results of a GERCOR and GISCAD phase III trial. J Clin Oncol 2005;23(15):3509–16.
16. Poplin E, Feng Y, Berlin J, et al. Phase III randomized study of gemcitabine and oxaliplatin versus gemcitabine (fixed dose rate infusion) compared with

gemcitabine (30-minute infusion) in patients with pancreatic carcinoma E6201: a trial of the Eastern Cooperative Oncology Group. J Clin Oncol 2009;27(23): 3778–85.

17. Chu E, DeVita V. Capecitabine: cancer chemotherapy drug manual 2009. Sudbury (MA): Jones and Bartlett; 2009. p. 64–70.

18. Stathopoulos GP, Syrigos K, Aravantinos G, et al. A multicenter phase III trial comparing irinotecan-gemcitabine (IG) with gemcitabine (G) monotherapy as first-line treatment in patients with locally advanced or metastatic pancreatic cancer. Br J Cancer 2006;95(5):587–92.

19. Heinemann V, Quietzsh D, Gieseler F, et al. Randomized phase III trial of gemcitabine plus cisplatin compared with gemcitabine alone in advanced pancreatic cancer. J Clin Oncol 2006;24(24):3946–52.

20. Saif MW, Kim R. Role of platinum agents in the management of advanced pancreatic cancer. Expert Opin Pharmacother 2007;8(16):2719–27.

21. Heinemann V, Labianca R, Hinke A, et al. Increased survival using platinum analog combined with gemcitabine as compared to single agent gemcitabine in advanced pancreatic cancer: pooled analysis of two randomized trials the GERCOR/GISCAD intergroup study and a German multicenter study. Ann Oncol 2007;18(10):1652–9.

22. Hermann R, Bodoky G, Ruhstaller B, et al. Gemcitabine plus capecitabine compared with gemcitabine alone in advanced pancreatic cancer. A randomized multicenter, phase III trial of the Swiss Group for Clinical Cancer research and the Central European Cooperative Oncology Group. J Clin Oncol 2007;25:2212–7.

23. Cunningham D, Chau I, Stocken D, et al. Phase III randomized comparison of gemcitabine (GEM) versus gemcitabine plus capecitabine (GEM-CAP) in patients with advanced pancreatic cancer. Eur J Cancer Suppl 2005;3:4.

24. Nieto J, Grossbard M, Kozuch P. Metastatic pancreatic cancer 2008: is the glass less empty? Oncologist 2008;13:562–76.

25. Mahalingam D, Kelly K, Swords R, et al. Emerging drugs in the treatment of pancreatic cancer. Expert Opin Emerg Drugs 2009;14(2):311–28.

26. Mahalingam D, Giles F. Challenges in developing targeted therapies for pancreatic adnenocarcinoma. Expert Opin Ther Targets 2008;12(11):1389–401.

27. Chu E, DeVita V. Erlotinib: cancer chemotherapy drug manual 2009. Sudbury (MA): Jones and Bartlett; 2009. p. 149–55.

28. Moore MJ, Goldstein D, Hamm J, et al. Erlotinib plus gemcitabine compared with gemcitabine alone in patients with advanced pancreatic cancer: a phase III trial of the National Cancer Institute of Canada Clinical Trials Group. J Clin Oncol 2007;25(15):1960–6.

29. Senderowicz A, Johnson J, Sridhara R, et al. Erlotinib/gemcitabine for first-line treatment of locally advanced or metastatic adenocarcinoma of the pancreas. Oncology (Williston Park). (FDA Approval Summary) 2007;21(14):1696–706.

30. Epelbaum R, Schnaider J, Gluzman A, et al. Erlotinib as a single agent therapy in patients with advanced pancreatic cancer. Presented at the 2007 ASCO GI Cancer Symposium. Orlando (FL), January 19–21, 2007.

31. Danovi SA, Wong HH, Lemoine NR. Targeted therapies for pancreatic cancer. Br Med Bull 2008;87:97–130.

32. Kindler HL, Niedzwiecki D, Hollis D, et al. Cancer and Leukemia group B A Double blind, placebo controlled randomized phase III trial of gemcitabine (G) plus bevacizumab (B) versus gemcitabine plus placebo (P) in pts with advanced pancreatic cancer (PC); a preliminary analysis of CALGB. J Clin Oncol 2007; 25(18s) (meeting abstracts) [abstract 4508].

33. Kindler HL, Friberg G, Singh DA, et al. Phase II trial of bevacizumab plus gemcitabine in patients with advanced pancreatic cancer. J Clin Oncol 2005;23: 8033–40.

34. Van Cutsem E, Ververnne WL, Bennouna J, et al. Phase III trial of bevacizumab in combination with gemcitabine and erlotinib in metastatic pancreatic cancer. J Clin Oncol 2009;27(13):2231–7.

35. Vervenne W, Bennouna Y, Humblet S, et al. A randomized, double-blind, placebo (P) controlled, multicenter phase III trial to evaluate the efficacy and safety of adding bevacizumab (B) to erlotinib (E) and gemcitabine (G) in patients (pts) with metastatic pancreatic cancer [abstract 4507]. 2008 ASCO Annual Meeting Proceedings. J Clin Oncol 2008;26(15S).

36. Wallace JA, Locker G, Nattam S, et al. Sorafenib plus gemcitabine for advanced pancreatic cancer (PC): a phase II trial of the University of Chicago Phase II Consortium. 2007 ASCO Annual Meeting Proceedings Part I [abstract 4608]. J Clin Oncol 2007;25(18S (Suppl 20)).

37. Michaelson MD, Schwarzberg A, Ryan DP, et al. Phase I dose findings study of sunitinib (SU) in combination with gemcitabine (G) in patients (pts) with advanced solid tumors [abstract 14522]. Clin Oncol 2008;26(Suppl 20).

38. Kindler HL, Bylow KA, Hoschester G, et al. A randomized phase II study of bevacizumab (B) and gemcitabine (G) plus cetuximab (C) or erlotinib (E) in patients (pts) with advanced pancreatic cancer (PC) [abstract 4502]. ASCO Annual Meeting Proceedings. J Clin Oncol 2006;26(15S).

39. El Kamar F, Grossbard M, Kozuch P. Metastatic pancreatic cancer; emerging strategies in chemotherapy and palliative care. Oncologist 2003;8:18–34.

40. Wolpin B, Hezel A, Abrams T, et al. Oral mTOR Inhibitor Everolimus in patients with gemcitabine-refractory metastatic pancreatic cancer. J Clin Oncol 2009; 27(2):193–8.

41. Javle MM, Xiong H, Reddy S, et al. Inhibition of mammalian target of rapamycin (mTOR) in advanced pancreatic cancer: the results of two prospective studies [abstract 4621]. ASCO Annual Meeting Proceedings. J Clin Oncol 2009;27(15S).

42. Phillip PA, Benedetti C, Fenoglio-Preiser M, et al. Phase III study of gemcitabine (G) plus cetuximab (C) versus gemcitabine in patients (pts) with locally advanced or metastatic pancreatic adenocarcinoma (PC): SWOG S0205 study [abstract LBA4509]. Annual Meeting Proceedings. J Clin Oncol 2007;25(18S).

43. Chu E, DeVita V. Cetuximab: cancer chemotherapy drug manual 2009. Sudbury (MA): Jones and Bartlett; 2009. p. 77–82.

44. Almhanna K, Kim R. Second-line therapy for gemcitabine-refractory pancreatic cancer: is there a standard? Oncology 2008;22(10):1176–83.

45. Pelzer U, Stieler J, Roll L, et al. Second-line therapy in refractory pancreatic cancer: results of a phase II study. Onkologie 2009;32(3):99–102.

46. Cereda S, Reni M. Weekly docetaxel as salvage therapy in patients with gemcitabine refractory metastatic pancreatic cancer. J Chemother 2008;20(4):509–12.

47. Ko AH, Dito E, Schillinger B, et al. Excess toxicity associated with docetaxel and irinotecan in patients with metastatic gemcitabine-refractory pancreatic cancer: results of a phase II study. Cancer Invest 2008;26(1):47–52.

Intraductal Papillary Mucinous Neoplasm: A Clinicopathologic Review

Toms Augustin, MD, MPH[a], Thomas J. VanderMeer, MD[b],*

KEYWORDS

• Intraductal papillary mucinous neoplasm • Pancreatic ducts
• Pancreatic neoplasm • Pancreatic cancer

Intraductal papillary mucinous neoplasm (IPMN) is an intraductal mucin-producing epithelial neoplasm that arises from the main pancreatic duct (MD-IPMN), secondary branch ducts (BD-IPMN), or both (mixed type; Mix-IPMN). These tumors are visible grossly and on imaging studies as cystic dilations of the pancreatic ducts, and are sometimes associated with papillary projections or mural nodules. Neoplastic progression from benign adenoma to invasive adenocarcinoma has not been proven but is generally thought to occur.[1] Unlike mucinous cystic neoplasms of the pancreas, however, IPMN can be multifocal or involve the pancreatic ductal epithelium diffusely, which has led to the notion that a field defect may exist in IPMN.[2]

After being first reported by Ohashi and colleagues[3] in 1982, IPMN is increasingly reported worldwide and accounts for about 5% of pancreatic neoplasms resected at referral centers.[2,4–7] In the past, IPMN has been referred to by many names including mucin-producing pancreatic cancer, intraductal papillary mucinous tumor, mucin-secreting carcinoma, intraductal mucin-hypersecreting neoplasm, villous adenoma of the main pancreatic duct, and mucinous duct ectasia.[8] The term intraductal papillary mucinous neoplasm is now widely accepted. The World Health Organization (WHO) has classified IPMN histologically into the following 3 categories:

IPMN adenoma: The epithelium is composed of tall columnar mucin-containing cells that show slight or no dysplasia.

IPMN borderline: IPMNs with moderate dysplasia are placed in the borderline category. The epithelium shows no more than moderate loss of polarity, nuclear crowding,

[a] Department of Surgery, Guthrie-Robert Packer Hospital, One Guthrie Square, Sayre, PA 18840, USA
[b] Department of Surgery, Guthrie Clinic, SUNY Upstate Medical University, One Guthrie Square, Sayre, PA 18840, USA
* Corresponding author. Department of Surgery Guthrie Clinic, SUNY Upstate Medical University, One Guthrie Square, Sayre, PA 18840.
E-mail address: vandermeer_thomas@guthrie.org

Surg Clin N Am 90 (2010) 377–398
doi:10.1016/j.suc.2009.12.008
0039-6109/10/$ – see front matter © 2010 Elsevier Inc. All rights reserved.
surgical.theclinics.com

nuclear enlargement, pseudostratification, and nuclear hyperchromatism. Papillary areas maintain identifiable stromal cores, but pseudopapillary structures may be present.

Intraductal papillary mucinous carcinoma (including carcinoma in situ): IPMNs with severe dysplastic epithelial change (carcinoma in situ) are designated as carcinoma even in the absence of invasion. They can be papillary or micropapillary. Cribriform growth and budding of small clusters of epithelial cells into the lumen support the diagnosis of carcinoma in situ. Severe dysplasia is manifest cytologically as loss of polarity, loss of differentiated cytoplasmic features including diminished mucin content, cellular and nuclear pleomorphism, nuclear enlargement, and the presence of mitosis (especially if suprabasal or luminal). Severely dysplastic cells may lack mucin.

From Hruban RH, Takaori K, Klimstra DS, et al. An illustrated consensus on the classification of pancreatic intraepithelial neoplasia and intraductal papillary mucinous neoplasms. Am J Surg Pathol 2004;28(8):977–87; with permission.

The natural history of IPMN, however, seems to vary depending on the anatomic distribution of the lesion and the degree of invasion. MD-IPMN is associated with a 57% to 92% risk of malignancy.[9] The risk of malignancy in BD-IPMN is much lower, with rates ranging from 6% to 46%.[9] Recurrence after resection of benign IPMN is rare, but the 5-year survival after resection of IPMN with invasive cancer is between 30% and 75%.[2,4,7,10–13]

With increasing recognition of IPMN, our understanding of the diagnosis and management of the tumors is evolving. At present, treatment options for patients with IPMN range from observation to pancreatic resection depending on the natural history of the lesion. This review focuses on currently available data that guide management decisions for patients with IPMN.

PATHOLOGY

IPMN is an intraductal proliferation of neoplastic mucinous epithelium. These lesions are characterized by papillary formations ranging from subtle areas of granularity to friable intraluminal masses. Clinically, IPMNs are classified based on the pattern of involvement of the pancreatic ducts and the degree of cellular atypia. Histopathologic classification systems describe epithelial subtypes and types of malignant lesions. Studies of genetic alterations and protein expression in IPMN suggest mechanisms of neoplastic progression that differ from pancreatic intraepithelial neoplasia (PanIN) and ductal adenocarcinoma. The common classification schemes are described as follows and are significant with regard to management and prognosis.

1. Based on the pattern of involvement of pancreatic ducts, IPMNs are classified as MD-IPMN, BD-IPMN, and Mix-IPMN.
2. Based on the degree of dysplasia, IPMNs can be classified into adenoma, borderline dysplasia, and carcinoma (including carcinoma in situ) (WHO classification, see preceding section).
3. Clinical studies classify IPMNs as
   a. Benign (adenoma, borderline) and malignant (carcinoma in situ, carcinoma)
   b. Noninvasive (adenoma, borderline, carcinoma in situ) and invasive (carcinoma)
4. Based on the histologic appearance of papillary epithelium, IPMNs are classified as intestinal type, gastric type, and pancreatobiliary type. Some investigators describe an oncocytic type.
5. Four phenotypes of adenocarcinoma are described in IPMN: colloid type, tubular type, mixed type, and anaplastic type.

Anatomic Classification

Grossly, IPMNs are classified based on the pattern of involvement of the pancreatic ducts into MD-IPMN, BD-IPMN, or Mix-IPMN (**Fig. 1**). MD-IPMN involves the main pancreatic duct and is characterized by segmental or diffuse dilatation of the main pancreatic duct, usually greater than 10 mm. BD-IPMN involves 1 or more of the branch ducts of the pancreas. BD-IPMN usually communicates with a nondilated main pancreatic duct. It is most commonly seen in the proximal pancreas (head and uncinate process).[2,14,15] About 40% of BD-IPMNs are multifocal.[14] Mix-IPMN involves both the main pancreatic duct and the side branches. The classification of IPMNs based on site of involvement predicts malignant potential. MD-IPMN is associated with malignancy (both in situ and invasive) in 57% to 92% of surgically resected cases, whereas BD-IPMN is associated with malignancy in 6% to 46% of resected cases.[2,9,10,16–18] Mix-IPMN is associated with malignancy in 35% to 40% of surgical specimens.[2,7]

Histopathology

Histologically, IPMNs are associated with a spectrum of neoplastic changes ranging from ectatic ducts lined by flat epithelium to florid papillae and invasive carcinoma. Varying degrees of cytoarchitectural atypia often coexist in the same tumor, a finding that supports the presence of an adenoma-carcinoma sequence in IPMN.[6,19]

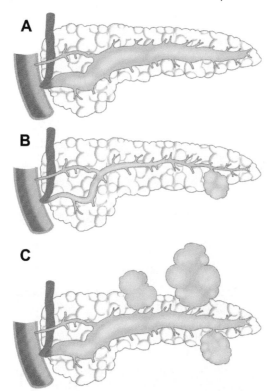

Fig. 1. Anatomic classification of IPMN. (*A*) Main duct IPMN with uniform dilatation of the duct of Wirsung. (*B*) Branch duct IPMN with cystic dilatation of a branch duct and communication with a nondilated duct of Wirsung. (*C*) Mixed IPMN with both main pancreatic duct dilatation and multifocal cystic dilatation of branch ducts.

WHO classified IPMNs based on the severity of epithelial atypia, into adenoma, borderline, or carcinoma (see list earlier in this article and **Fig. 2**). In the WHO classification, carcinomas include both carcinoma in situ and invasive carcinoma, and are called malignant IPMN in many clinical studies.[2,7] Clinically, IPMNs are classified as noninvasive (benign, borderline, carcinoma in situ) and invasive (invasive carcinoma) because of the excellent prognosis following resection of noninvasive IPMN. Clinical

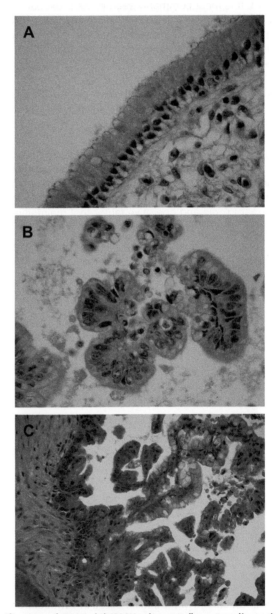

Fig. 2. WHO classification of IPMN. (*A*) IPMN adenoma (hematoxylin-eosin, original magnification ×200). (*B*) Borderline IPMN (hematoxylin-eosin, original magnification ×200). (*C*) IPMN carcinoma in situ (hematoxylin-eosin, original magnification ×100).

studies also refer to IPMNs as benign (adenoma and borderline) or malignant (carcinoma in situ and invasive carcinoma) based on implications for clinical management.[2,4,6,7,9,20–31]

IPMNs demonstrate different epithelial subtypes that have been described as intestinal type (~35%), gastric type(~31%), and pancreatobiliary type (~22%).[32,33] An oncocytic variant has also been described by some investigators.[34] Intestinal-type IPMNs have well-formed villous structures lined by columnar cells resembling villous adenomas of the intestine, and are associated with moderate or high-grade dysplasia. The intestinal epithelial subtype is seen in 73% of MD-IPMNs.[33,35,36] Invasive carcinomas developing from the intestinal type are frequently colloid adenocarcinoma.[32] Gastric-type IPMN has flat epithelium or papillae resembling gastric foveolar epithelium (**Fig. 3**).[35] This type of IPMN is most commonly associated with adenomas and invasive carcinoma is rarely seen in association with gastric epithelium.[32,35] Pancreatobiliary epithelium is more complex, with thick papillae that resemble papillary neoplasms of the biliary tract. The pancreatobiliary epithelial subtype is associated with more severe degrees of nuclear atypia. Most of the invasive cancers developing from pancreatobiliary type are tubular carcinoma, which carries a worse prognosis than colloid carcinoma.[32]

Four types of adenocarcinoma are described in IPMN: colloid carcinoma, tubular carcinoma, mixed type, and anaplastic type. Colloid-type invasive carcinoma is characterized by large pools of extracellular mucin containing relatively scant strips, clusters, and individual neoplastic cells. About 40% of invasive carcinomas arising from IPMNs are of the colloid type and almost all colloid carcinomas of the pancreas are associated with an IPMN.[11,37] Tubular carcinomas resemble conventional infiltrating ductal adenocarcinoma with predominantly tubular neoplastic glands associated with a desmoplastic stroma in the absence of significant stromal mucin. Patients with tubular-type carcinoma have been reported to have a much worse 5-year survival compared with colloid carcinoma (24%–50% vs 70%–83%).[2,6,11]

Genetics

Genetic alterations that have been described in IPMN include mutations of K-ras,[38] p53,[39] STK11/LKB1,[40] PIK3CA, and BRAF,[41] and loss of heterozygosity in CDKN2A/p16.[42] Gene expression studies suggest that the mechanisms of tumorigenesis may differ between IPMN and ductal adenocarcinoma. For example, inactivation of tumor suppressor genes such as CDKN2A/p16, p53 and DPC4 (MADH4, SMAD4), K-ras mutations, and inactivation of the Peutz-Jeghers gene (STK11/LKB1) are less common in IPMN than in ductal adenocarcinoma of the pancreas.[40,43,44] PIK3CA mutation is reported in 10% of IPMNs but not in ductal adenocarcinoma.[45] Sato and colleagues[46] found that IPMNs overexpress gastric-related genes such as MUC5AC, pepsinogen C, claudin-18, and cathepsin E that are associated with a better prognosis in patients with ductal adenocarcinoma. There also appear to be different pathways of carcinogenesis between different subtypes of IPMN.[47] Adsay and colleagues[32] suggested that the progression of intestinal-type IPMN to colloid carcinoma occurs via a distinct pathway of carcinogenesis involving intestinal-related genes CDX2 and MUC2. Other genes known to be important in tumor invasion and metastasis such as Claudin 4, CXCR4, S100A4, and mesothelin have been shown to be overexpressed selectively in the intraductal components of invasive IPMN.[46]

Variable patterns of mucin expression have been noted in IPMN as well. Mucins are a heterogeneous family of glycoproteins, some of which are located in the cell membrane, and others prepared as secretory products and excreted. MUC1 has been found to be a marker of an aggressive phenotype and is present uniformly in

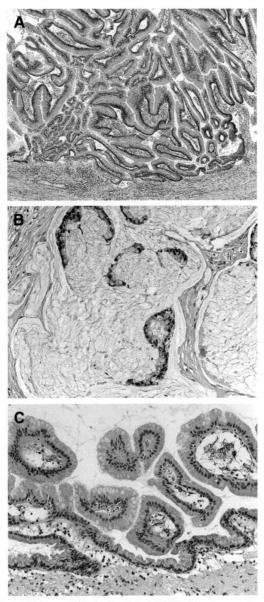

Fig. 3. Histopathology of IPMN. (*A*) Intestinal-type IPMN demonstrating well-formed villous structures lined by columnar cells resembling villous adenomas of the intestine. The florid papillary areas seen in this example may be associated with more aggressive clinical behavior (hematoxylin-eosin, original magnification ×40). (*B*) Colloid carcinoma demonstrating characteristic large pools of extracellular mucin containing relatively scant strips, clusters, and individual neoplastic cells. Invasive IPMN is most commonly colloid carcinoma, which carries a better prognosis than ductal adenocarcinoma of the pancreas (hematoxylin-eosin, original magnification ×100). (*C*) Gastric-type IPMN with flat epithelium and less papillary formation. The gastric epithelial subtype is associated with benign adenomas (hematoxylin-eosin, original magnification ×100). (*Courtesy of* N. Adsay Volkan, MD, Atlanta, GA.)

infiltrating ductal adenocarcinoma.[32] MUC2 is a secretory type of mucin produced almost exclusively in goblet cells and functions as a protective barrier in the intestinal epithelium.[32] MUC2 is a marker for indolent behavior.[32,48–52] Most intestinal-type IPMNs express MUC2 but not MUC1, and most pancreatobiliary-type IPMNs express MUC1 but not MUC2.[32] Thus, MUC1-positive IPMNs are associated with tubular carcinoma and may have a worse prognosis than MUC2-positive IPMNs that are associated with colloid carcinoma.[48,52]

IPMN is associated with extrapancreatic neoplasms in about 30% of cases.[7,53,54] The primary sites reported have included colon, breast, stomach, rectum, lung, and liver.[9] Gastric adenocarcinoma and colorectal adenocarcinoma were the most common neoplasms in one study.[53] The explanation for this finding is not clear but IPMN has been associated with a variety of germline mutations in some familial genetic syndromes. The Peutz-Jeghers gene (STK11/LKB1) is inactivated in up to one-third of IPMNs.[40] IPMN has also been described in patients with familial adenomatous polyposis coli.[55] In Lynch syndrome, identical staining profiles with loss of expression of MSH2 and MSH6 proteins and high levels of microsatellite instability have been described in adenocarcinoma of the colon as well as IPMN.[56]

NATURAL HISTORY

IPMNs are thought to progress from benign adenomas to invasive cancer in a manner similar to adenomatous colon polyps.[1] This concept is supported by the common histologic finding that varying degrees of dysplasia often coexist in one tumor and the clinical observation that IPMNs in older patients have a higher risk of harboring invasive cancer.[1,15,19] One study noted that the risk of malignancy is 45% in patients younger than 60 years old and 73% in patients older than 60.[5] The average age at diagnosis of malignant IPMN is about 5 years older than patients with benign IPMN.[2,10]

Malignancy is also observed much more frequently in patients with MD-IPMN (about 70%) than BD-IPMN (about 25%).[9] Levy and colleagues[15] noted that 58% of patients with MD-IPMN had developed malignancy within 2 years of the first sign of IPMN. The actuarial risk of malignancy in BD-IPMN was only 15% within 5 years of the first sign of IPMN.[15] Thus, it would seem that the mechanism and risk of neoplastic progression varies among and between the morphologic types of IPMN. As described previously, 3 distinct epithelial patterns have been described that are associated with different genetic and immunohistochemical phenotypes. These classifications seem to have biologic significance and may help explain the variability observed in the clinical behavior of IPMN. Further work will be necessary to stratify risk based on these pathologic factors.

Controversy exists about the concept that the entire pancreatic ductal epithelium may be at risk for neoplastic transformation in patients with IPMN. The notion of a field defect is supported by the observation that BD-IPMN is multifocal in about 40%[14] of patients and that recurrence in the pancreatic remnant is seen in about 8% of patients with resected benign IPMN.[4] Although it is difficult to distinguish local recurrence from metachronous IPMN, recurrences occur even after margin-negative resection and benign IPMN may recur as malignant or metastatic IPMN. In one study, recurrence following resection of benign IPMN was 8% after partial pancreatectomy and no recurrences were observed in the 29 patients undergoing total pancreatectomy.[7]

CLINICAL PRESENTATION

Most series have noted that males are affected with IPMN more often than females (ratio 1.4:1).[2,7] The age at presentation is most commonly in the sixth decade and patients with malignant IPMN tend to be about 5 years older than those with benign

IPMN.[2,15] About 30% of patients with IPMN are asymptomatic.[10,57] In these patients, IPMN is detected incidentally as a pancreatic cyst on cross-sectional imaging or ultrasound. The most common presenting complaint is abdominal pain, which is present in 50% to 70% of symptomatic patients.[2,7,10,11,15,16] Symptoms of chronic pancreatitis such as diarrhea, new-onset or worsening diabetes, and intermittent acute pancreatitis are also common presenting symptoms related to chronic obstruction of the pancreatic duct with mucin.[2,7,10,11,15,16] Weight loss, obstructive jaundice, diabetes, short duration of symptoms, and elevated liver function tests have been found to be associated with malignant IPMN.[2,5,10,18,58,59] The absence of symptoms, however, is not a sensitive marker for benignity, as up to 40% of patients with malignant IPMN are asymptomatic.[6,9,10,57,60]

DIAGNOSIS

The diagnosis of IPMN is usually based on cross-sectional imaging such as multidetector computed tomography (MDCT) scans and magnetic resonance cholangiopancreatography (MRCP). These studies readily demonstrate dilatation of the duct of Wirsung with mucin in MD-IPMN and a grapelike cluster of cysts that usually communicates with a nondilated duct of Wirsung in BD-IPMN. Endoscopic ultrasound (EUS) with fine-needle aspiration (EUS-FNA) is useful in confirming the diagnosis, gathering fluid for analysis, and differentiating cystic lesions of the pancreas.

MDCT demonstrates ductal abnormalities in 97% of patients with IPMN.[61] Diffuse or segmental dilatation of the main pancreatic duct is readily seen on MDCT in patients with MD-IPMN. MDCT is very sensitive for BD-IPMN, although small lesions may not demonstrate the classic clustering of cysts or communication with the main pancreatic duct. Mix-IPMN will show features of both varieties of IPMN (**Fig. 4**). CT scan features associated with malignancy include bulging papilla, presence of solid lesion, diffuse or multifocal involvement or attenuating or calcified intraluminal contents, local invasion, and mural nodule (**Fig. 5**).[18,61–64] In addition, CT may demonstrate signs of invasive cancer such as dilatation of the common bile duct, areas of abnormal attenuation in the surrounding parenchyma, and local invasion.[62]

MRCP is an excellent modality for demonstrating the pancreatic ductal architecture, delineating cystic lesions, and defining the extent of the tumor.[65–69] MRCP may be more accurate than a CT scan in delineating the communication between BD-IPMN and the main pancreatic duct, especially in small tumors.[63,70] The features of malignancy seen on MRCP are similar to those seen on MDCT. The overall sensitivity, specificity, and accuracy of MRCP for the diagnosis of malignancy in IPMN have been reported to be 70%, 92%, and 80%, respectively.[66] Intravenous administration of secretin prior to MRCP (S-MRCP) may improve the quality of the study by increasing pancreatic exocrine secretion, thus improving the visualization of the pancreatic duct. However, the role of S-MRCP in the evaluation of IPMN is still evolving.

EUS is an excellent modality for demonstrating the pancreatic ductal dilatation, papillary projections, and mural nodules that are characteristic of IPMN (**Fig. 6**).[71] Mucin is usually present in the cyst fluid aspirate and its presence is very helpful in the diagnosis of IPMN. One large study showed that a cyst fluid carcinoembryonic antigen (CEA) level greater that 192 ng/mL was 79% sensitive for distinguishing mucinous from nonmucinous tumors.[72] Amylase content is generally higher in the cyst fluid of IPMN than in other cystic neoplasms such as serous cystadenoma, but it is not accurate in differentiating cystic lesions of the pancreas.[72] The accuracy of cytologic evaluation of cyst fluid is only 59%, but can be diagnostic when mucin-producing goblet cells arranged in a papillary pattern are identified within thick

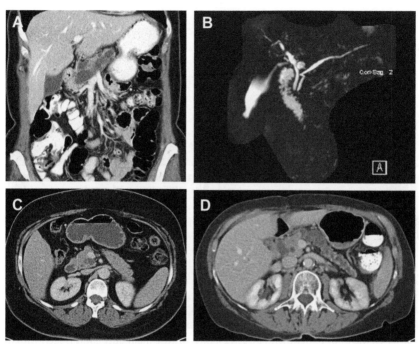

Fig. 4. Cross-sectional imaging of patients with IPMN. (*A*) MDCT of patient with main duct IPMN. In this case the main pancreatic duct is diffusely dilated. (*B*) MRCP of patient with small branch duct IPMN. Characteristic grapelike clusters and communication with a nondilated pancreatic duct are seen. (*C*) MDCT of patient with small branch duct IPMN. A small cyst is seen in the uncinate process without clear-cut clusters or communication with the main pancreatic duct. (*D*) MDCT of patient with mixed-type IPMN. The main duct IPMN is seen in the body and tail of the pancreas. The lesion near the neck of the pancreas shows clusters of cysts typical for branch duct IPMN.

viscous mucus.[73,74] Papillary fragments, parachromatin clearing, atypical clusters, hypercellularity, necrosis, and inflammation may be seen and are suggestive of malignancy.[75] EUS-FNA–guided biopsy of solid components can also be performed and is useful for histopathologic evaluation.[76] Overall, EUS-FNA has a sensitivity of 68% to 91% and an accuracy of about 85% in the diagnosis of malignant IPMN.[7,71,77,78] Identification of accurate cyst fluid markers for the diagnosis and prognosis of IPMN is the subject of considerable investigation.[71,77]

Endoscopic retrograde cholangiopancreatography is not used routinely in the diagnosis of IPMN but can be useful for demonstrating some of the features of IPMN, such as the presence of mucus at a patulous papilla in MD-IPMN and ductal communication in BD-IPMN.[7,26,77] It is not uncommon, however, for viscid mucus to limit the opacification of the pancreatic duct. Peroral pancreatoscopy (POPS) and intraductal ultrasound (IUS) are emerging modalities that may be useful in the diagnosis of IPMN.[79] The combination of POPS and IUS had a sensitivity and specificity of 91% and 82% in differentiating malignant and benign IPMN in one study.[23] Pancreatic duct lavage cytology is noted to have a sensitivity and specificity of 78% and 93%, respectively, in differentiating benign from malignant BD-IPMN disease.[80] The role of positron emission tomography (PET) and PET-CT has not been established in the diagnosis of IPMN.

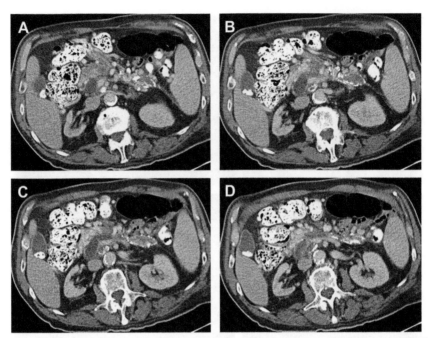

Fig. 5. (*A–D*) MDCT of patient with invasive IPMN. Diffuse main duct IPMN is seen with dilatation of the main pancreatic duct and a solid mass in the body of the pancreas. The mass invades and occludes the superior mesenteric vein. The duct in the tail of the pancreas has intraluminal calcifications.

IPMN is readily differentiated from mucinous cystic neoplasm of the pancreas (MCN) on cross-sectional imaging because MCN is a round unifocal tumor that rarely communicates with the pancreatic duct.[9] Patients with MCN are almost always female, generally in the fourth or fifth decade of life.[9] More than 95% of MCNs are located in the body and tail of the pancreas as opposed to IPMN, which is most commonly located in the head of the pancreas.[81–83] Both IPMN and MCN are mucinous neoplasms and the cyst fluid CEA is elevated in both tumors.[72] Histologically, MCN contains ovarian-type stroma, which is absent in IPMN and other pancreatic neoplasms.[84,85]

In general, the diagnosis of IPMN is based on cystic dilatation of more than 10 mm of the duct of Wirsung (in MD-IPMN) or the communication of a cystic lesion with the duct of Wirsung (in BD-IPMN) along with other features such as mural nodules, papillary projections, and the presence of mucin and CEA higher than 192 ng/mL in the cyst fluid. Findings concerning for malignancy include MD-IPMN, solid mass, biliary obstruction, mural nodules, intraluminal calcification, symptoms, and positive cytology.

MANAGEMENT

Once the diagnosis is established, the management of IPMNs is based on the risk of malignancy (**Fig. 7**). Because MD-IPMN and Mix-IPMN have a significant risk of malignancy, resection is recommended for patients who are surgical candidates. The decision to proceed with surgery is frequently based on imaging studies alone or on diagnostic testing as outlined previously. For patients with BD-IPMN, the decision to recommend surgery or surveillance is based on factors that predict malignant behavior.

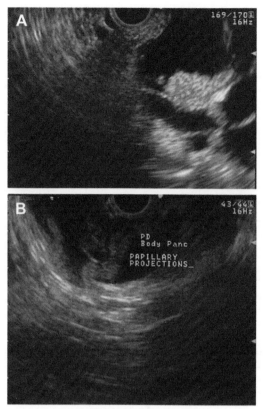

Fig. 6. Endoscopic ultrasound of IPMN shows a mural nodule (*A*) and papillary projections (*B*). (*Courtesy of* Assad Ullah, MD, Rochester, NY.)

MD-IPMN

Because clinical and radiologic predictors of malignancy such as mural nodules, symptoms, and positive cytology are absent in about 30% of patients with malignant MD-IPMN,[10] resection is recommended for all patients with MD-IPMN and Mix-IPMN who are candidates for surgery. MDCT and EUS are useful diagnostic modalities for MD-IPMN but MRCP may be more useful in preoperative planning, as it more accurately demonstrates the extent of main duct involvement and the presence of small BD-IPMNs.[70] Typical pancreatic resection techniques (Whipple, distal pancreatectomy, and total pancreatectomy) are performed to remove the involved portion of the pancreas with negative margins. When the main pancreatic duct is involved diffusely, however, it is difficult to determine whether the ductal dilatation in the left pancreas is attributable to the presence of tumor or distal obstruction. In these cases, MRCP can be helpful in evaluating the left pancreas for signs of neoplasia such as mural nodules, multifocality, and side branch involvement. In the absence of these findings, many surgeons will perform a Whipple procedure with evaluation of the margin to determine the need for extended resection. If the initial margin is positive, a negative margin often can be obtained by resecting additional pancreatic parenchyma. In some cases, however, total pancreatectomy is necessary to obtain a negative margin or to completely resect diffuse MD-IPMN. Although the quality of life after total pancreatectomy has improved with the use of basal insulin, long-term morbidity

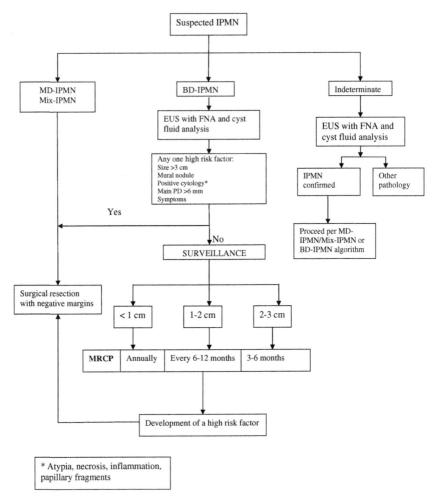

Fig. 7. Algorithm for management of IPMN.

may be experienced by a significant number of patients and the decision to perform a total pancreatectomy should be individualized based on careful assessment of the risk of recurrence and postoperative quality of life.[86]

Intraoperative Margin

Neoplastic involvement frequently extends microscopically beyond the grossly and radiographically visible extent of IPMN. For this reason, frozen section analysis plays an important role in the intraoperative management of IPMN.[87] The International Association of Pancreatology (IAP) consensus management guidelines classify frozen section findings into 3 categories: "IPMN Adenoma," "IPMN with Borderline Atypia," and "IPMN with CIS [carcinoma in situ] or Invasive Carcinoma."[9]

The IAP guidelines suggest no further resection for normal epithelium, hyperplasia, mucinous metaplasia, or adenoma at the resection margin. It should be noted, however, that a recurrence rate of 2% to 8% has been reported in patients with noninvasive IPMN and negative margins on final pathology.[2,4,7,10,88] It is not clear from these studies if these recurrences were caused by local recurrence at the margin or metachronous IPMN in the pancreatic remnant. However, MD-IPMN is not thought to be multicentric and recurrences may represent inadequate surgical margins or synchronous skip lesions. Other investigators have made the point that MD-IPMN adenoma may undergo malignant transformation and, ideally, efforts should be made to completely resect these lesions until no evidence of IPMN, even adenomatous change, remains in the pancreatic remnant.[1] In one older study, noninvasive IPMN was identified at the surgical margin in 24% of patients with noninvasive IPMN and their 5-year survival rate was only 77%.[2] In a more recent study where the rate of noninvasive IPMN at the margin was 7%, the 5-year survival was 96%.[7]

Borderline IPMN at the surgical margin is generally considered noninvasive IPMN and the risk of recurrence is similar to adenoma. The IAP guidelines suggest that "florid papilla formation (with villous-intestinal or pancreatobiliary patterns) may require further attention."[9] These epithelial subtypes may exhibit more aggressive behavior because they are associated with tubular carcinoma. At this point, however, no clinical studies have demonstrated a higher recurrence rate with borderline IPMN at the resection margin, and recurrence rates after resection of borderline IPMN appear to be similar to IPMN adenoma.

Severe dysplasia, carcinoma in situ, or invasive carcinoma at the resection margin are generally considered a positive margin and additional resection is recommended. If the margin remains positive after resection of additional pancreatic parenchyma, total pancreatectomy may be required. When the frozen section reveals denuded epithelium, the margin status cannot be adequately evaluated and it is often prudent to repeat the biopsy of the margin. It should be noted that pancreatic intraepithelial neoplasia (PanIN) is a distinct epithelial neoplasm of the pancreatic duct that can be seen in conjunction with IPMN. PanIN-3 lesions are significant risk factors for ductal adenocarcinoma, and this finding at the initial resection margin should prompt an intraoperative evaluation for coexisting ductal adenocarcinoma and additional resection.[9] PanIN-1 and -2 demonstrate less nuclear atypia, are considered incidental findings, are not associated with ductal adenocarcinoma, and do not require further resection.[9,19]

BD-IPMN

The IAP recommendations for management of BD-IPMN were based on 7 recent studies that found that the average risk of malignancy was 25%.[2,16–18,58,89–91] In these studies, invasive malignancy was uncommon in patients with small, asymptomatic tumors without mural nodules. Consensus guidelines were developed that recommended surveillance for patients with BD-IPMN with the following features:

- Size smaller than 3 cm
- No high-risk features such as the following:
  ○ Mural nodules
  ○ Dilated main pancreatic duct (>6 mm)
  ○ Positive cytology
- No symptoms such as the following:
  ○ Pancreatitis
  ○ Abdominal pain
  ○ Jaundice
  ○ Constitutional symptoms of cancer.

Subsequently, a retrospective study of 147 patients with BD-IPMN analyzed the predictive value of these guidelines.[14] The incidence of malignancy was 15% when at least 1 risk factor was present. In the patients with no risk factors, malignancy was not identified. Thus, the sensitivity and negative predictive value of the guidelines were 100%. However, the specificity was only 23%. Similar findings have been reported by several other investigators (**Table 1**).[57,94,95] Size alone has been found to be a poor predictor of malignancy in BD-IPMN.[12,96] Schmidt and colleagues[12] reported the experience with BD-IPMN at Indiana University and noted malignancy in 17% of patients with lesions smaller than 1 cm. It should be noted that more than 90% of these patients were symptomatic and, therefore, would have met IAP guidelines for resection. The IAP guidelines, therefore, seem to be sufficiently sensitive to detect and treat patients with malignant BD-IPMN. However, the low specificity of these guidelines leads to pancreatic resection in many patients with benign BD-IPMN, and the natural history of theses lesions is not well defined. Neither the IAP guidelines nor existing studies define the importance of growth during follow-up or the management of patients with multifocal BD-IPMN. Further studies of clinical and pathologic features will be necessary to improve risk stratification of patients with BD-IPMN.

BD-IPMN is multifocal in up to 40% of patients.[9] The behavior of multifocal BD-IPMN appears similar to unifocal BD-IPMN, with rates of malignancy between 15% and 25%.[12,14] Considering these findings and the safety of the IAP guidelines, it seems reasonable to manage each lesion separately using the IAP guidelines. Lesions that do not satisfy criteria for surveillance should be resected, and other lesions that do satisfy criteria for surveillance can be followed postoperatively.

The aim of surgery for BD-IPMN is to resect the tumor to a negative margin, as outlined previously. Typical pancreatic resections are generally performed but the small size of many of the lesions allows for more limited resections such as central pancreatectomy, duodenum-preserving pancreatic head resection, pancreatic head resection with second portion duodenectomy, ventral pancreatectomy, and so forth. Experience with these procedures is limited and concerns about margin status and postoperative complications have limited their widespread use.

Table 1
Studies of patients with branch duct intraductal mucin-producing epithelial neoplasm

Authors, Year	N	Percent Initially Resected	Percent Initially Observed	Resection Criteria[a,b]	Percent Malignant at Initial Resection	Percent Requiring Surgery on Follow-up	Percent Malignant on Follow-up
Pelaez-Luna et al, 2007[14]	147	45	55	1–8	15	14	0
Rodriguez et al, 2007[57]	145	100	0	NA	22	NA	NA
Salvia et al, 2007[92]	109	18	82	1, 4, 5, 8	15	6	0
Tanno et al, 2008[93]	82	0	100	5, 7	0	8	1
Woo et al, 2009[94]	190	45	55	1, 3, 5, 7, 9	16	15	1.5

Abbreviation: NA, not available.
    [a] Includes resection criteria used in patients who underwent resection initially as well patients who underwent resection during follow-up.
    [b] (1) Symptoms attributable to the cyst, (2) MPD dilatation ≥ 10 mm, (3) cyst size ≥ 30 mm, (4) cyst size ≥ 35 mm, (5) presence of intramural nodules, (6) cyst fluid cytology suspicious or positive for malignancy, (7) multifocality, (8) increase in cyst size on follow-up, (9) increased serum CA19-9.

The IAP guidelines for surveillance of patients with BD-IPMN suggest evaluation with MDCT or MRI annually for lesions smaller than 10 mm, at 6- to 12-month intervals for lesions 1 to 2 cm, and at 3- to 6-month intervals for lesions 2 to 3 cm. Resection is indicated if the lesion demonstrates any of the risk factors noted previously. The safety of this surveillance program was evaluated in a subsequent retrospective study that found that 13% of patients with initial criteria for surveillance went on to resection.[14] None of these patients had malignancy on final pathology. Ten patients were resected who would have qualified for surveillance under the IAP guidelines. All of these patients had benign BD-IPMN.[14]

Outcomes After Resection

Recurrence after partial pancreatectomy for noninvasive IPMN (adenoma, borderline, and carcinoma in situ) occurs in about 8% of patients. Recurrences occur in the pancreatic remnant with a significant number progressing to invasive IPMN, especially if the original tumor was carcinoma in situ. Recurrence rates appear to be similar in MD-IPMN and BD-IPMN. As noted previously, a significant number of these recurrences occur in patients after partial pancreatectomy with negative margins. This pattern of recurrence suggests a field defect in IPMN with the entire ductal epithelium potentially involved, although this concept remains controversial. Although not specifically addressed in most studies, the authors could find no report of a recurrence after total pancreatectomy for noninvasive IPMN. Overall 5-year survival rate for resected noninvasive IPMN is 77% to 100% (**Table 2**).

Recurrence after resection of invasive IPMN occurs in 50% to 60% of patients and 5-year survival is between 30% and 75%. Recurrence rates appear to be similar in invasive MD-IPMN and invasive BD-IPMN. Survival and recurrence rates for invasive IPMN appear to be similar following partial pancreatectomy with intent to achieve negative margins and total pancreatectomy.[1,4,7,10] Positive lymph nodes, vascular invasion, and perineural invasion are associated with a significantly worse prognosis.[2,10,11] The pattern of recurrence is similar to that of ductal adenocarcinoma. Most of the recurrences after resection of invasive IPMN present with distant metastatic disease (60%–74%), with the liver being the most common site.[4,7,11] Many studies have found that the overall survival following resection of invasive IPMN is superior to that of ductal adenocarcinoma. Many have postulated that this is because of the high proportion of colloid carcinoma seen in invasive IPMN. However, Schnelldorfer and colleagues[7] found that stage-matched survival was similar. These investigators found that invasive IPMN was resected at an earlier stage than a comparable group of patients with ductal adenocarcinoma. Other investigators noted that 5-year survival for stage I invasive IPMN was 67% compared with 21% for ductal adenocarcinoma.[6]

Follow-up After Pancreatic Resection

The IAP guidelines recommend yearly follow-up with MDCT or MRI for patients with resected noninvasive IPMN. EUS is used to evaluate suspicious lesions. Tumor markers have not been shown to be useful in the follow-up of these patients. As mentioned previously, the recurrence rate in these patients is about 8%, occurs in the pancreatic remnant, and can be resected for cure. Surveillance after resection for invasive IPMN is similar to ductal adenocarcinoma. Follow-up should be performed for many years because recurrences have been detected at least 11 years after resection.[7] During follow-up, it is not uncommon for additional primary neoplasms to be diagnosed because about 30% of patients with IPMN will develop an extrapancreatic malignancy.[7,53,54]

Table 2
Studies of patients with resected intraductal mucin-producing epithelial neoplasms only

Authors, Year	N	Percent MD-IPMN	Percent BD-IPMN	IPMN Percent Malignant	IPMN Percent Invasive	MD-IPMN Percent Malignant	BD-IPMN Percent Malignant	Invasive IPMN 5-Year Survival (%)	Noninvasive IPMN 5-Year Survival (%)	Invasive IPMN Recurrence Rate (%)	Noninvasive IPMN Recurrence Rate (%)
Chari et al, 2002[4]	113	Not stated	Not stated	50	35	Not stated	Not stated	36	84	65	8
Sohn et al, 2004[2]	136	28	46	48	38	50[a]	30[a]	43	77	Not stated	Not stated
Salvia et al, 2004[10]	140	100	NA	60	42	60	NA	60	100	12	<1
D'Angelica et al, 2004[11]	63	69	31	76	48	Not stated	Not stated	58	91	30	9
Wada et al, 2005[13]	100	Not stated	Not stated	Not stated	25	Not stated	Not stated	46	100	46	1
Schmidt et al, 2007[12]	156	33	66	32	19	56	19	Not stated	Not stated	Not stated	Not stated
Schnelldorfer et al, 2008[7]	208	64	18	39	30	64	18	31	94	58	8

Abbreviations: BD-IPMN, branch duct intraductal mucin-producing epithelial neoplasm; IPMN, intraductal mucin-producing epithelial neoplasm; MD-IPMN, main duct intraductal mucin-producing epithelial neoplasm.
[a] Does not include carcinoma in situ. Only includes invasive IPMN.

SUMMARY

IPMN is a neoplastic proliferation of mucinous epithelium that arises from the main pancreatic duct (MD-IPMN), secondary branch ducts (BD-IPMN), or both (mixed type; Mix-IPMN). These lesions are discovered on CT or MRI incidentally in about 40% of cases. Neoplastic progression along an adenoma-carcinoma sequence is thought to occur, and malignancy is present in about 70% of patients with MD-IPMN. Resection with negative margins is recommended for patients with MD-IPMN who are surgical candidates. Patients with BD-IPMN are managed selectively based on the risk of malignancy as suggested by the consensus guidelines of the IAP. Recurrence rates after resection of noninvasive IPMN (adenoma, borderline, and carcinoma in situ) are about 8% and generally occur in the pancreatic remnant. This finding supports the notion of a field defect in IPMN. After resection of invasive IPMN (carcinoma), the recurrence rate is about 50% and the 5-year survival is 30% to 60%. Further studies are needed to improve our understanding of the natural history of IPMN. Increased specificity of clinical and pathologic prognostic markers could lead to a more tailored operative approach to patients with BD-IPMN and better informed decisions about the extent of resection in all forms of IPMN.

REFERENCES

1. Bassi C, Sarr MG, Lillemoe KD, et al. Natural history of intraductal papillary mucinous neoplasms (IPMN): current evidence and implications for management. J Gastrointest Surg 2008;12(4):645–50.
2. Sohn TA, Yeo CJ, Cameron JL, et al. Intraductal papillary mucinous neoplasms of the pancreas: an updated experience. Ann Surg 2004;239(6):788–97 [discussion: 797–9].
3. Ohashi K, Murakami Y, Mardyama M, et al. Four cases of "mucin producing" cancer of the pancreas on specific findings of the papilla of Vater. Prog Dig Endsc 1982;20:348–51.
4. Chari ST, Yadav D, Smyrk TC, et al. Study of recurrence after surgical resection of intraductal papillary mucinous neoplasm of the pancreas. Gastroenterology 2002;123(5):1500–7.
5. Bernard P, Scoazec JY, Joubert M, et al. Intraductal papillary-mucinous tumors of the pancreas: predictive criteria of malignancy according to pathological examination of 53 cases. Arch Surg 2002;137(11):1274–8.
6. Maire F, Hammel P, Terris B, et al. Prognosis of malignant intraductal papillary mucinous tumours of the pancreas after surgical resection. Comparison with pancreatic ductal adenocarcinoma. Gut 2002;51(5):717–22.
7. Schnelldorfer T, Sarr MG, Nagorney DM, et al. Experience with 208 resections for intraductal papillary mucinous neoplasm of the pancreas. Arch Surg 2008;143(7):639–46 [discussion: 646].
8. Tollefson MK, Libsch KD, Sarr MG, et al. Intraductal papillary mucinous neoplasm: did it exist prior to 1980? Pancreas 2003;26(3):e55–8.
9. Tanaka M, Chari S, Adsay V, et al. International consensus guidelines for management of intraductal papillary mucinous neoplasms and mucinous cystic neoplasms of the pancreas. Pancreatology 2006;6(1–2):17–32.
10. Salvia R, Fernandez-del Castillo C, Bassi C, et al. Main-duct intraductal papillary mucinous neoplasms of the pancreas: clinical predictors of malignancy and long-term survival following resection. Ann Surg 2004;239(5):678–85 [discussion: 685–7].

11. D'Angelica M, Brennan MF, Suriawinata AA, et al. Intraductal papillary mucinous neoplasms of the pancreas: an analysis of clinicopathologic features and outcome. Ann Surg 2004;239(3):400–8.
12. Schmidt CM, White PB, Waters JA, et al. Intraductal papillary mucinous neoplasms: predictors of malignant and invasive pathology. Ann Surg 2007; 246(4):644–51 [discussion: 651–4].
13. Wada K, Kozarek RA, Traverso LW. Outcomes following resection of invasive and noninvasive intraductal papillary mucinous neoplasms of the pancreas. Am J Surg 2005;189(5):632–6 [discussion: 637].
14. Pelaez-Luna M, Chari ST, Smyrk TC, et al. Do consensus indications for resection in branch duct intraductal papillary mucinous neoplasm predict malignancy? A study of 147 patients. Am J Gastroenterol 2007;102(8):1759–64.
15. Levy P, Jouannaud V, O'Toole D, et al. Natural history of intraductal papillary mucinous tumors of the pancreas: actuarial risk of malignancy. Clin Gastroenterol Hepatol 2006;4(4):460–8.
16. Kobari M, Egawa S, Shibuya K, et al. Intraductal papillary mucinous tumors of the pancreas comprise 2 clinical subtypes: differences in clinical characteristics and surgical management. Arch Surg 1999;134(10):1131–6.
17. Terris B, Ponsot P, Paye F, et al. Intraductal papillary mucinous tumors of the pancreas confined to secondary ducts show less aggressive pathologic features as compared with those involving the main pancreatic duct. Am J Surg Pathol 2000;24(10):1372–7.
18. Sugiyama M, Izumisato Y, Abe N, et al. Predictive factors for malignancy in intraductal papillary-mucinous tumours of the pancreas. Br J Surg 2003;90(10): 1244–9.
19. Hruban RH, Takaori K, Klimstra DS, et al. An illustrated consensus on the classification of pancreatic intraepithelial neoplasia and intraductal papillary mucinous neoplasms. Am J Surg Pathol 2004;28(8):977–87.
20. Sugiyama M, Atomi Y, Kuroda A. Two types of mucin-producing cystic tumors of the pancreas: diagnosis and treatment. Surgery 1997;122(3):617–25.
21. Sugiyama M, Atomi Y. Intraductal papillary mucinous tumors of the pancreas: imaging studies and treatment strategies. Ann Surg 1998;228(5):685–91.
22. Suzuki Y, Atomi Y, Sugiyama M, et al. Cystic neoplasm of the pancreas: a Japanese multiinstitutional study of intraductal papillary mucinous tumor and mucinous cystic tumor. Pancreas 2004;28(3):241–6.
23. Hara T, Yamaguchi T, Ishihara T, et al. Diagnosis and patient management of intraductal papillary-mucinous tumor of the pancreas by using peroral pancreatoscopy and intraductal ultrasonography. Gastroenterology 2002;122(1):34–43.
24. Cuillerier E, Cellier C, Palazzo L, et al. Outcome after surgical resection of intraductal papillary and mucinous tumors of the pancreas. Am J Gastroenterol 2000; 95(2):441–5.
25. Kimura W, Makuuchi M, Kuroda A. Characteristics and treatment of mucin-producing tumor of the pancreas. Hepatogastroenterology 1998;45(24): 2001–8.
26. Cellier C, Cuillerier E, Palazzo L, et al. Intraductal papillary and mucinous tumors of the pancreas: accuracy of preoperative computed tomography, endoscopic retrograde pancreatography and endoscopic ultrasonography, and long-term outcome in a large surgical series. Gastrointest Endosc 1998;47(1): 42–9.
27. Traverso LW, Peralta EA, Ryan JA Jr, et al. Intraductal neoplasms of the pancreas. Am J Surg 1998;175(5):426–32.

28. Sohn TA, Yeo CJ, Cameron JL, et al. Intraductal papillary mucinous neoplasms of the pancreas: an increasingly recognized clinicopathologic entity. Ann Surg 2001;234(3):313–21 [discussion: 321–2].

29. Yamao K, Ohashi K, Nakamura T, et al. The prognosis of intraductal papillary mucinous tumors of the pancreas. Hepatogastroenterology 2000;47(34): 1129–34.

30. Raimondo M, Tachibana I, Urrutia R, et al. Invasive cancer and survival of intraductal papillary mucinous tumors of the pancreas. Am J Gastroenterol 2002; 97(10):2553–8.

31. Nakagohri T, Asano T, Kenmochi T, et al. Long-term surgical outcome of noninvasive and minimally invasive intraductal papillary mucinous adenocarcinoma of the pancreas. World J Surg 2002;26(9):1166–9.

32. Adsay NV, Merati K, Basturk O, et al. Pathologically and biologically distinct types of epithelium in intraductal papillary mucinous neoplasms: delineation of an "intestinal" pathway of carcinogenesis in the pancreas. Am J Surg Pathol 2004; 28(7):839–48.

33. Ishida M, Egawa S, Aoki T, et al. Characteristic clinicopathological features of the types of intraductal papillary-mucinous neoplasms of the pancreas. Pancreas 2007;35(4):348–52.

34. Adsay NV, Adair CF, Heffess CS, et al. Intraductal oncocytic papillary neoplasms of the pancreas. Am J Surg Pathol 1996;20(8):980–94.

35. Ban S, Naitoh Y, Mino-Kenudson M, et al. Intraductal papillary mucinous neoplasm (IPMN) of the pancreas: its histopathologic difference between 2 major types. Am J Surg Pathol 2006;30(12):1561–9.

36. Katabi N, Klimstra DS. Intraductal papillary mucinous neoplasms of the pancreas: clinical and pathological features and diagnostic approach. J Clin Pathol 2008;61(12):1303–13.

37. Adsay NV, Conlon KC, Zee SY, et al. Intraductal papillary-mucinous neoplasms of the pancreas: an analysis of in situ and invasive carcinomas in 28 patients. Cancer 2002;94(1):62–77.

38. Z'Graggen K, Rivera JA, Compton CC, et al. Prevalence of activating K-ras mutations in the evolutionary stages of neoplasia in intraductal papillary mucinous tumors of the pancreas. Ann Surg 1997;226(4):491–8 [discussion: 498–500].

39. Sasaki S, Yamamoto H, Kaneto H, et al. Differential roles of alterations of p53, p16, and SMAD4 expression in the progression of intraductal papillary-mucinous tumors of the pancreas. Oncol Rep 2003;10(1):21–5.

40. Sato N, Rosty C, Jansen M, et al. STK11/LKB1 Peutz-Jeghers gene inactivation in intraductal papillary-mucinous neoplasms of the pancreas. Am J Pathol 2001; 159(6):2017–22.

41. Schonleben F, Qiu W, Remotti HE, et al. PIK3CA, KRAS, and BRAF mutations in intraductal papillary mucinous neoplasm/carcinoma (IPMN/C) of the pancreas. Langenbecks Arch Surg 2008;393(3):289–96.

42. Biankin AV, Biankin SA, Kench JG, et al. Aberrant p16(INK4A) and DPC4/Smad4 expression in intraductal papillary mucinous tumours of the pancreas is associated with invasive ductal adenocarcinoma. Gut 2002;50(6):861–8.

43. Hruban RH, Petersen GM, Ha PK, et al. Genetics of pancreatic cancer. From genes to families. Surg Oncol Clin N Am 1998;7(1):1–23.

44. Iacobuzio-Donahue CA, Klimstra DS, Adsay NV, et al. Dpc-4 protein is expressed in virtually all human intraductal papillary mucinous neoplasms of the pancreas: comparison with conventional ductal adenocarcinomas. Am J Pathol 2000; 157(3):755–61.

45. Schonleben F, Qiu W, Ciau NT, et al. PIK3CA mutations in intraductal papillary mucinous neoplasm/carcinoma of the pancreas. Clin Cancer Res 2006;12(12): 3851–5.

46. Sato N, Fukushima N, Maitra A, et al. Gene expression profiling identifies genes associated with invasive intraductal papillary mucinous neoplasms of the pancreas. Am J Pathol 2004;164(3):903–14.

47. Chadwick B, Willmore-Payne C, Tripp S, et al. Histologic, immunohistochemical, and molecular classification of 52 IPMNs of the pancreas. Appl Immunohistochem Mol Morphol 2009;17(1):31–9.

48. Luttges J, Zamboni G, Longnecker D, et al. The immunohistochemical mucin expression pattern distinguishes different types of intraductal papillary mucinous neoplasms of the pancreas and determines their relationship to mucinous noncystic carcinoma and ductal adenocarcinoma. Am J Surg Pathol 2001;25(7):942–8.

49. Nakamura A, Horinouchi M, Goto M, et al. New classification of pancreatic intraductal papillary-mucinous tumour by mucin expression: its relationship with potential for malignancy. J Pathol 2002;197(2):201–10.

50. Terris B, Dubois S, Buisine MP, et al. Mucin gene expression in intraductal papillary-mucinous pancreatic tumours and related lesions. J Pathol 2002;197(5):632–7.

51. Yonezawa S, Nakamura A, Horinouchi M, et al. The expression of several types of mucin is related to the biological behavior of pancreatic neoplasms. J Hepatobiliary Pancreat Surg 2002;9(3):328–41.

52. Yonezawa S, Taira M, Osako M, et al. MUC-1 mucin expression in invasive areas of intraductal papillary mucinous tumors of the pancreas. Pathol Int 1998;48(4): 319–22.

53. Choi MG, Kim SW, Han SS, et al. High incidence of extrapancreatic neoplasms in patients with intraductal papillary mucinous neoplasms. Arch Surg 2006;141(1): 51–6 [discussion: 56].

54. Sugiyama M, Atomi Y. Extrapancreatic neoplasms occur with unusual frequency in patients with intraductal papillary mucinous tumors of the pancreas. Am J Gastroenterol 1999;94(2):470–3.

55. Maire F, Hammel P, Terris B, et al. Intraductal papillary and mucinous pancreatic tumour: a new extracolonic tumour in familial adenomatous polyposis. Gut 2002; 51(3):446–9.

56. Sparr JA, Bandipalliam P, Redston MS, et al. Intraductal papillary mucinous neoplasm of the pancreas with loss of mismatch repair in a patient with Lynch syndrome. Am J Surg Pathol 2009;33(2):309–12.

57. Rodriguez JR, Salvia R, Crippa S, et al. Branch-duct intraductal papillary mucinous neoplasms: observations in 145 patients who underwent resection. Gastroenterology 2007;133(1):72–9 [quiz: 309–10].

58. Kitagawa Y, Unger TA, Taylor S, et al. Mucus is a predictor of better prognosis and survival in patients with intraductal papillary mucinous tumor of the pancreas. J Gastrointest Surg 2003;7(1):12–8 [discussion: 18–19].

59. Yamaguchi K, Ogawa Y, Chijiiwa K, et al. Mucin-hypersecreting tumors of the pancreas: assessing the grade of malignancy preoperatively. Am J Surg 1996; 171(4):427–31.

60. Sugiura H, Kondo S, Islam HK, et al. Clinicopathologic features and outcomes of intraductal papillary-mucinous tumors of the pancreas. Hepatogastroenterology 2002;49(43):263–7.

61. Taouli B, Vilgrain V, Vullierme MP, et al. Intraductal papillary mucinous tumors of the pancreas: helical CT with histopathologic correlation. Radiology 2000;217(3): 757–64.

62. Ogawa H, Itoh S, Ikeda M, et al. Intraductal papillary mucinous neoplasm of the pancreas: assessment of the likelihood of invasiveness with multisection CT. Radiology 2008;248(3):876–86.
63. Fukukura Y, Fujiyoshi F, Hamada H, et al. Intraductal papillary mucinous tumors of the pancreas. Comparison of helical CT and MR imaging. Acta Radiol 2003;44(5): 464–71.
64. Kawamoto S, Lawler LP, Horton KM, et al. MDCT of intraductal papillary mucinous neoplasm of the pancreas: evaluation of features predictive of invasive carcinoma. AJR Am J Roentgenol 2006;186(3):687–95.
65. Sugiyama M, Atomi Y, Hachiya J. Intraductal papillary tumors of the pancreas: evaluation with magnetic resonance cholangiopancreatography. Am J Gastroenterol 1998;93(2):156–9.
66. Sahani DV, Kadavigere R, Blake M, et al. Intraductal papillary mucinous neoplasm of pancreas: multi-detector row CT with 2D curved reformations—correlation with MRCP. Radiology 2006;238(2):560–9.
67. Yamada Y, Mori H, Matsumoto S. Intraductal papillary mucinous neoplasms of the pancreas: correlation of helical CT and dynamic MR imaging features with pathologic findings. Abdom Imaging 2008;33(4):474–81.
68. Koito K, Namieno T, Ichimura T, et al. Mucin-producing pancreatic tumors: comparison of MR cholangiopancreatography with endoscopic retrograde cholangiopancreatography. Radiology 1998;208(1):231–7.
69. Onaya H, Itai Y, Niitsu M, et al. Ductectatic mucinous cystic neoplasms of the pancreas: evaluation with MR cholangiopancreatography. AJR Am J Roentgenol 1998;171(1):171–7.
70. Waters JA, Schmidt CM, Pinchot JW, et al. CT vs MRCP: optimal classification of IPMN type and extent. J Gastrointest Surg 2008;12(1):101–9.
71. Pais SA, Attasaranya S, Leblanc JK, et al. Role of endoscopic ultrasound in the diagnosis of intraductal papillary mucinous neoplasms: correlation with surgical histopathology. Clin Gastroenterol Hepatol 2007;5(4):489–95.
72. Brugge WR, Lewandrowski K, Lee-Lewandrowski E, et al. Diagnosis of pancreatic cystic neoplasms: a report of the cooperative pancreatic cyst study. Gastroenterology 2004;126(5):1330–6.
73. Recine M, Kaw M, Evans DB, et al. Fine-needle aspiration cytology of mucinous tumors of the pancreas. Cancer 2004;102(2):92–9.
74. Layfield LJ, Cramer H. Fine-needle aspiration cytology of intraductal papillary-mucinous tumors: a retrospective analysis. Diagn Cytopathol 2005;32(1): 16–20.
75. Michaels PJ, Brachtel EF, Bounds BC, et al. Intraductal papillary mucinous neoplasm of the pancreas: cytologic features predict histologic grade. Cancer 2006;108(3):163–73.
76. Jhala NC, Jhala DN, Chhieng DC, et al. Endoscopic ultrasound-guided fine-needle aspiration. A cytopathologist's perspective. Am J Clin Pathol 2003;120(3): 351–67.
77. Maire F, Couvelard A, Hammel P, et al. Intraductal papillary mucinous tumors of the pancreas: the preoperative value of cytologic and histopathologic diagnosis. Gastrointest Endosc 2003;58(5):701–6.
78. Brandwein SL, Farrell JJ, Centeno BA, et al. Detection and tumor staging of malignancy in cystic, intraductal, and solid tumors of the pancreas by EUS. Gastrointest Endosc 2001;53(7):722–7.
79. Yamao K, Ohashi K, Nakamura T, et al. Efficacy of peroral pancreatoscopy in the diagnosis of pancreatic diseases. Gastrointest Endosc 2003;57(2):205–9.

80. Sai JK, Suyama M, Kubokawa Y, et al. Pancreatic duct lavage cytology for the diagnosis of branch duct-type intraductal papillary mucinous neoplasm of the pancreas. Pancreas 2008;36(2):216–7.

81. Reddy RP, Smyrk TC, Zapiach M, et al. Pancreatic mucinous cystic neoplasm defined by ovarian stroma: demographics, clinical features, and prevalence of cancer. Clin Gastroenterol Hepatol 2004;2(11):1026–31.

82. Zamboni G, Scarpa A, Bogina G, et al. Mucinous cystic tumors of the pancreas: clinicopathological features, prognosis, and relationship to other mucinous cystic tumors. Am J Surg Pathol 1999;23(4):410–22.

83. Thompson LD, Becker RC, Przygodzki RM, et al. Mucinous cystic neoplasm (mucinous cystadenocarcinoma of low-grade malignant potential) of the pancreas: a clinicopathologic study of 130 cases. Am J Surg Pathol 1999; 23(1):1–16.

84. Tanaka M. International consensus guidelines for the management of IPMN and MCN of the pancreas. Nippon Shokakibyo Gakkai Zasshi 2007;104(9):1338–43.

85. Crippa S, Salvia R, Warshaw AL, et al. Mucinous cystic neoplasm of the pancreas is not an aggressive entity: lessons from 163 resected patients. Ann Surg 2008; 247(4):571–9.

86. Billings BJ, Christein JD, Harmsen WS, et al. Quality-of-life after total pancreatectomy: is it really that bad on long-term follow-up? J Gastrointest Surg 2005;9(8): 1059–66 [discussion: 1066–57].

87. Eguchi H, Ishikawa O, Ohigashi H, et al. Role of intraoperative cytology combined with histology in detecting continuous and skip type intraductal cancer existence for intraductal papillary mucinous carcinoma of the pancreas. Cancer 2006; 107(11):2567–75.

88. White R, D'Angelica M, Katabi N, et al. Fate of the remnant pancreas after resection of noninvasive intraductal papillary mucinous neoplasm. J Am Coll Surg 2007;204(5):987–93 [discussion: 993–5].

89. Choi BS, Kim TK, Kim AY, et al. Differential diagnosis of benign and malignant intraductal papillary mucinous tumors of the pancreas: MR cholangiopancreatography and MR angiography. Korean J Radiol 2003;4(3):157–62.

90. Doi R, Fujimoto K, Wada M, et al. Surgical management of intraductal papillary mucinous tumor of the pancreas. Surgery 2002;132(1):80–5.

91. Matsumoto T, Aramaki M, Yada K, et al. Optimal management of the branch duct type intraductal papillary mucinous neoplasms of the pancreas. J Clin Gastroenterol 2003;36(3):261–5.

92. Salvia R, Crippa S, Falconi M, et al. Branch-duct intraductal papillary mucinous neoplasms of the pancreas: to operate or not to operate? Gut 2007;56(8): 1086–90.

93. Tanno S, Nakano Y, Nishikawa T, et al. Natural history of branch duct intraductal papillary-mucinous neoplasms of the pancreas without mural nodules: long-term follow-up results. Gut 2008;57(3):339–43.

94. Woo SM, Ryu JK, Lee SH, et al. Branch duct intraductal papillary mucinous neoplasms in a retrospective series of 190 patients. Br J Surg 2009;96(4):405–11.

95. Sadakari Y, Ienaga J, Kobayashi K, et al. Cyst size indicates malignant transformation in branch duct intraductal papillary mucinous neoplasm of the pancreas without mural nodules. Pancreas 2009. [Epub ahead of print].

96. Walsh RM, Vogt DP, Henderson JM, et al. Management of suspected pancreatic cystic neoplasms based on cyst size. Surgery 2008;144(4):677–84 [discussion: 684–5].

Diagnostic Evaluation of Pancreatic Cystic Malignancies

Grant Hutchins, MD[a], Peter V. Draganov, MD[b],*

KEYWORDS

- Pancreas • Pancreatic cyst • Cystic neoplasms
- Pancreatic malignancy

Pancreatic cystic neoplasms despite increased recognition remain rare and represent approximately 10% to 15% of primary cystic masses of the pancreas.[1–3] Many pancreatic cysts are discovered incidentally during the workup for abdominal pain, diarrhea, and other nonspecific gastrointestinal symptoms and represent a frequent clinical referral in tertiary academic centers with pancreatic expertise. Not surprisingly the increase in the diagnosis of a pancreatic cystic mass parallels that of the improved number and type as well as the improved overall sensitivity of cross-sectional imaging studies used in routine practice today.[4] It is important for today's practicing physician to be aware of these increasingly recognized neoplasms on radiologic imaging and more importantly to understand the potential for the presence or development of pancreatic malignancy in a certain subset of these lesions, particularly in those presenting with symptoms or in whom symptoms develop.

CLASSIFICATION

The classification of cystic pancreatic neoplasms has its roots in the surgical, radiologic, and perhaps most importantly in the clinical pathologic literature and dates from the mid to late 1970s.[5,6] The distinction between serous and mucinous cystic neoplasms was first realized at that time and despite many modifications and attempts at radiologic,[7] endoscopic,[8] and more recently with newer laboratory-based analysis using techniques such as mass spectrometry[9] and DNA analysis,[10] remains intact and a solid initial clinical approach to these neoplastic lesions even today. Our understanding of mucinous cystic neoplasms has evolved and since the early 1980s

Funding support: none.
[a] University of Nebraska, 982000 Nebraska Medical Center, Omaha, NE 68198-2000, USA
[b] Division of Gastroenterology, Hepatology and Nutrition, University of Florida, 1600 SW Archer Road, Room HD 602, PO Box 100214, Gainesville, FL 32610, USA
* Corresponding author.
E-mail address: dragapv@medicine.ufl.edu

Surg Clin N Am 90 (2010) 399–410
doi:10.1016/j.suc.2010.01.003
0039-6109/10/$ – see front matter © 2010 Elsevier Inc. All rights reserved.

surgical.theclinics.com

the clinical entity we now recognize as intraductal papillary mucinous neoplasm (IPMN) was first described in the literature.[11] IPMN remains an important "lesion of clinical distinction" when evaluating pancreatic cystic neoplasms and is recognized as a distinct histopathologic entity in the World Health Organization histologic classification system (**Table 1**).[12] Indeed, awareness regarding IPMN recognition and diagnosis has increased so much in recent years that the entity originally known as the IPMN is now further subdivided into main and side-branch IPMN lesions, respectively, each with different clinical, endoscopic, and radiologic presentation, and perhaps most importantly, with different biologic behavior, particularly involving malignant transformation.

MALIGNANT POTENTIAL OF PANCREATIC CYSTIC NEOPLASMS

The incidentally discovered pancreatic cystic neoplasm not only represents an alarming clinical discovery but for the affected patient in many instances represents a precancerous condition with a great deal of uncertainty regarding management. The discussion regarding malignant potential focuses mainly on the distinction between IPMNs and mucinous cystic neoplasms (MCNs). Serous cystadenomas are largely benign lesions although case reports of malignant transformation do exist and as such are often managed nonsurgically. Solid pseudopapillary tumors have a fairly well-defined behavior and malignant risk and are often managed surgically.

The distinction between IPMN lesions and MCN lesions remains a controversial topic and relies on several clinical and pathologic factors. Clinical factors include patient age, location of the cyst, cyst characteristics, and relationship to the main pancreatic duct. As is described in more detail later, main duct IPMNs are found most often in male patients in their 60 or 70s and are more often than not found in the pancreatic head/neck region, whereas side-branch IPMN lesions are not sex specific and tend to be well distributed throughout the pancreas. Main-branch IPMNs appear grapelike on imaging including EUS and appear as individual cysts rather than the cyst within a cyst characteristic seen in MCNs. IPMN lesions also communicate with the pancreatic duct, a feature not seen in MCNs. MCNs in comparison are often seen in women in the 40- to 50 -year age range and are located most often in the pancreatic body and tail regions.

Pathologically, the best-studied differentiation criterion involves the presence of ovarian-type stroma on histologic analysis.[5,13] The presence of ovarian-type stroma

Table 1	
Histologic classification of neoplastic pancreatic cysts	
Serous cystic tumors	Serous cystadenoma
	Serous cystadenocarcinoma (rare)
Mucinous cystic tumors	Mucinous cystadenoma
	Mucinous cystadenoma with moderate dysplasia
	Mucinous cystadenocarcinoma
	Noninfiltrating
	Infiltrating
	Intraductal papillary mucinous adenoma
	IPMN with moderate dysplasia
	Intraductal papillary mucinous carcinoma
	Noninfiltrating
	Infiltrating
Solid pseudopapillary tumors	

is strongly suggestive of an MCN lesion although nonovarian stroma MCNs are reported in the literature. The distinction between MCN and IPMN lesions is clinically important as the malignant potential and resultant management are often based on these differences and permit an individualized care plan rather than pursuing a "remove all mucinous neoplastic process" management style.

The malignant potential of the various cystic neoplasms of the pancreas are important for the clinician and are best understood by dividing IPMNs into main-branch versus side-branch lesions and comparing/contrasting these with the MCN. Main-branch IPMN lesions carry the highest percentage of malignancy ranging in most studies between 60% and 92%.[14–19] Invasive malignancy, defined as noncarcinoma in situ, is also more common in these lesions and approaches 60% in some studies. Side-branch IPMN lesions in comparison are less often malignant with a range of malignancy in reported studies between 6% and 46% and are also less likely to be invasive with the highest reported percentage in the 30% range. In comparison with IPMN lesions, MCNs have a malignant potential ranging from as low as 6% to as high as 36%.[20–22] A better understanding of the malignant potential of MCN lesions is likely to improve with further acceptance of the ovarian-type stroma as a diagnostic criterion for these lesions.

PRESENTATION/EPIDEMIOLOGY

The exact prevalence of pancreatic cysts is difficult to measure because many patients are entirely asymptomatic but it has been estimated to be approximately 20% in patients undergoing radiologic imaging for nonpancreatic diseases/indications.[23] The asymptomatic nature of these cystic lesions (estimated at 40%–75%) in some studies[24] make further epidemiologic studies a clinically difficult task. Data analysis from a large midwestern tertiary care center with recent EUS-FNA capability revealed 45 cases out of 425 being referred for a pancreatic cyst indication. In addition, autopsy series from Japan estimated the prevalence of pancreatic cysts at 25% with an increasing prevalence paralleling advanced patient age.[25] Regardless, the proportion of pancreatic cysts felt to be primary cystic neoplasms is well documented and in the range of 10% to 15%, with most of the remaining cysts found to be pseudocysts.[26] This percentage draws attention to the importance of ruling out the presence of a pancreatic pseudocyst using a combination of historical questioning and in many cases of cystic sampling usually done via EUS.

DIAGNOSIS AND DIFFERENTIAL DIAGNOSIS OF PANCREATIC CYSTIC LESIONS

Once the presence of a pancreatic cyst has been established by some type of imaging modality, the cornerstone of management is to differentiate whether the lesion is a pseudocyst or cystic neoplasm. If a pseudocyst has been effectively excluded, a prudent clinical strategy regarding pancreatic cyst is the division into serous versus mucinous neoplasms. During the evaluation of a pancreatic cyst, it is important for the clinician to have an understanding of the different cyst types, their typical location in the pancreas, and their biologic behavior. Serous cystic neoplasms (SCNs) represent approximately 30% of primary cystic neoplasms of the pancreas[27] with the largest subset being the serous cystadenoma (SCA). The mucinous neoplasms are primarily subdivided into MCNs, which represent approximately 45% to 50% of primary cystic neoplasms of the pancreas,[27] and IPMNs, which make up approximately 25% of primary cystic neoplasms.[28]

It is of great clinical importance at this point of the workup to consider the clinical background of the patient with a newly discovered pancreatic cystic neoplasm.

Remembering the large proportion of pancreatic cysts found to be pseudocystic in nature, a thorough review of the history for episodes of definable pancreatitis in conjunction with risk factors for pancreatitis such as chronic alcohol ingestion, family history of pancreatic diseases as often described by patients and their families, and autoimmune disease is always a good clinical starting point. A clear history of a well-documented episode of pancreatitis strongly suggests that the cystic pancreatic lesion is a pseudocyst but occasionally an attack of pancreatitis is the clinical presentation of a neoplastic cystic lesion particularly main-branch IPMNs.[29] Side-branch IPMN lesions tend to be less symptomatic, however recent studies[30] point to a trend in increased episodes of cyst-related pancreatitis. Patient demographics, including age, sex, presence or absence of symptoms, and the location of the cyst, are important considerations while a diagnosis is being sought. For example MCNs tend to be a middle-age, female predominant disease with most, but not all lesions located in the pancreatic body or tail.[21] SCAs in contrast, although present most often in middle-aged women, are evenly distributed throughout the pancreatic gland; IPMNs have an elderly male predominance and are predominantly located, but not confined to, the pancreatic head region.[29,31] Solid pseudopapillary tumors of the pancreas (SPNs) are a pathologically distinct, rare clinical entity occurring predominately in young women.[32] A comparative index involving the different pancreatic cystic neoplasms and pancreatic pseudocysts is shown in **Table 2** and the usual location of pancreatic cystic lesions in **Fig. 1**.[33]

The discovery of a lesion felt to represent a possible pancreatic cystic neoplasm is often made incidentally by computed tomography (CT) scan performed for other clinical reasons. With this in mind, a thorough understanding of the different imaging modalities, radiologic and if available endoscopic, is needed to construct a diagnostic algorithm to best care for these patients. The availability of endoscopic retrograde cholangiopancreatography (ERCP) and perhaps most importantly EUS plus/minus FNA and cystic fluid analysis has led to much improved understanding and characterization of these lesions.

RADIOLOGIC IMAGING STUDIES

Traditionally 3 imaging modalities have been used to evaluate pancreatic lesions: transabdominal ultrasound (US), CT scanning, and magnetic resonance imaging

Table 2
Typical characteristics of pancreatic cystic lesions

Cyst Type	Pseudocyst	SCA	MCN	IPMN	SPN
Age	Variable	Middle-aged	Middle-aged	Elderly	Young
Sex	M>F	F>M	Female	M>F	Female
Pancreatitis history[a]	Yes	No	No	Yes[b]	No
Location	Evenly	Evenly	Body/tail	Head	Evenly
Malignant potential	None	Rarely	Moderate to high	Low to high	Low
Biliary obstruction	Yes, uncommon	No	No	Yes, uncommon	No

[a] A history of pancreatitis episodes and pancreatic risk factors including alcohol abuse, gallstones, and complications, or family history of pancreatitis is often given.
[b] Pancreatitis caused by IPMN is predominately of the main pancreatic duct subtype.

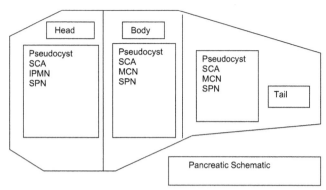

Fig. 1. Typical location of pancreatic cystic lesions.

(MRI)/magnetic resonance cholangiopancreatography (MRCP). Transabdominal US, although it has the advantage of being inexpensive and readily available, is operator dependent and is limited in its ability to visualize the entire pancreas. Furthermore, the presence of significant bowel gas limits the sensitivity of US for characterization of pancreatic cystic processes.

CT scanning, particularly with intravenous contrast enhancement, is a widely available, relatively inexpensive imaging modality and is often the first imaging procedure ordered when a diagnosis of a pancreatic cystic neoplasm is being considered. A review of the diagnostic accuracy of CT scanning has recently been performed[33] with a reported range between 20% and 90%. Differences in study design, characterization of lesions, especially those with atypical features,[34,35] and the ultimate study goal (ie, specific cyst type[36–39] vs differentiation of benign and malignant cyst types[8]) all were felt to contribute to the wide range in diagnostic accuracy.

The typical appearance of a given cystic neoplasm is reported in many ways via CT. Size (ie, microcystic [<2 cm] vs macrocystic [>2 cm]), uni- versus multilocularity, pancreatic duct communication and/or dilation, and the presence of a mass or mural nodule remain the most important imaging characteristics seen on routine CT scans. Serous cystadenomas are characteristically microcystic with many small cysts within the larger cyst creating a honeycomb type pattern. A central stellate scar is often seen at the center of a serous cystadenoma and is considered pathognomonic. Pancreatic duct communication is rarely seen and dilation of the pancreatic duct is also uncommon. MCNs are in comparison most often macrocystic although microcystic lesions do occur and characteristically are multilocular with an orange fruit type appearance. Dilation of the pancreatic duct is uncommon as is communication with the main pancreatic duct. IPMN lesions in contrast are often described as a bag of grapes and contain numerous smaller cysts. Pancreatic duct communication is common and in main-branch IPMN lesions pancreatic duct dilation is seen and predictive of an invasive nature. Associated mural nodules and/or masses are most often observed in IPMN lesions and to a lesser extent MCNs. The presence of a mural nodule is significant as this is often predictive of an invasive cystic neoplasm.

MRI of the abdomen when combined with MRCP is a rapidly emerging imaging modality with widespread availability with wonderful potential to add to our understanding of pancreatic cystic lesions. MRI/MRCP is rivaled only by EUS in its ability to obtain quality images of not only the pancreatic parenchyma but also of the pancreatic and biliary ductal structures.[39–42] MRCP does remain inferior to ERCP in terms of diagnostic accuracy but the gap is narrowing and in addition MRCP offers a noninvasive means of diagnosis compared with ERCP and its complications, most notably post-ERCP pancreatitis.

ENDOSCOPIC STUDIES

The role of endoscopy, specifically ERCP and EUS, in the evaluation and diagnosis of pancreatic cystic neoplasms is a study in evolution that continues today. ERCP remains the most sensitive diagnostic modality for detecting communication between the main pancreatic duct and a given cystic lesion.[43,44] In addition, in a minority of cases an endoscopic diagnosis of an IPMN can be established if a patulous papilla with mucin extrusion, also sometimes referred to as the "fish-eye" ampulla is visualized.[31] The use of ERCP as a primary diagnostic tool in pancreatic cystic neoplasms is not routinely recommended. In most cases the correct diagnosis can be achieved with a higher-yield less-invasive test.

Since its introduction as an endoscopic technology in the late 1970s and early 1980s, EUS has become an increasingly available tool in the diagnosis, management, and in some cases therapy for pancreatic cystic neoplasms. The ability to better describe/characterize pancreatic cystic neoplasms, in particular those lesions felt to be premalignant or frankly malignant, make the use of EUS, with and without FNA, an attractive option in the cystic neoplastic workup. EUS criteria for mucinous/malignant neoplasms are still being developed but include size greater than 2 cm, pancreatic duct dilation, the presence of wall calcifications, and perhaps most importantly the presence of a frank mass or mural nodule. Recent studies have also suggested the presence of a thick cyst wall, intracystic growth, and the presence of a long string sign as potential markers of aggressiveness, however further validation is needed.[45] The growth of a pancreatic cystic neoplasm on serial cross-sectional imaging is also sometimes associated with a more aggressive cystic lesion, necessitating close follow-up of patients with a combination of cross-sectional imaging and repeat EUS. Despite initial enthusiasm, however,[44] several studies[46–50] have reported a wide range of diagnostic accuracy of EUS imaging alone ranging from 40% to 96%. Although many factors including study design, number of patients enrolled, goals of a particular study, and interobserver EUS agreement contribute to this discrepancy, a single, prospective study[50] achieved a diagnostic accuracy of approximately 51%. Clearly, larger, prospective, multicenter studies are needed to better define the role of EUS in the diagnostic workup of a pancreatic cystic neoplasm.

EUS, in addition to its imaging capabilities outlined earlier, allows direct sampling of cystic contents and the cyst wall in an effort to better determine what type of cyst is present. The performance of fine-needle aspirate does, however, remain limited to larger, tertiary centers with extensive experience in EUS. In addition, analysis of cystic fluid is often subject to local cytologic and laboratory expertise with a definite learning curve present for accurate analysis of cystic contents and in some cases by the small volume of aspirate obtained at FNA.

Ideally, an aspirated pancreatic cystic neoplasm should be evaluated for cytologic diagnosis and for the presence of specific intracystic proteins such as amylase and carcinoembryonic antigen (CEA). The cytologic evaluation includes specific testing for the presence of columnar epithelial cells, which stain for mucin (MCNs, IPMNs), or cuboidal epithelial cells, which stain for glycogen (SCAs). Several studies have appeared in the literature regarding the analysis of pancreatic cystic fluid. Several larger studies involving cystic fluid cytologic analysis[32,51,52] reflect a sensitivity of approximately 50%, a low but reproducible percentage, although a more recent study by Moparty and colleagues[53] revealed a cytologic sensitivity of approximately 93% in the differentiation of mucinous and nonmucinous pancreatic neoplasms. The cytologic analysis of cystic fluid continues to be an area of intense research.

Amylase level is routinely checked in the cyst fluid aspirate and may be of some diagnostic value. It is uniformly increased in pseudocysts and IPMNs and frequently increased in MCNs but consistently low in SCAs. The analysis of specific, intracytstic, aspirated proteins continues to evolve. Several proteins including CA19-9, CEA, CA125, and CA72-4 have been studied. The best studied and that currently used most often in routine practice is the level of CEA. The basic differentiation involving the CEA level is which lesions are mucinous (usually but not always increased CEA levels) and which are serous (low CEA levels).[52,54,55] A low CEA level (ie, <5 ng/mL) has been shown in pooled data[45,50,52,56] to have a sensitivity between 50% and 100% with a specificity of 77% to 95% to differentiate mucinous and serous lesions. The degree of CEA level required to best distinguish mucinous and serous lesions continues to be debated in the pancreatic literature with CEA cutoff levels deemed diagnostically sensitive ranging between 20 and 800 ng/mL.[51,54,57–60] The wide range of reported CEA levels lends confusion to the analysis of cystic pancreatic fluid. By increasing the cutoff value of the CEA level considered diagnostic for mucinous lesions the specificity of the test increases at the expense of decreased sensitivity. Currently no standardized cutoff level for CEA exists, however many centers particularly in the United States use a CEA level of 192 ng/mL as established by Brugge and colleagues[51] as diagnostically sensitive (75%) and specific (84%). At present, aspirated cystic fluid should be evaluated for cytologic and biochemical analysis. The biochemical tests that should be routinely ordered are CEA level and amylase. If not enough fluid is available (eg, small cyst or very viscous fluid) CEA level should be obtained first with cytology and amylase level ordered only if there is a sufficient amount of fluid left for analysis.

Newer advances in the study of pancreatic cystic fluid analysis have begun to appear in the literature and represent a potentially exciting and useful avenue to help differentiate mucinous and nonmucinous pancreatic cysts as well as the potential to help differentiate premalignant and malignant pancreatic cysts. The pancreatic cyst fluid DNA analysis in evaluating pancreatic cysts (PANDA) group recently added DNA analysis to the diagnostic algorithm/spectrum. Molecular analysis of pancreatic cystic contents has been reported previously,[61,62] however the recent data by Khalid and colleagues[61] raise several issues regarding analysis of DNA in a given pancreatic cystic neoplasm. During this study the investigators used DNA parameters such as the presence of K-ras mutation, alleleic loss amplitude, and amount and quality of DNA, separate and combined with cyst CEA level, to help differentiate mucinous and nonmucinous cysts and in combination with cytologic analysis to help in the detection of malignant cysts. Despite significant selection bias and nonblinding of physicians to the results during the study, several important findings can be gleaned from the study.

The confirmation of K-ras as an important but not singularly causative mutation in the tumorigenesis of pancreatic cystic neoplasms is an important finding of the PANDA study group. In addition, the use of K-ras in pancreatic cysts without increased CEA (ie, <192 ng/mL) was shown with a high degree of specificity (96%) to be helpful in differentiation/identification of MCNs. In patients with negative cytologic results at FNA it was suggested that the presence of a high-amplitude K-ras mutation followed by allelic loss was specific (ie, 96%) for malignancy. Clearly, progress is being made in the molecular arena, however larger, randomized, controlled studies are needed especially in the small, endoscopically and radiologically defined cyst thought to represent the most benign end of the pancreatic cystic neoplastic spectrum.

DIAGNOSTIC ALGORITHM

The diagnosis and prospective management of a pancreatic cystic neoplasm involves coordination on several levels ranging from the initial discovery to possible surgical

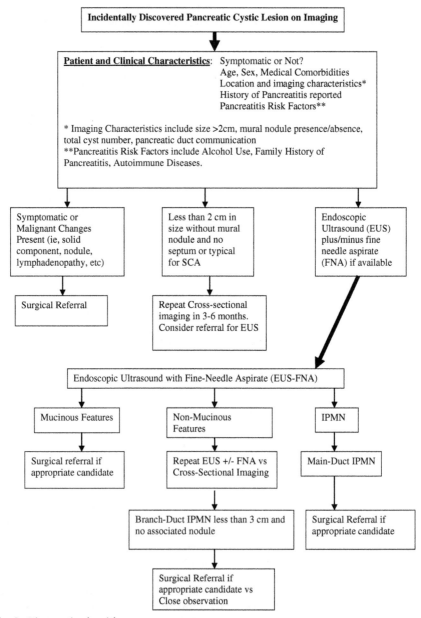

Fig. 2. Diagnostic algorithm.

referral if a frankly malignant or premalignant pancreatic cystic neoplasm is suspected. A proposed diagnostic algorithm beginning with the incidentally discovered pancreatic lesion is presented in **Fig. 2.**

SUMMARY

The evaluation of cystic lesions of the pancreas remains a process in evolution. Significant advances have been made in expanding our understanding of these lesions and in the refinement of our diagnostic approach. A comprehensive diagnostic strategy that incorporates data from patient history, lesion imaging, EUS, and cyst fluid analysis provides an accurate diagnosis in most cases.

REFERENCES

1. Fernandez-del Castillo C, Warshaw AL. Cystic neoplasms of the pancreas. Pancreatology 2001;1:641–7.
2. Mulkeen AL, Yoo PS, Cha C. Less common neoplasms of the pancreas. World J Gastroenterol 2006;12(20):3180–5.
3. Sakorafas GH, Sarr MG. Cystic neoplasms of the pancreas; what a clinician should know. Cancer Treat Rev 2005;31:507–35.
4. Megibow AJ, Lombardo FP, Guiarise A, et al. Cystic masses: cross-sectional imaging observations and serial follow-up. Abdom Imaging 2001;26:640–7.
5. Compagno J, Oertel JE. Mucinous cystic neoplasms of the pancreas with overt and latent malignancy (cystadenocarcinoma and cystadenoma). A clinicopathologic study of 41 cases. Am J Clin Pathol 1978;69:573–80.
6. Compagno J, Oertel JE. Microcystic adenomas of the pancreas (glycogen-rich cystadenomas): a clinicopathologic study of 34 cases. Am J Clin Pathol 1978; 69:289–98.
7. Sahani DV, Kadavigere R, Saokar A, et al. Cystic pancreatic lesions: a simple imaging-based classification system for guiding management. Radiographics 2005;25:1471–84.
8. Gerke H, Jaffe TA, Mitchell RM, et al. Endoscopic ultrasound and computer tomography are inaccurate methods of classifying cystic pancreatic lesions. Dig Liver Dis 2006;38(1):39–44.
9. Scarlett CJ, Samra JS, Xue A, et al. Classification of pancreatic cystic lesions using SELDI-TOF mass spectrometry. ANZ J Surg 2007;77(8):648–53.
10. Khalid A, Zahid M, Finkelstein SD, et al. Pancreatic cyst fluid DNA analysis in evaluating pancreatic cysts: a report of the PANDA study. Gastrointest Endosc 2009;69(6):1095–102.
11. Ohhashi K, Murakami Y, Takekoshi T, et al. Four cases of mucin producing cancer of the pancreas on specific findings of the papilla of Vater. Prog Dig Endosc 1982; 20:348–51.
12. Kloppel G, Solia E, Longnecker DS, et al. World Health Organization International histologic classification of tumours. 2. Histologic typing of tumours of the exocrine pancreas. Berlin: Springer-Verlag; 1996.
13. Izumo A, Yamaguchi K, Eguchi T, et al. Mucinous cystic tumor of the pancreas: immunohistochemical assessment of 'ovarian-type stroma'. Oncol Rep 2003;10: 515–25.
14. Kobari M, Egawa S, Shibuya K, et al. Intraductal papillary mucinous tumors of the pancreas comprise 2 clinical subtypes: differences in clinical characteristics and surgical management. Arch Surg 1999;134:1131–6.

15. Terris B, Ponsot P, Paye F, et al. Intraductal papillary mucinous tumors of the pancreas confined to secondary ducts show less aggressive pathologic features as compared with those involving the main pancreatic duct. Am J Surg Pathol 2000;24:1372–7.

16. Doi R, Fujimoto K, Wada M, et al. Surgical management of intraductal papillary mucinous tumor of the pancreas. Surgery 2002;132:80–5.

17. Kitagawa Y, Unger TA, Taylor S, et al. Mucus is a predictor of better prognosis and survival in patients with intraductal papillary mucinous tumor of the pancreas. J Gastrointest Surg 2003;7:12–9.

18. Sugiyama M, Izumisato Y, Abe N, et al. Predictive factors for malignancy in intraductal papillary-mucinous tumors of the pancreas. Br J Surg 2003;90:1244–9.

19. Sohn TA, Yeo CJ, Cameron JL, et al. Intraductal papillary mucinous neoplasms of the pancreas: an updated experience. Ann Surg 2004;239:788–99.

20. Reddy RP, Smyrk TC, Zapiach M, et al. Pancreatic mucinous cystic neoplasm defined by ovarian stroma: demographics, clinical features, and prevalence of cancer. Clin Gastroenterol Hepatol 2004;2:1026–31.

21. Thompson LD, Becker RC, Przygodzki RM, et al. Mucinous cystic neoplasm (mucinous cystadenocarcinoma of low-grade malignant potential) of the pancreas: a clinicopathologic study of 130 cases. Am J Surg Pathol 1999;23:1–16.

22. Tanaka M, Chari S, Adsay V, et al. International consensus guidelines for management of intraductal papillary mucinous neoplasms and mucinous cystic neoplasms of the pancreas. Pancreatology 2006;6:17–32.

23. Zhang XM, Mitchell DG, Dohke M, et al. Pancreatic cysts: depiction on single-shot fast spin-echo MR images. Radiology 2002;223:547–53.

24. Sarr MG, Murr M, Smyrk T, et al. Primary cystic neoplasms of the pancreas: neoplastic disorders of emerging importance – current state-of-the-art and unanswered questions. J Gastrointest Surg 2003;7:417–28.

25. Kimura W, Nagai H, Kuroda A, et al. Analysis of small cystic lesions of the pancreas. Int J Pancreatol 1995;18:197–206.

26. Warshaw AL, Rutledge PL. Cystic tumors mistaken for pancreatic pseudocysts. Ann Surg 1987;205:393–8.

27. Fernandez-del Castillo C, Warshaw AL. Cystic tumors of the pancreas. Surg Clin North Am 1995;75:1001–16.

28. Loftus EV Jr, Olivares-Pakzad BA, Batts KP, et al. Intraductal papillary-mucinous tumors of the pancreas: clinicopathologic features, outcome, and nomenclature. Gastroenterology 1996;110:1909–18.

29. Salvia R, Fernandez-del Castillo C, Bassi C, et al. Main duct intraductal papillary mucinous neoplasms of the pancreas: clinical predictors of malignancy and long-term survival following resection. Ann Surg 2004;239:678–85.

30. Ringold DA, Shroff P, Sikka SK, et al. Pancreatitis is frequent among patients with side-branch intraductal papillary mucinous neoplasia diagnosed by EUS. Gastrointest Endosc 2009;70(3):488–94.

31. Scheiman JM. Cystic lesion of the pancreas. Gastroenterology 2005;128:463–9.

32. Azar C, Van de Stadt J, Rickaert F, et al. Intraductal papillary mucinous tumours of the pancreas. Clinical and therapeutic issues in 32 patients. Gut 1996;39:457–64.

33. Pettinato G, Di Vizio D, Manivel JC, et al. Solid-pseuodopapillary tumor of the pancreas: a neoplasm with distinct and highly characteristic cytological features. Diagn Cytopathol 2002;27:325–34.

34. Oh HC, Kim MH, Hwang CY, et al. Cystic lesions of the pancreas: challenging issues in clinical practice. Am J Gastroenterol 2008;103:229–39.

35. Johnson CD, Stephens DH, Charboneau JW, et al. Cystic pancreatic tumors: CT and sonographic assessment. AJR Am J Roentgenol 1988;151:1133–8.
36. Curry CA, Eng J, Norton KM, et al. CT of primary cystic pancreatic neoplasms: can CT be used for patient triage and treatment? AJR Am J Roentgenol 2000; 175:99–103.
37. Procacci C, Biasiutti C, Carbognin G, et al. Characterization of cystic tumors of the pancreas: CT accuracy. J Comput Assist Tomogr 1999;23:906–12.
38. Le Borgne J, de Calan L, Partensky C. Cystadenomas and cystadenocarcinomas of the pancreas: a multiinstitutional retrospective study of 398 cases. French Surgical Association. Ann Surg 1999;230:152–61.
39. Bassi C, Salvia R, Molinari E, et al. Management of 100 consecutive cases of pancreatic serous cystadenoma: wait for symptoms and see at imaging or vice versa? World J Surg 2003;27:319–23.
40. Koito K, Namieno T, Nagakawa T, et al. Solitary cystic tumor of the pancreas: EUS-pathologic correlation. Gastrointest Endosc 1997;45:268–76.
41. Gress F, Gottlieb K, Cummings O, et al. Endoscopic ultrasound characteristics of mucinous cystic neoplasms of the pancreas. Am J Gastroenterol 2000;95: 961–5.
42. Koito K, Namieno T, Ichimura T, et al. Mucin-producing pancreatic tumors: comparison of MR cholangiopancreatography with endoscopic retrograde cholangiopancreatography. Radiology 1998;208:231–7.
43. Sahani D, Prasad S, Saini S, et al. Cystic pancreatic neoplasms evaluation by CT and magnetic resonance cholangiopancreatography. Gastrointest Endosc Clin N Am 2002;12:657–72.
44. Fukukura Y, Fujiyoshi F, Hamada H, et al. Intraductal papillary mucinous tumors of the pancreas. Comparison of helical CT and MR imaging. Acta Radiol 2003;44: 464–71.
45. Leung KK, Ross WA, Evans D, et al. Pancreatic cystic neoplasm: the role of cyst morphology, cyst fluid analysis, and expectant management. Ann Surg Oncol 2009;16:2818–24.
46. Yamao K, Nakamura T, Suzuki T, et al. Endoscopic diagnosis and staging of mucinous cystic neoplasms and intraductal papillary mucinous tumors. J Hepatobiliary Pancreat Surg 2004;10:142–6.
47. O'Toole D, Palazzo L, Hammel P, et al. Macrocystic pancreatic cystadenoma: the role of EUS and cyst fluid analysis in distinguishing mucinous and serous lesions. Gastrointest Endosc 2004;59:823–9.
48. Sedlack R, Affi A, Vazquez-Sequeiros E, et al. Utility of EUS in the evaluation of cystic pancreatic lesions. Gastrointest Endosc 2002;56:543–7.
49. Ahmad NA, Kochman ML, Brensinger C, et al. Interobserver agreement among endosonographers for the diagnosis of neoplastic versus non-neoplastic pancreatic cystic lesions. Gastrointest Endosc 2003;58:59–64.
50. Hernandez LV, Mishra G, Forsmark C, et al. Role of endoscopic ultrasound (EUS) and EUS-guided fine needle aspiration in the diagnosis and treatment of cystic lesions of the pancreas. Pancreas 2002;25:222–8.
51. Brugge WR, Lewandrowski K, Lee-Lewandrowski E, et al. Diagnosis of pancreatic cystic neoplasms: a report of the cooperative pancreatic cyst study. Gastroenterology 2004;126:1330–6.
52. Walsh RM, Henderson JM, Vogt DP, et al. Prospective preoperative determination of mucinous pancreatic cystic neoplasms. Surgery 2002;132:628–33 [discussion: 633–4].

53. Moparty B, Logrono R, Nealon WH, et al. The role of endoscopic ultrasound and endoscopic ultrasound-guided fine-needle aspiration in distinguishing pancreatic cystic lesions. Diagn Cytopathol 2007;35(1):18–25.

54. van der Waaij LA, van Dullemen HM, Porte RJ, et al. Cyst fluid analysis in the differential diagnosis of pancreatic cystic lesions: a pooled analysis. Gastrointest Endosc 2005;62:383–9.

55. Federle MP, McGrath KM. Cystic neoplasms of the pancreas. Gastroenterol Clin North Am 2007;36:365–76.

56. Ryu JK, Woo SM, Hwang JH, et al. Cyst fluid analysis for the differential diagnosis of pancreatic cysts. Diagn Cytopathol 2004;31:100–5.

57. Frossard JL, Amouyal P, Amouyal G, et al. Performance of endosonography-guided fine needle aspiration and biopsy in the diagnosis of pancreatic cystic lesions. Am J Gastroenterol 2003;98:1516–24.

58. Hammel P, Voitot H, Vilgrain V, et al. Diagnostic value of CA 72-4 and carcinoembryonic antigen determination in the fluid of pancreatic cystic lesions. Eur J Gastroenterol Hepatol 1998;10:345–8.

59. Sperti C, Pasquali C, Pedrazzoli S, et al. Expression of mucin-like-carcinoma-associated antigen in the cyst fluid differentiates mucinous from nonmucinous pancreatic cysts. Am J Gastroenterol 1997;92:672–5.

60. Hammel PR, Forgue-Lafitte ME, Levy P, et al. Detection of gastric mucins (M1 antigens) in cyst fluid for the diagnosis of cystic lesions of the pancreas. Int J Cancer 1997;74:286–90.

61. Khalid A, McGrath KM, Zahid M, et al. The role of pancreatic cyst fluid molecular analysis in predicting cyst pathology. Clin Gastroenterol Hepatol 2005;3:967–73.

62. Sawhney MS, Devarajan S, O'Farrel P, et al. Comparison of carcinoembryonic antigen and molecular analysis in pancreatic cyst fluid. Gastrointest Endosc 2009;69(6):1106–10.

Pancreatic Cystic Neoplasms

Jennifer E. Verbesey, MD[a],*, J. Lawrence Munson, MD[b]

KEYWORDS

- Pancreatic cystic neoplasms • Serous cystadenoma
- Mucinous cystic neoplasms
- Intraductal papillary mucinous neoplasm

Cystic neoplasms of the pancreas have been recognized for almost two centuries. In 1830, Becourt's first description noted a tumor "the size of a child's head and composed of very strong fibrous walls."[1] Soon after, Gross published the first report of a cystic neoplasm in the United States. It took 50 years for Bozeman to understand in 1872 that aspiration alone would not cure this type of tumor, and he accomplished the first successful resection of a tumor with survival of the patient. In 1900, Reginald Fitz acknowledged the malignant potential of such tumors. Much progress in terms of the understanding of etiology, diagnosis, treatment, and prognosis has been accomplished since then. In 1978, Compagno and Oertel[2] divided cystic tumors into 2 types: benign serous neoplasms and mucinous cystic tumors that harbored a malignancy. In 1982, Ohashi described what one would now call an intraductal papillary mucinous neoplasm (IPMN), which he initially described as a "mucin-producing cancer."[3]

Over 70% of cystic neoplasms are found in asymptomatic patients, usually as an incidental finding on scans obtained for another reason. In an autopsy study published in 1995, the investigators found that almost half of the 300 deceased patients studied had small cystic lesions.[4] Older age was directly related to the probability of finding a lesion. Most published studies agree that the ratio of benign to malignant lesions is approximately 2:1. Cystic neoplasms are found in females at a ratio of 2:1 to 3:1 compared with males. Ferrone and colleagues[5] looked at 401 patients with pancreatic cystic lesions and found that 61% were women with a median age of 62 years.

Given the malignant potential of cystic neoplasms, it is important that this entity be differentiated from pancreatic pseudocysts. Postinflammatory cystic collections, especially pseudocysts, represent the vast majority of cystic lesions (as much as 90%). Pancreatic pseudocysts lack an epithelial lining and will, many times, follow an illness, particularly a bout of pancreatitis. Radiologic imaging plays a large role in

a Department of Transplantation, Lahey Clinic Medical Center, 41 Mall Road, Burlington, MA 01805, USA
b Department of General Surgery, Lahey Clinic Medical Center, 41 Mall Road, Burlington, MA 01805, USA
* Corresponding author.
E-mail address: jennifer.verbesey@lahey.org

Surg Clin N Am 90 (2010) 411–425
doi:10.1016/j.suc.2009.12.006
0039-6109/10/$ – see front matter © 2010 Elsevier Inc. All rights reserved.
surgical.theclinics.com

diagnosis. Evidence of chronic pancreatitis make a pseudocyst more likely. On the other hand, calcification in the wall of the cyst, septations, or solid components can point one more in the direction of a cystic neoplasm.[6] Communication with the pancreatic duct can be seen in both pseudocysts and some forms of mucinous cystic lesions, so this does not confirm a diagnosis. Abdominal and endoscopic ultrasound has proven very helpful in differentiation between these 2 entities. The type of cyst wall seen, presence of a multilocular versus unilocular cyst, appearance of septations or solid components, and simultaneous lymphadenopathy can all help make an accurate diagnosis.[7,8] A recent study showed that presence of internal dependent debris was a highly specific magnetic resonance imaging (MRI) finding indicating the diagnosis of pseudocyst.[9] In cases that remain difficult to diagnose despite radiologic studies, cyst fluid analysis can help. Analysis includes cyst epithelial cell staining, stains for mucin, amylase levels, and tumor markers carcinoembryonic antigen (CEA) and carbohydrate antigen 19-9 (CA19-9).[6] The positive predictive value of such tests is very high, but negative results are unreliable and cannot be used to rule out malignancy. In a minority of cases, differentiating between a pseudocyst and pancreatic cystic neoplasm proves impossible before going to the operating room. However, in general a combination of the patient's history, radiologic studies, and laboratory tests will allow the physician to feel confident in choosing the differential diagnosis.

WORLD HEALTH ORGANIZATION CLASSIFICATION OF CYSTIC NEOPLASMS

The World Health Organization (WHO) first published a classification system for cystic neoplasms in 1996, and a revision in 2000. This classification system divided pancreatic cystic neoplasms into 3 categories: malignant tumors (in situ or invasive), borderline (uncertain malignant potential), and benign (adenomas).[10,11] Microcystic, glycogen-rich, serous tumors are almost universally benign, and macrocystic, mucinous tumors accepted as either malignant or premalignant.

Malignant tumors include serous cystadenocarcinomas, mucinous cystadenocarcinomas, intraductal papillary mucinous carcinomas, invasive papillary mucinous carcinomas, and acinar cell cystadenocarcinomas. Borderline tumors consist of mucinous cystic tumors with moderate dysplasia, IPMN with moderate dysplasia, and solid pseudopapillary tumors. Benign or adenomatous tumors are serous cystadenomas, mucinous cystadenomas, and certain IPMNs.

SEROUS TUMORS: SEROUS CYSTADENOMA AND SEROUS CYSTADENOCARCINOMAS

Serous tumors represent approximately 1% to 2% of pancreatic neoplasms and almost 25% of all cystic tumors.[12] Serous neoplasms are distributed evenly throughout the pancreas. These tumors are almost universally found incidentally when a computed tomography (CT) scan is obtained for another reason. The tumors cause symptoms only if they are very large (>15 cm), usually compressive symptoms from a mass effect. Although extremely rare, the most common symptoms would be either jaundice or gastric outlet obstruction, caused by extrinsic pressure on adjacent structures. Serous tumors tend to be found more often in older women (average age 61 years). A mean diameter of 5 to 8 cm is most common.

Serous neoplasms will stain negative for mucin. It is generally believed that they carry no risk of invasive cancer; however, there are several case reports in the literature describing serous cystadenomas that presented with metastases, now more correctly termed a serous cystadenocarcinoma.[13–16] Serous neoplasms have glycogen-rich clear cytoplasm that stains positive with a PAS test (periodic acid-Schiff stain) and uniform, cuboidal epithelium. Serous neoplasms are microcystic and can have thin-walled septae that produce the typical "honeycomb appearance." On CT scan, these neoplasms will have a thin wall and a typical sunburst pattern of calcification with a central, late-enhancing scar (**Figs. 1** and **2**). The tumor will appear grossly to be grapelike, with 6 or more uniformly sized cysts 2 cm or smaller. Small septae and internal debris may be seen in the individual cysts (**Figs. 3–5**). The capsule is usually poorly developed, and there is often a poor distinction between tumor and surrounding pancreatic parenchyma. Serous neoplasms never communicate with the main pancreatic duct.

MUCINOUS CYSTIC TUMORS: MUCINOUS CYSTADENOMAS AND MUCINOUS CYSTADENOCARCINOMAS

Mucinous tumors represent approximately 2% of all pancreatic neoplasms and one-third of all cystic neoplasms.[12] Mucinous tumors are almost all found in the body or tail of the pancreas, most frequently in women in their fifth or sixth decade of life. Mucinous tumors range in size from 6 to 35 cm. The contents of the tumor are usually thick, but may be hemorrhagic, watery, or necrotic.[17] The tumors are circumscribed unilocular or multilocular cysts with no communication with the pancreatic duct (with rare exceptions) (**Fig. 6**). CT scan will show a cyst with a thick wall and possible calcification within the wall (**Fig. 7**). Mucinous neoplasms rarely, if every, recur after complete resection.[18]

Mucinous neoplasms are thought to behave in a way similar to other cancers, in that there seems to a progression from atypia to frank malignancy. Malignancy risk is directly related to an increase in size and duration of existence. Approximately 65% of the epithelium is composed of mucin-producing cells, and it is in these cells that malignant deterioration occurs. In a study conducted at Massachusetts General Hospital, 64% of all mucinous tumors found proved to be malignant, 33% had metastases, and only 63% were resectable. Of those resected 76% were cured, which represented 48% of the total. All of the patients who were unresectable died of the disease.[19]

Ovarian-like stroma that usually stains positive histologically for estrogen and progesterone receptors is found.[20] It is suspected that mucinous neoplasms may arise

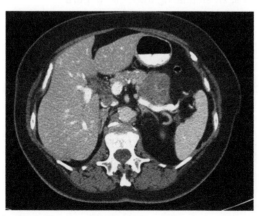

Fig. 1. Contrast-enhanced CT scan demonstrating a large cystic mass in the tail of the pancreas consistent with a serous cystadenoma.

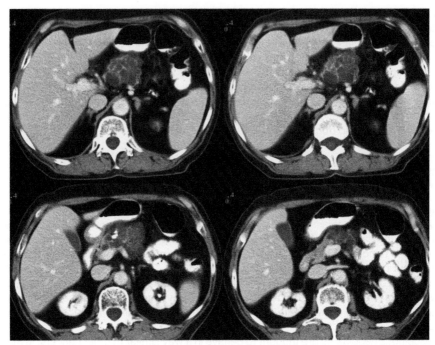

Fig. 2. Contrast-enhanced CT scan showing 4 axial sections of cystic mass in body and tail of pancreas. Pathology confirmed the presence of a serous cystadenoma.

from ovarian rests in the pancreas. Tanaka and colleagues[11] evaluated the hypothesis that ovarian-type stroma is a histologic requirement for diagnosing a mucinous cystic neoplasm (MCN). Their hypothesis was confirmed when they found that women older than 60 years and also men had ovarian-type stroma, and they concluded that ovarian-type stroma is a prerequisite for the diagnosis of a MCN.

Mucinous ductal ectasia is a premalignant finding. Pathology demonstrates papillary hyperplasia and mucin overproduction along the pancreatic duct. The pancreatic duct can become obstructed by filling with mucin, and can lead to pancreatitis. At times, mucus can be seen emanating from the ampulla.[19]

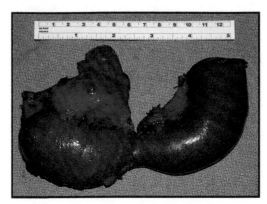

Fig. 3. Resected pancreatic head and duodenum (Whipple procedure) for serous cystadenoma.

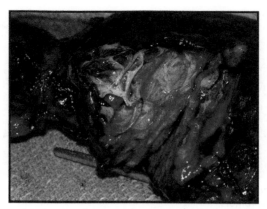

Fig. 4. Freshly removed and opened pancreatic serous cystadenoma. Septations and "honey-combing" evident.

INTRADUCTAL PAPILLARY MUCINOUS NEOPLASMS

The WHO defined an IPMN as a papillary mucin-producing neoplasm that arises in the main pancreatic duct or major branches. This entity was first described by Ohashi and colleagues[3] in 1982. IPMNs represent approximately 1% of all pancreatic neoplasms and 25% of cystic neoplasms.[12] IPMNs have direct communication with either the main pancreatic duct or the smaller branch ducts, and are most commonly found in the head or proximal region of the pancreas (**Fig. 8**). It was traditionally thought that IPMNs were more common in men older than 70 years.[21] However, recent studies by Salvia, Sohn, D'Angelica and colleagues[22–24] showed a more equal distribution between sexes. IPMNs are divided into main duct IPMNs or branch duct IPMNs; mixed type (which is present approximately 40% of the time) are considered main duct for the purpose of prognosis and treatment. Branch duct tumors are more commonly found in younger patients and have a lower malignant potential. Noninvasive IPMNs are divided into low-grade dysplasia (adenoma), moderate dysplasia (borderline IPMN), and high-grade dysplasia or carcinoma in situ. Malignancy is found in a reported 58% to 92% of main duct tumors. Malignancy is much less common in branch duct tumors, with a reported presence of 6% to 46%.[25] Fujino and

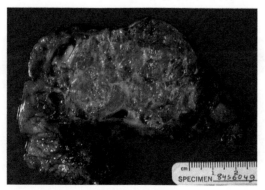

Fig. 5. Pathologic specimen after resection of pancreatic serous cystadenoma. Microcystic nature, "grapelike" form, and small septations can be seen.

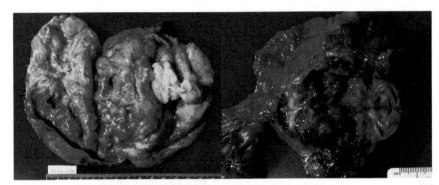

Fig. 6. Resected pancreatic mucinous cystic neoplasms. Both of these tumors were multilo-culated, macrocystic tumors.

colleagues[26] found main duct type tumors in 55% of their patients, and 8.6% were adenomas whereas 91.4% were carcinomas. Consistent with past studies, 45% were branch type tumors, of which 62% were adenomas and only 38% carcinomas. Woo and colleagues[25] studied 190 patients and found malignancy was more common in diabetic patients, and showed an even lower prevalence of invasive cancer in branch duct tumors (6.3%).

Multiple studies have shown an average lag time of approximately 5 years from age at presentation of IPMN with low-grade dysplasia to the point at which it becomes an invasive carcinoma. In their published study, Sohn and colleagues[23] showed that the average age of patients with low-grade dysplasia was 63.2 years and that of those with invasive cancer was 68.2 years. In addition, several studies have showed that patients with IPMNs have a higher risk of synchronous or metachronous primary ex-trapancreatic tumors, including 25% of patients that had cancers of the stomach, colon, rectum, lung, breast, or liver.[27,28]

On histologic examination, IPMNs are grossly visible. Tall, columnar, mucin-con-taining epithelium with cytoarchitectural atypia is found. There are 2 subtypes: intes-tinal subtype, which exhibits abundant extracellular mucin and typically has a high survival rate after resection, and pancreatobiliary subtype, which is the form that typi-cally evolves into ductal adenocarcinoma and leads to a very poor survival rate. A third subtype can be found in branch type tumors that is described as a gastric foveolar subtype, which rarely progresses to malignancy.[17] The spectrum of atypia ranges

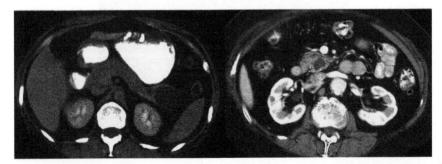

Fig. 7. CT scans from 2 different patients showing mucinous cystic neoplasms in the tail and body of the pancreas.

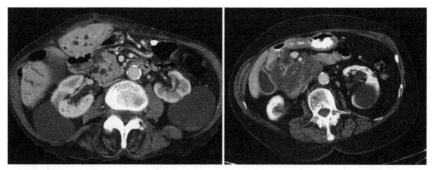

Fig. 8. Contrast-enhanced CT scans of pancreatic IPMNs. Patients can often have multiple IPMNs along the length of the pancreas.

from hyperplasia (adenoma) to low-grade dysplasia to invasive carcinoma. Mucinous ductal ectasia is sometimes present. Mucin accumulation leads to ductal dilatation.

A summary of common characteristics of pancreatic pseudocysts, serous neoplasms, MCNs, and IPMNs is found in **Table 1**.

CLINICAL PRESENTATION

In most cases of pancreatic cystic neoplasm, symptoms are due to mass effect of the tumor on adjacent structures. Looking at all patients with a cystic neoplasm, most have a history of no trauma or alcoholic pancreatitis. The vast majority feel, at some point, epigastric fullness or ache. Fifty percent will have palpable mass. A patient rarely will complain of weight loss, steatorrhea, and back pain, or show signs of jaundice. Serous neoplasms are most commonly found incidentally, so are therefore most often asymptomatic.

With MCNs, some patients may complain of vague abdominal pain or discomfort. Weight loss or anorexia is associated with malignancy. In contrast to most serous and mucinous lesions, IPMNs are most often discovered in association with symptoms (75%). The clinical scenario most often mimics that of pancreatitis, with vague epigastric pain and occasional steatorrhea. For the most part, patients have no history of trauma or alcohol abuse. Laboratory values are normal outside of an acute attack of pancreatitis. Jaundice is usually only present if invasive cancer exists.

DIAGNOSIS

Multiple radiologic modalities can be used to make the diagnosis of a pancreatic cystic neoplasm including ultrasound, CT, MRI/magnetic resonance cholangiopancreatography (MRCP), endoscopic retrograde cholangiopancreatography (ERCP), arteriography, and endoscopic ultrasound. CT scanning is widely accepted as the best initial diagnostic tool. CT can be used to evaluate the important qualities of the cystic lesion, such as size, multi- or unilocular composition, solid components, and presence of calcifications. In addition, it can be used to evaluate the relationship of the mass to the celiac axis, superior mesenteric artery, superior mesenteric vein, and portal vein, and assess the resectability of the tumor. Septations can be visualized in mucinous neoplasms, "sunburst" calcifications in serous cystadenomas, and peripheral calcification in cystadenocarcinomas. Finally, CT can be used to differentiate main duct from branch duct type IPMNs. Nodules in the main duct system or dilatation of the main duct to greater than 1 cm is suggestive of a main duct IPMN,

Table 1
Comparison of common characteristics of various pancreatic cystic lesions

	Pseudocyst	Serous Neoplasm	Mucinous Cystic Neoplasm	IPMN
Demographics	Any age	Females Average age 61	Females 20:1 Average age 45	Males or 1:1 Average age 50–60s
Symptoms	Early satiety Pain	Asymptomatic unless very large	Usually asymptomatic	Occasional pain
Location	Throughout	More often in body/tail	Body/tail (>90%)	Head (2/3)
CT Findings	Thick Wall	Thin wall Sunburst/honeycomb	Thick wall	Cystic +/– solid components
ERCP/MRCP	+/– Communication with pancreatic duct	No communication with pancreatic duct	No communication with pancreatic duct	Connection with main or branch pancreatic ducts
Aspiration quality	Thin, dark, opaque, nonmucinous	Serous fluid No mucin	Clear, thick, mucin-rich fluid	Mucinous fluid
Tumor markers in cyst fluid	Not elevated	Not elevated	Possibly elevated	Possibly elevated
Cancer risk	None	None	6%–36%	Main Duct 70% Branch Duct 25%
Gross appearance			Orangelike	Grapelike
Surgery	If symptomatic or large	If >4 cm or symptoms	Resect all	Resect all main duct neoplasms Resect branch duct if large or suspicious findings (see text)
Recurrence risk in noninvasive tumors		Zero	Near zero	Continued risk in remaining pancreas
Recurrence risk if invasive			Significant risk	Significant risk

Abbreviations: CT, computed tomography; ERCP, endoscopic retrograde cholangiopancreatography; IPMN, intraductal papillary mucinous neoplasm; MRCP, magnetic resonance cholangiopancreatography.

whereas a mucinous cyst that communicates with the ductal system in the context of a main duct with a normal diameter is probably a branch duct IPMN.

MRI/MRCP is a useful adjunct in that it can identify the cyst and show its relationship to the ductal anatomy (**Fig. 9**), which is particularly useful in identifying IPMNs and visualizing small connections to the ductal system. MRCP may also be a good way to follow IPMNs postoperatively. ERCP is the true gold standard for evaluating pancreatic ductal anatomy and communication between cyst and duct, and in addition there is the added advantage of being able to obtain cytology (**Fig. 10**). ERCP is the most definitive test for IMPNs in that intraductal mucin or mucin leakage from a patulous or dilated ampulla is pathognomonic for an IPMN.[25] However, of importance is that once the tumor has become invasive, mucin can block the communication so that most IPMNs will not have mucin emanating from the papilla. A positive finding of mucin at the ampulla is highly sensitive for the presence of an IPMN; however, a negative finding in no way rules out its presence. ERCP can also be helpful in revealing ductal stricturing, displacement, or obstruction.

Least invasive of all tests is an abdominal ultrasound that can be used to evaluate septations and debris in the cyst. In addition, mural nodularity and vascular flow can be evaluated. Endoscopic ultrasound (EUS) is increasingly viewed as the best modality to stage tumors for resection, identify nodal involvement, and show presence or absence of vascular invasion; it is also one of the best ways to obtain cytologic sampling. EUS can be used to follow up on vague findings on other studies or to help differentiate benign from malignant. Kubo and colleagues[29] found that a dilated main pancreatic duct, branch type tumors that are greater than 30 mm with irregular septa, or mural nodules indicate malignancy. Multiple other studies have demonstrated that predictors of malignancy include Type III or IV mural nodules or irregularities of the pancreatic duct.[30,31]

Arteriography is rarely used at the present time during the workup of cystic lesions. In the past, if performed, one could find a hypervascular blush with serous cysts and draping or displacement of vessels by mucinous tumors.

CYTOLOGY

CEA is a glycoprotein found in embryonic endodermal epithelium. Mucinous cysts are lined by endoderm-derived columnar epithelium that secretes CEA. Nonmucinous cysts are lined by simple cuboidal epithelium that should not have any CEA.[32] This

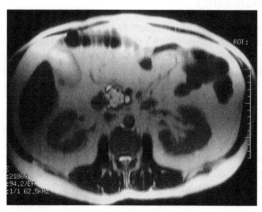

Fig. 9. MRI showing presence of IPMN in body of pancreas.

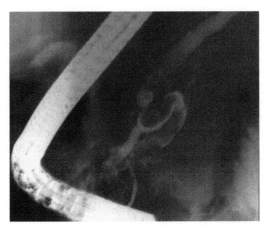

Fig. 10. ERCP of IPMN. Communication with the main pancreatic duct is visualized.

situation makes CEA, along with other tumor markers such as CA19-9 and CA-125, helpful in diagnosis. Pseudocysts will often have an elevated amylase and lipase, but negligible tumor markers. Fluid aspirated from MCNs will often exhibit low amylase and lipase levels, but high CEA, CA19-9, and CA-125 levels. On the other hand, IPMNs show variable levels of amylase and lipase but also higher levels of CEA and CA19-9. However, because these values are often not consistent, the true benefit of fine-needle aspiration is controversial.[33] Sawhney and colleagues[32] showed very poor agreement between CEA levels and molecular analysis (DNA quantity, k-ras 2 point mutation or 2 or more allelic imbalance mutations, and pathologic analysis of cyst) for diagnosis of mucinous neoplasms. Their study showed a sensitivity of 82% for CEA and 77% for molecular analysis, but 100% combined sensitivity.

Cytologic contribution to diagnosis and prognosis should certainly be a major focus of future research. Recent studies such as the one published by Fritz and colleagues[33] showed how using array comparative genomic hybridization (CGH) to look for recurrent mutations in IPMNs to help differentiate these from pancreatic adenocarcinomas can be helpful with diagnosis and prognosis. Future studies will need to focus on the usefulness of molecular tumor markers and mutations in the care of these patients.

PREDICTORS OF MALIGNANCY

One would optimally wish to be able to identify tumors with an extremely low chance of malignancy so that those patients can pursue more conservative or observational therapy and avoid aggressive surgical intervention. Given the vastly improving ability of radiologic examinations to pick up even the smallest abnormality, and the increasing number of incidental findings, it is of paramount importance that there be criteria to determine which lesions are most likely to be malignant.

A large number of studies have been published that detail numerous factors found to be independent predictors of malignancy. In general, irregularity of borders, mixed solid and cystic components, or symptomatic lesions are all ominous signs. Nearly all tumors with radiologic calcification are malignant. Many MCNs that are malignant demonstrate peripheral calcification, a thickened cyst wall, papillary proliferations, and a hypervascular pattern, and may show vascular involvement.[17] In addition, Garcea and colleagues demonstrated that the earliest change in malignant cells of a mucinous neoplasm is a mutation of the Kras2 oncogene on chromosome 12p.

This mutation is found in 89% of MCNs with carcinoma in situ (compared with 20% of adenomas).[17]

Multiple studies have confirmed predictors of malignancy for IPMNs. These factors include the type of IPMN (main duct type has higher malignant potential), larger tumor size (tumor diameter >30 mm), proximal location, involvement of a dilated main pancreatic duct larger than 7 mm, presence of mural nodules, protruding lesions in dilated branch ducts, thick cyst wall, a patulous papilla with mucin leakage from the ampulla of Vater, and increased CA19-9 level. Other independent risk factors are older age, presence of jaundice, diabetes, and pancreatitis.[17,22,25,26,30,34] In partial conflict with other reports, Fujino and colleagues[26] showed that the following factors were not significant predictors of malignancy: gender, location, mural nodules, abdominal pain, the presence of other tumors, history of pancreatitis, cyst size, serum CEA, and serum amylase. A low level of CA19-9 does not distinguish between invasive and noninvasive IPMNs. IPMN malignancies have very different biologic behavior to invasive ductal adenocarcinomas. IPMNs tend to grow less aggressively, have a lower incidence of nodal positivity, and have lower rates of perineural and vascular invasion.[18,23]

TREATMENT

There are certain basic principles for the surgical treatment of cystic neoplasms. While not all tumors will be amenable to resection, surgery can be curative for many. Growth by displacement, which is usually the case, instead of invasion into adjacent structures, favors resection. A distal pancreatectomy is the traditional treatment for body and tail lesions. A Whipple procedure (pancreaticoduodenectomy) is usually needed for head lesions. Total pancreatectomy can be considered for IMPNs with diffuse dysplasia. Central pancreatectomy can be performed for body lesions, particularly at the neck, with pancreaticoenteric reconstruction. A variety of limited pancreatectomies have been proposed, but there are no long-term data verifying the efficacy of these procedures. In past years, it was recommended that all cystic neoplasms be resected due to the difficulty in predicting which lesions were malignant. At present, given the large number of tumors that are incidental findings and studies that have demonstrated that many tumors have a very low malignant potential, other treatment strategies need to be considered at times.

SEROUS NEOPLASMS

Surgical treatment is not indicated for serous neoplasms unless the patient has obstructive symptoms or symptoms from local compression of surrounding structures. Acceptable growth of serous neoplasms is approximately 0.6 cm per year. Larger tumors that are more than 4 cm in size may increase as much as 2 cm per year and start to cause local symptoms. Therefore, in excellent surgical candidates without significant comorbidities, surgical resection is a reasonable option for tumors that are 4 cm or greater.[12]

MUCINOUS NEOPLASMS

All MCNs must be considered premalignant and can undergo malignant transformation at any time. Their progression toward malignancy is thought to mirror that of pancreatic intraepithelial neoplasia, albeit at a much more indolent rate. Therefore, the general recommendation is to resect all mucinous tumors, given the patient is an acceptable surgical risk. Because more than 90% of mucinous neoplasms are found in the body or tail of the pancreas, a distal pancreatectomy is the usual treatment, with intraoperative frozen section of the pancreatic margin. Cameron and colleagues[34] report that a laparoscopic pancreatectomy is appropriate if there is a low risk of invasive cancer, the cyst is small (<3 cm), and there is no evidence of mural nodules or calcifications. The authors have found laparoscopic distal pancreatectomy with or without splenectomy safe and acceptable for these lesions.

INTRADUCTAL PAPILLARY MUCINOUS NEOPLASMS

Because the main duct variant of IPMNs has a much greater tendency to become malignant, a more aggressive surgical approach is indicated. In general, all main duct IPMNs should be resected. A pancreaticoduodenectomy or distal pancreatectomy is the proper treatment based on tumor location. A total pancreatectomy should be avoided because recurrence rates are similar to partial resection,[18,35,36] and it carries the additional risk of endocrine and exocrine insufficiency. In high risk surgical patients, if other predictors of malignancy are not present, the main pancreatic duct is smaller than 15 mm, and there are no visible mural nodules on either CT or EUS, observation may be a better choice for treatment. On the other hand, smaller branch type IPMNs may lend themselves to duodenum sparing resection, uncinatectomy, or conservative/observational therapy. In 2006, the International Association of Pancreatology published revised guidelines for the management of IPMNs in which they listed the following indications for surgery: (1) main pancreatic duct type IPMN (includes mixed type tumors); (2) branch duct IPMNs with cyst diameters of over 30 mm or cyst diameter of 10 to 30 mm with a mural nodule; (3) IPMNs with a dilated main pancreatic duct; and (4) cytology-positive IPMN.[11,34]

Multiple studies have evaluated conservative treatment of smaller branch duct tumors. Most agree that close observation is appropriate for branch duct IPMNs smaller than 30 mm, without symptoms, suspicious radiologic findings, or mural nodules. Simple increase in size of cyst is not a reliable predictor of malignancy.[25] Small branch duct lesions rarely progress to invasive disease (0%–5%).[34] If conservative management is chosen, resection should be performed as soon as there is evidence of progression such as progressive growth, new symptoms, new intramural nodules, cyst size greater than 30 mm, or dilation of main pancreatic duct to greater than 6 mm.

FROZEN SECTIONS

Intraoperative frozen sections are not usually necessary with MCNs, as they usually have discernible borders and microscopic extension is not likely. Frozen sections can be used to rule out invasive cancer if the margins are firm and abnormal appearing. On the other hand, frozen sections are recommended during the resection of IPMNs. In the case of IPMNs, microscopic extension beyond visible disease is common. In addition, IPMNs are frequently multiple and can be spread throughout pancreas in a noncontiguous fashion. Tanaka and colleagues[11] published these guidelines for treatment of positive margins on frozen section: (1) IPM adenoma—no further resection due to minimal risk of progression; (2) IPMN with borderline atypia—further resection if feasible; and (3) IPMN with carcinoma in situ or invasive cancer—complete resection whenever feasible.

FOLLOW-UP

Resection of a serous neoplasm should be 100% curative, so long-term follow-up is not necessary. After resection, a benign MCN should similarly have zero risk of recurrence and requires no follow-up. A resected, malignant MCN has a much higher risk of recurrence and should therefore be followed every 6 months using CT or MRI.

Resected, benign IPMNs carry a small risk of recurrence and should be followed yearly with CT or MRI. This follow-up interval can be spaced out to longer periods if nothing is found over a time span of several years. On the other hand, resected, malignant IPMNs carry a very significant risk of recurrence and need to be reevaluated every 6 months with radiologic imaging. CEA and CA19-9 levels have had no proven value in the follow-up of IPMNs.

Branch duct IPMNs that have not been resected should be followed very closely. For lesions between 10 and 20 mm, CT or MRI should be obtained every 6 to 12 months. For cystic lesions larger than 20 mm, radiologic imaging should be evaluated every 3 to 6 months.[11] In addition, on each occasion patients should be reassessed for any symptoms that can be attributed to the tumor.

Given the high rate of synchronous extrapancreatic tumors in patients with IPMNs, care should be taken to screen these patients for other malignant neoplasms on a periodic basis.

PROGNOSIS

The prognosis for cystic pancreatic neoplasms is much better than ductal pancreatic adenocarcinoma, for which 5-year survival rates are 20% to 25% in the most optimistic studies. Serous neoplasms are not malignant and therefore have a 100% 5-year survival rate. Benign MCNs and benign IPMNs have a 95% to 100% 5-year survival rate, with benign MCNs having a recurrence risk of near zero. Multiple investigators have agreed that survival rate for a malignant IPMN is between 60% and 70%.[10,22,34,37–42] The worst prognosis is for malignant MCNs, which have a 5-year predicted survival rate of 50% to 60%.[43,44]

ACKNOWLEDGMENTS

All CT and MRI scans are courtesy of Dr Francis Scholz, Lahey Clinic.

REFERENCES

1. Becourt PJ. Recherches sur le pancreas: ses foncions et ses alterations organiques. Strasbourg, France: Levrault; 1830.
2. Compagno J, Oertel JE. Mucinous cystic neoplasms of the pancreas with overt and latent malignancy (cystadenocarcinoma and cystadenoma). A clinicopathologic study of 41 cases. Am J Clin Pathol 1980;74(1):1–11.
3. Ohashi K, Mirukami Y, Muruyama M, et al. Four cases of mucus secreting pancreas cancer. Prog Dig Endosc 1982;20:348–51.
4. Kimura W, Nagai H, Kuroda A, et al. Analysis of small cystic lesions of the pancreas. Int J Pancreatol 1995;18:197–206.
5. Ferrone CR, Correa-Gallego C, Warshaw AL, et al. Current trends in pancreatic cystic neoplasms. Arch Surg 2009;144(5):448–54.
6. Sand J, Nordback I. The differentiation between pancreatic neoplastic cysts and pancreatic pseudocyst. Scand J Surg 2005;94:161–4.
7. Hernandez LV, Mishra G, Forsmark C, et al. Role of endoscopic ultrasound (EUS) and EUS-guided fine needle aspiration in the diagnosis and treatment of cystic lesions of the pancreas. Pancreas 2002;25:222–8.

8. Ahmad NA, Kochman ML, Lewis JD, et al. Can EUS alone differentiate between malignant and benign cystic lesion of the pancreas? Am J Gastroenterol 2001;96: 3295–300.

9. Macari M, Finn ME, Bennett GL, et al. Differentiating pancreatic cystic neoplasms from pancreatic pseudocysts at MR imaging: value of perceived internal debris. Radiology 2009;251:77–84.

10. Kloppel G, Solcia E, Longnecker DS, et al. Histological typing of tumors of the exocrine pancreas. In: World Health Organization. International histological classification of tumors. 2nd edition. Berlin: Springer; 1996. p. 15–21.

11. Tanaka M, Chari S, Adsay V, et al. International consensus guidelines for management of intraductal papillary mucinous neoplasms and mucinous cystic neoplasms of the pancreas. Pancreatology 2006;6:17–32.

12. Phillips K, Fleming JB, Tamm EP, et al. Unusual pancreatic tumors. In: Cameron JL, editor. Current surgical therapy. 9th edition. Philadelphia: Moby Elsevier; 2008. p. 524–9.

13. Klug JC, Ng TT, White SC, et al. Pancreatic serous cystadenocarcinoma: a case report and review of the literature. J Gastrointest Surg 2009;13:1864–8.

14. George DH, Murphy F, Michalski R, et al. Serous cystadenocarcinoma of the pancreas: a new entity? Am J Surg Pathol 1989;13:61–6.

15. Kamei K, Funabiki T, Ochiai M, et al. Multifocal pancreatic serous cystadenoma with atypical cells and focal perineural invasion. Int J Pancreatol 1991;10: 161–72.

16. Eriguchi N, Aoyagi S, Nakayama T, et al. Serous cystadenocarcinoma of the pancreas with liver metastases. J Hepatobiliary Pancreat Surg 1998;383:56–61.

17. Garcea G, Ong SL, Rajesh A, et al. Cystic lesions of the pancreas: a diagnostic and management dilemma. Pancreatology 2008;8:236–51.

18. Fritz S, Warshaw AL, Thayer S. Management of mucin-producing cystic neoplasms of the pancreas. Oncologist 2009;14(2):125–36.

19. Warshaw AL, Compton CC, Lewandrowski K, et al. Cystic tumors of the pancreas—new clinical, radiologic, and pathologic observations in 67 patients. Ann Surg 1990;212(4):432–43.

20. Volkan Adsay N. Cystic lesions of the pancreas. Mod Pathol 2007;20(Suppl 1): S71–93.

21. Woodside KJ, Riall TS. Intraductal papillary mucinous neoplasms of the pancreas. In: Cameron JL, editor. Current surgical therapy. 9th edition. Philadelphia: Moby Elsevier; 2008. p. 530–4.

22. Salvia R, Fernandez-del Castillo C, Bassi C, et al. Main-duct intraductal papillary mucinous neoplasms of the pancreas: clinical predictors of malignancy and long-term survival following resection. Ann Surg 2004;239:678–85 [discussion: 685–7].

23. Sohn TA, Yeo CH, Cameron JL, et al. Intraductal papillary mucinous neoplasms of the pancreas: an updated experience. Ann Surg 2004;239:788–97 [discussion: 797–9].

24. D'Angelica M, Brennan MF, Suriawinata AA, et al. Intraductal papillary mucinous neoplasms of the pancreas: an analysis of clinicopahtologic features and outcome. Ann Surg 2004;239:400–8.

25. Woo SM, Ryu JK, Lee SH, et al. Branch duct intraductal papillary mucinous neoplasms in a retrospective series of 190 patients. Br J Surg 2009;96:405–11.

26. Fujino Y, Matsumoto I, Ueda T, et al. Proposed new score predicting malignancy of intraductal papillary mucinous neoplasms of the pancreas. Am J Surg 2007; 194:304–7.

27. Yamaguchi K, Yokohata K, Noshiro H, et al. Mucinous cystic neoplasm of the pancreas or intraductal papillary-mucinous tumour of the pancreas. Eur J Surg 2000;166:141–8.
28. Eguchi H, Ishikawa O, Ohigashi H, et al. Patients with pancreatic intraductal papillary mucinous neoplasms are at high risk of colorectal cancer development. Surgery 2006;139:749–54.
29. Kubo H, Chijiiwa Y, Akahoshi K, et al. Intraductal papillary-mucinous tumors of the pancreas: differential diagnosis between benign and malignant tumors by endoscopic ultrasonography. Am J Gastroenterol 2001;96:1429–34.
30. Sugiyama M, Atomi Y. Intraductal papillary mucinous tumors of the pancreas: imaging studies and treatment strategies. Ann Surg 1998;228:684–91.
31. Ohno E, Hirooka Y, Itoh A, et al. Intraductal papillary mucinous neoplasms of the pancreas: differentiation of malignant and benign tumors by endoscopic ultrasound findings of mural nodules. Ann Surg 2009;249:628–34.
32. Sawhney MS, Devarajan S, O'Farrel P, et al. Comparison of carcinoembryonic antigen and molecular analysis in pancreatic cyst fluid. Gastrointest Endosc 2009;69:1106–10.
33. Fritz S, Fernandez-del Castillo C, Mino-Kenudson M, et al. Global genomic analysis of intraductal papillary mucinous neoplasms of the pancreas reveals significant molecular differences compared with ductal adenocarcinoma. Ann Surg 2009;249:440–7.
34. Cameron JL, Riall TS, Coleman J, et al. One thousand consecutive pancreaticoduodenectomies. Ann Surg 2006;244:10–5.
35. Jang JY, Kim SW, Ahn YJ, et al. Multicenter analysis of clinicopathologic features of intraductal papillary mucinous tumor of the pancreas: is it possible to predict the malignancy before surgery? Ann Surg Oncol 2005;12:124–32.
36. Maire F, Hammel P, Terris B, et al. Prognosis of malignant intraductal papillary mucinous tumours of the pancreas after surgical resection. Comparison with pancreatic ductal adenocarcinoma. Gut 2002;51:717–22.
37. Yamao K, Nakamura T, Suzuki T, et al. Endoscopic diagnosis and staging of mucinous cystic neoplasms and intraductal papillary-mucinous tumors. J Hepatobiliary Pancreat Surg 2003;10:142–6.
38. Brugge WR, Lewandrowski K, Lee-Lewandrowski E, et al. Diagnosis of pancreatic cystic neoplasms: a report of the cooperative pancreatic cyst study. Gastroenterology 2004;126:1330–6.
39. Allen PJ, Jaques DP, D'Angelica M, et al. Cystic lesions of the pancreas: selection criteria for operative and nonoperative management in 109 patients. J Gastrointest Surg 2003;7:970–7.
40. Izumo A, Yamaguchi K, Eguchi T, et al. Mucinous cystic tumor of the pancreas: immunohistochemical assessment of "ovarian-type stroma". Oncol Rep 2003;10:515–25.
41. Sarr MG, Carpenter HA, Praghaka LP, et al. Clinical and pathologic correlation of 84 mucinous cystic neoplasms of the pancreas: can one reliably differentiate benign from malignant (or premalignant) neoplasms? Ann Surg 2000;231:205–12.
42. Wilentz RE, Albores-Saavedra J, Zahurak M, et al. Pathologic examination accurately predicts prognosis in mucinous cystic neoplasms of the pancreas. Am J Surg Pathol 1999;23:1320–7.
43. Hruban RH, Takaori K, Klimstra DS, et al. An illustrated consensus on the classification of pancreatic intraepithelial neoplasia and intraductal papillary mucinous neoplasms. Am J Surg Pathol 2004;28:977–87.
44. Wilentz RE, Albores-Saavedra J, Hruban RH. Mucinous cystic neoplasms of the pancreas. Semin Diagn Pathol 2000;17:31–42.

Laparoscopic Management of Pancreatic Malignancies

David A. Kooby, MD[a],*, Carrie K. Chu, MD[b]

KEYWORDS

- Minimally invasive surgery • Pancreas • Laparoscopic
- Enucleation • pancreaticoduodenectomy
- Distal pancreatectomy

Since the results of the COST trial, the role of minimally invasive surgery (MIS) has grown dramatically in the management of abdominal malignancies.[1] MIS for pancreatic resection has progressed slowly compared with applications of laparoscopy in other organs such as the colon, adrenal glands, kidneys, and liver, for several reasons: the pancreas is in a retroperitoneal location surrounded by large vessels and other crucial structures, making it less accessible to the laparoscopic approach; the organ itself can be unforgiving if mishandled; many pancreatic tumors are located in the head of the gland require pancreaticoduodenectomy (PD), which remains difficult to perform laparoscopically; pancreatic adenocarcinoma is an aggressive malignancy that may not be appropriate for laparoscopic management; and many pancreatic surgeons were not traditionally exposed to MIS during their training and have been slower to adopt these methods.

Early pioneers in laparoscopic pancreatic surgery first used MIS to diagnose and stage pancreatic cancers.[2–4] Currently, some centers routinely perform diagnostic laparoscopy before opening patients for pancreatic cancer to identify occult metastases not confirmed by preoperative imaging.[5–7] This approach is geared toward preventing unnecessary laparotomy, thereby expediting transition to palliative chemotherapy. Other investigators have used laparoscopic techniques to bypass intestinal and biliary obstructions in patients with pancreatic tumors.[8–10]

More recently, the number of pancreatic resections being performed laparoscopically has increased substantially.[11] Recent data support improved perioperative

Funding: Supported by the Georgia Cancer Coalition.
[a] Division of Surgical Oncology, Department of Surgery, Emory University School of Medicine and the Winship Cancer Institute, 1365C Clifton Road, NE, 2nd Floor, Atlanta, GA 30322, USA
[b] Department of Surgery, Emory University School of Medicine, 1364 Clifton Road, NE, H120, Atlanta, GA 30322, USA
* Corresponding author.
E-mail address: dkooby@emory.edu

outcomes following laparoscopic compared with open distal (left) pancreatectomy, with similar incidence in pancreatic fistula, with shorter hospital stays.[12] As a result, this approach is becoming standard at many centers. Increasing series of pancreaticoduodenectomies,[13–15] enucleations,[16–19] and central pancreatic resections[20] are also appearing in the literature.

Data concerning cancer outcomes (adequacy of resection and survival) for laparoscopic resection of pancreatic malignancies remain limited. All existing reports addressing laparoscopic resection of pancreatic cancer are retrospective and small, making this area of exploration almost uncharted. This article examines existing data for laparoscopic management of pancreatic malignancies. Areas discussed are the common procedures being performed, tumor biology as it pertains to laparoscopic pancreatectomy, short-term cancer outcomes such as adequacy of tumor margins and node dissection, and long-term cancer survival.

DIAGNOSIS AND STAGING

Early reports of MIS for pancreatic cancers focused on staging.[2–4] A report from Warshaw and colleagues[3] demonstrated that diagnostic laparoscopy before exploration for pancreatic adenocarcinoma helped identify radiologically occult metastatic disease in 35% of the 40 patients studied. More recently, with the use of pancreatic protocol helical computerized tomography (CT) imaging with fine cuts, the diagnostic yield of staging laparoscopy before open resection of pancreatic cancer is at 5% to 15%,[21] and other groups have limited the application of staging laparoscopy to high-risk cases: patients with CT scans with indeterminate liver lesions, patients with high preoperative CA19-9 serum levels, and patients in marginal health for pancreatectomy.[22,23]

Another aspect of staging is that of vascular tumor involvement and local resectability. Diagnostic laparoscopy can be used to assess this issue, and a few reports have examined this approach.[22,24] Borderline tumors can be assessed laparoscopically with the addition of intraoperative laparoscopic ultrasonography,[25–27] but no comparative data exist describing the advantages of this approach over that of staging CT. The authors find that laparoscopic ultrasonography to assess vascular involvement provides little benefit over dedicated pancreatic protocol CT.

Potentially more challenging than staging is the issue of diagnosis. A tissue diagnosis is required in cases for which preoperative or palliative chemotherapy is being considered. For patients without obvious distant metastases, the pancreatic primary is the target for biopsy. The options for tissue acquisition include endoscopic retrograde cholangiopancreatography (ERCP), image-guided fine needle aspirate (FNA), or endoscopic ultrasonography (EUS) FNA. Based on the existing literature, EUS-FNA is the most reliable and accurate method of obtaining tissue.[28,29]

PALLIATION

Patients with unresectable pancreatic cancer are subject to gastrointestinal and biliary obstruction, both of which can be managed laparoscopically. Some small series have compared the laparoscopic and open approaches to gastrojejunostomy.[8,30] The most recent compared 10 laparoscopic with 10 open procedures. Despite the 5-day difference in hospital stay (8 vs 14 days, $P = .14$), the result was not statistically different given the small sample size.[8] The largest series of 26 cases of palliative laparoscopic biliary bypasses included benign and malignant disease. The average hospital stay was 12.6 ($\pm$11.5) days, and the major complication rate was 23%, making the value of this approach questionable. Currently, the combination of ERCP-placed biliary stent with endoscopically placed duodenal stent obviates the need for the laparoscopic approaches, and most patients can be managed without general anesthetic and laparoscopy in the palliative setting.[7] Another recently described palliative procedure is the laparoscopic celiac plexus block.[31] The procedure is well described within the report, and patients may derive a substantial pain-control benefit at the same setting as the diagnostic laparoscopy; however, the success of this approach is unclear, as percutaneous methods are now standard and no comparison with the laparoscopic approach has been performed.

RESECTIONS

In this section the 3 most common types of pancreatic resections performed for neoplastic disease (distal pancreatectomy, tumor enucleation, and PD) are discussed with respect to perioperative outcomes. Particular attention is given to distal (left) pancreatectomy, as this is the most thoroughly evaluated procedure. If available, data comparing the laparoscopic and open approaches are highlighted. Some common variations of these procedures are also reviewed.

Distal (Left) Pancreatectomy

Distal (left) pancreatectomy is the most commonly performed laparoscopic pancreatic resection. The earliest descriptions of this procedure were by Sussman and collegues.[32] They used an ultrasound probe to localize an insulinoma and a linear surgical staple to divide the pancreas. Later that year, Gagner and colleagues[33] published a report describing 8 laparoscopic distal pancreatectomies for islet cell tumors. A few small reports and 1 large multicenter experience from Europe were subsequently published demonstrating the feasibility of this approach, but it was nearly a decade before larger series were published showing comparative perioperative results with open distal pancreatectomy (**Table 1**).

The steps of laparoscopic distal pancreatectomy are described in detail elsewhere.[11] Common variations include the hand-access approach versus the straight laparoscopic method, spleen preserving with or without splenic vessel preservation versus splenopancreatectomy, and the radical antegrade modular pancreatectomy described by Strasberg and colleagues[42] geared at obtaining improved radial resection margins, which can also be performed laparoscopically.

Splenic preservation

When anatomically and biologically possible, splenic preservation during left pancreatectomy has been shown to be associated with reduced postoperative overall and infectious complications.[43] The proportion of cases with splenic preservation is greater for those patients having laparoscopic distal pancreatectomy than for those having open resections in the 2 largest comparative series to date (40.8% vs 5.7% and 30% vs 12%).[12,44] Proponents of the laparoscopic approach support improved visualization of the lesser sac and retropancreatic space as provided by angled cameras, and some have attributed the increased rates of splenic preservation to this and the inherent magnification associated with laparoscopy.

Spleen-preserving distal pancreatectomy can be a tedious procedure in which division of the numerous small arterial and venous connections between the pancreas and the splenic vessels is performed. In 1988, Warshaw[45] described a more expedient technique of splenic preservation in which the splenic vessels are ligated and divided at the pancreatic transection line and at the splenic hilum. In this approach, splenic viability is maintained via the short gastric vessels. Splenic infarction and gastric variceal hemorrhage are concerns of using this approach.

Table 1
Reported published reports of laparoscopic left (distal) pancreatectomy including 25 or more cases

Study	Cases	Multi-Institutional	Mean Operative Time (min)	Mean Blood Loss (mL)	Mean Length of Stay (d)	Conversion Rate (%)	Splenic Preservation (%)	Overall Morbidity (%)	Pancreatic Fistula Rate (%)	Mortality (%)
Park et al 2002[34]	25	Yes	222	274	4	8	48	16	4	0
Mabrut et al 2005[35]	96	Yes	200[a,c] 195[b,c]	NR	7	10	71	53	16	0
Melotti et al 2007[36]	58	Yes	165[c]	NR	9[c]	0	55	53	27.5	0
Eom et al 2008[37]	31	No	218	NR	11.5	0	42	36	10	0
Fernandez-Cruz et al 2007[38]	82	No	NR	NR	7[c]	7	64	20	9	0
Taylor et al 2008[39]	46	Yes	157[c]	200[c]	7[c]	26	48	39	15	0
Laxa et al 2008[40]	32	Yes	238	221	5	6	19	34	19	0
Sa Cunha et al 2008[41]	31	No	200[a,c] 246[b,c]	100[c,d]	12.7[d]	19	80	31[d]	20[a] 45[b]	0
Kooby et al 2008[12]	167	Yes	230	357	5.9	13	31	40	11	0

Abbreviation: NR, not reported.
[a] With splenic preservation.
[b] With splenectomy.
[c] Median reported rather than mean.
[d] Reported for all laparoscopic pancreatic resections in series, not individually reported for laparoscopic left pancreatectomy.

Long-term studies evaluating splenic function after sacrifice of the splenic vessels and value of splenic preservation are lacking, and no data exist elucidating the effect of spleen preservation in cases of pancreatic malignancy. One study from Fernandez-Cruz and colleagues[38] in Barcelona addresses perioperative outcomes for a large number of patients who underwent laparoscopic pancreatic resections. Of these, 82 had distal pancreatectomy and 52 had their spleens preserved with or without splenic vessel preservation. Overall complications were higher in the splenic preservation group (25.2% vs 16.7%, $P<.05$) primarily due to splenic infarction, particularly in those cases in which the splenic vessels were sacrificed. In the absence of level 1 data demonstrating a particular benefit, spleen preservation can be considered a matter of surgical preference. It is not recommended in cases of suspected or confirmed adenocarcinoma of the pancreatic body/tail, or in the case of pancreatic endocrine tumors in which the splenic vessels are involved.

Laparoscopic management of the pancreatic stump and perioperative complications

One of the ongoing debates regarding MIS pancreatic resection is that of pancreatic stump control after laparoscopic distal pancreatectomy. Pancreatic fistula is a common and potentially devastating complication following distal pancreatectomy, and detractors of the laparoscopic approach question the ability to seal the pancreatic stump adequately via the laparoscope. Clinical manifestations of postoperative pancreatic fistula range from asymptomatic amylase-rich fluid in surgical drains to life-threatening sepsis requiring reoperation as defined by the International Study Group on Pancreatic Fistula Definition (ISGPF).[46] In open distal pancreatectomy, the fistula rate ranges between 5% and 18%.[12,47,48] Management of the pancreatic stump, the presumed source of leak after left pancreatectomy, has therefore received much attention, with varied proponents of main duct suture ligation, oversewing of the pancreatic stump, linear stapled closure with or without staple-line reinforcement, electrocautery, ultrasound coagulation, radiofrequency, omental patch, fibrin glue application, enteric anastomosis, octreotide administration, or various combinations of the listed techniques.

Studies comparing these techniques provide mixed results, with some analyses identifying reduced fistula rates after stapling,[49] some reporting more favorable results using hand suturing,[48] and still others showing no difference between the 2 methods.[50] The multi-institutional DISPACT trial, an ongoing randomized controlled study, aims to compare hand-sewn and stapled techniques in left pancreatectomy.[51] Still other investigators have evaluated the usefulness of staple-line reinforcement. A recent series of patients who had transection with staple-line reinforcement (n = 29) compared with patients who did not (n = 23) suggested an 84% reduction in pancreatic fistula when reinforcement was used ($P = .04$).[52] However, another retrospective institutional assessment found no difference in rate of fistula formation after stapled transection with (n = 45) or without (n = 41) staple-line reinforcement (33% vs 24%, $P>.05$).[53]

Perhaps more important than the method of transection is the identification and selective suture ligation of the main pancreatic duct; in an analysis of 126 patients over a span of 9 years, fistula rates were 9.6% in the 74 cases of duct ligation and 34% in the 53 cases without duct ligation ($P<.001$). Absence of selective ligation was the only clinicopathologic and operative factor that maintained association with increased risk of pancreatic fistula development (odds ratio 5.0, 95% confidence interval 2.0–10.0).[54] Some have suggested that selective ligation may be more difficult to achieve during laparoscopic resection, and may therefore contribute to increased fistula rates.[35]

Comparison of the open and laparoscopic approaches has not shown increased rates of fistula formation after laparoscopic resection. In the largest published study of laparoscopic and open left pancreatectomy, 142 laparoscopic and 200 case-matched open cases were compared; similar overall fistula rates were reported (26% laparoscopic vs 32% open, $P = .28$). When only clinically significant fistula were considered (ISGPF grades B/C), there was a nonsignificant trend toward increased fistula formation in open pancreatectomy (11% laparoscopic vs 18% open, $P = .01$).[12] Comparison analyses between laparoscopic and open left pancreatectomy are summarized in **Table 2**.

Review of trends from comparison studies between laparoscopic and open left pancreatectomy reveals that, despite equivalent or somewhat increased operative time, the laparoscopic technique is associated with a reduction in blood loss and postoperative length of stay. Overall perioperative morbidity and mortality seem similar with both approaches. These existing data suggest that, compared with the open approach, laparoscopic left pancreatectomy is feasible and safe, and may be associated with reduced blood loss, shorter hospital length of stay, reduced postoperative pain, and greater likelihood of splenic preservation.

The Central Pancreas Consortium (CPC) evaluated 219 consecutive laparoscopic distal pancreatectomies performed over an 8-year span at 9 specialized pancreatic surgical centers and devised a clinical risk score for predicting which patients were likely to suffer complications after laparoscopic distal pancreatectomy.[60] Major complications were seen in 11% of this cohort and 10% had type B/C pancreatic fistulae. Factors identified for importance in predicting these adverse events were patient body mass index greater than 27, pancreatic specimen length greater than 8 cm, and operative blood loss greater than 150 mL. This information is helpful in counseling patients before surgery.

Pancreatic Enucleation

Technical considerations
Some benign lesions and low-grade malignancies of the pancreas may be suitable for enucleation. In this approach, the lesion is shelled out and the surrounding pancreatic parenchyma is preserved. Key elements of consideration are tumor size, biology, and location with respect to the main pancreatic duct. Smaller, encapsulated tumors with indolent behavior (such as insulinoma), located away from the main duct, are ideal for this approach.

The first reports of laparoscopic pancreatic enucleation were published by Amikura and colleagues[61] in 1995 for treatment of an adrenocorticotropic hormone-producing pancreatic tumor and Gagner and colleagues[33] in 1996 for insulinoma. Since then, several small series have been published, mostly reporting on solitary insulinomas, the most commonly occurring functional pancreatic neuroendocrine tumor (**Table 3**).[27,38,45–53] Typically, the technique is applied to lesions in the body and tail, although superficial tumors of the anterior head and neck have also been successfully enucleated.[16,63,66] The technique is described elsewhere.[69]

As with left pancreatectomy, pancreatic fistula formation is a concern. Several methods for managing the tumor resection bed are described. Oversewing, omental patching, cauterization, and fibrin application are all reported, sometimes in combination with prophylactic octreotide administration.[16,63] Despite these maneuvers, rates of fistula formation after laparoscopic enucleation range from 0% to 78% (see **Table 3**). In one of the largest reported series of laparoscopic enucleation for

Table 2
Comparisons of laparoscopic and open left (distal) pancreatectomy

Study	Cases		Mean Operative Time (min)		Mean Blood Loss (mL)		Splenic Preservation (%)		Mean Length of Stay (d)		Overall Morbidity (%)		Fistula Rate (%)		Mortality (%)	
	LLP	OLP	LLP	OLP	LLP	OLP	LLP	OLP	LLP	OLP	LLP	OLP	LLP	OLP	LLP	OLP
Velanovich 2006[a,55]	15	15	NR	NR	NR	NR	0	0	5.0[b]	8.0[b]	20	27	13	13	0	0
Misawa et al 2007[56]	8	9	255[b]	205[b]	14[b]	307[b]	12.5	0	10.0[b]	16.0[b]	NR	NR	0	22	0	0
Teh et al 2007[57]	12	16	278	212	193	609	62	17	6.2	10.6	17	56	8	6	0	0
Eom et al 2008[a,37]	31	62	218	195	NR	NR	42	NR	11.5	13.5	36	24	9.7	6.5	0	0
Kim et al 2008[44]	93	35	195[b]	190[b]	110	110	40.8	5.7	10[b]	16[b]	25	29	8.6	14.3	0	0
Matsumoto et al 2008[58]	14	19	291	213	247	400	7	NR	12.9	23.8	NR	NR	0	10.5	0	0
Kooby et al 2008[a,12]	142	200	230	216	357	588	30	12	5.9	9.0	40	57	11	18	0	1
Nakamura et al 2009[59]	21	16	308	282	249	714	35	31	10.0	25.8	0	19	0	12.5	0	0

Abbreviations: LLP, laparoscopic left pancreatectomy; OLP, open left pancreatectomy; NR, not reported.
[a] Case-controlled series.
[b] Median reported rather than mean.

Table 3
Recent published series describing successful laparoscopic enucleation of pancreatic tumors

Study	Cases	Pathology	Conversion Rate (%)	Mean Tumor Size (cm)	Tumor Location	Use of Intraoperative Ultrasound (%)	Mean Operative Time (min)	Mean Blood Loss (mL)	Mean Length of Stay (d)	Overall Morbidity (%)	Pancreatic Fistula Rate (%)	Mortality (%)
Patterson et al 2001[62]	4	Islet cell tumors	NR	NR	Body and tail	100	NR	NR	NR	NR	25	0
Ayav et al 2005[63]	19	Insulinomas	10.5	1.5	4 head; 1 isthmus; 9 body; 3 tail	NR	115	NR	NR	NR	42	0
Mabrut et al 2005[35]	22	NR	4.5	NR	NR	NR	120[a]	NR	NR	NR	29	0
Toniato et al 2006[64]	4	Insulinomas	NR	NR	NR	100	NR	NR	NR	NR	NR	0
Liu et al 2007[65]	9	Insulinomas	33.3	1.5[b]	4 body; 2 tail	NR	159[b]	77[b]	11.8[b]	28[b]	17	0
Schraibman et al 2007[18]	5	Insulinomas	0	1.3–2.0	Body and tail	NR	130	Minimal	3	NR	0	0

Sweet et al 2007[17]	9	Insulinomas	22.2	NR	NR	66.7	NR	NR	2.3	NR	77.8	0
Fernandez-Cruz et al 2008[66]	21	15 insulinoma; 6 nonfunctioning PNET	4.8	3.0	4 head; 1 neck; 12 body and tail	NR	120	<220	5.5	42.8	38	0
Roland et al 2008[67]	10	Insulinomas	20	NR	NR	NR	NR	NR	NR	NR	12.5	0
Luo et al 2009[16]	18	Insulinomas	11.1	NR	4 head; 1 uncinate; 2 neck; 9 body	NR	85[a]	255[a]	NR	NR	25	0
Martinez-Isla et al 2009[68]	14	Insulinomas	7.1	NR	4 head; 6 body; 3 tail	NR	NR	NR	NR	NR	7.7	0

Abbreviations: PNET, pancreatic neuroendocrine tumor; NR, not reported or not individually reported for laparoscopic enucleations.
[a] Median reported rather than mean.
[b] Includes 1 case of laparoscopic left pancreatectomy.

pancreatic neuroendocrine tumors, Fernandez-Cruz and colleagues[66] used ISGPF criteria to identify a 38% (8/21) fistula rate, of which half were clinically significant (ISGPF B/C). In contrast, laparoscopic left pancreatectomy resulted in an 8.7% (2/23) fistula rate; neither case was clinically significant (ISGPF A) (P<.001). In a separate analysis evaluating all laparoscopic resections of pancreatic tumors, the same group from Barcelona found that, in addition to increased fistula rates, laparoscopic enucleation was associated with fistulas of greater clinical severity compared with laparoscopic left pancreatectomy.[38] This finding parallels the published experience with open enucleation and left pancreatectomy.[19,70] Comparisons of the various methods of tumor bed management have not shown any definitive superiority.[38,52]

Although conventionally enucleation is reserved for smaller tumors, retrospective series have not identified a significant size cutoff for insulinoma patients successfully undergoing left pancreatectomy versus enucleation.[63] Despite the increased risk for pancreatic fistula formation with enucleation, the degree to which pancreatic complications affect clinical course seems to parallel those occurring after left pancreatectomy; postoperative length of stay after enucleation seems to be shorter than or equivalent to left pancreatectomy.[17,66] Potential advantages in reduced endocrine and exocrine insufficiency associated with minimal removal of unaffected pancreatic parenchyma have only recently been evaluated.[70] Based on existing evidence, laparoscopic enucleation seems to be a feasible and safe technique for management of benign, superficial pancreatic tumors without proximity to ductal and vascular structures. Further prospective studies are necessary to compare associated efficacy and outcome with those of laparoscopic left pancreatectomy and open enucleation in the same subset of pancreatic tumor patients.

Pancreaticoduodenectomy

PD is a more challenging technical endeavor than enucleation or distal pancreatectomy, owing to the complexity of dissection and necessity for reconstruction with several critical anastomoses (intestinal, biliary, and pancreatic). Laparoscopic PD is still in its infancy despite its initial description more than a decade ago.[71] Larger series are emerging reporting margin-negative laparoscopic resections of pancreatic head tumors with seemingly acceptable morbidity (**Table 4**).[13–15,72–74] Detailed descriptions of preferred surgical techniques are available within these reports,[13–15,71] but one main variation lies in the degree to which hand assistance is used during dissection, resection, and subsequent reconstruction.

The earliest series of 2 patients by Gagner and Pomp[71] in 1994 describes use of a right subcostal hand port during initial trocar placement to facilitate retraction, palpation, and dissection. In the report by Dulucq and colleagues,[74] completely laparoscopic resection was performed followed by intracorporeal anastomoses in 6 patients and via small midline laparotomy incisions in 4. Others completed extracorporeal anastomoses after incision extension for specimen removal.[59] In the largest published series by Palanivelu and colleagues,[15] spanning 1998 to 2006, all 45 patients underwent intracorporeal laparoscopic reconstruction. In this series, there were no conversions to open procedure, blood loss was low, operative time was slightly more than 6 hours and mean length of hospital stay was approximately 10 days (see **Table 4**). No other series to date has achieved such excellent outcomes, especially with regard to length of hospital stay.

Before attempting laparoscopic PD, consideration is generally given to patient comorbidities, body habitus, surgical history, suspected pathology, lesion size, and degree of local invasion.[14] Conversion to the open approach is common despite the scrutiny of patient selection, with difficulty of dissection and hemorrhage cited as

Table 4
Recent published series describing successful laparoscopic PD

Study	Cases	Pathology	Conversion Rate (%)	Use Hand-Assist port (%)	Mean Operative Time (min)	Mean Blood Loss (mL)	Mean length of Stay (d)	Pancreatic Fistula Rate (%)	Overall Morbidity (%)	Mortality (%)	Mean Nodes Procured (range)	Positive Margins (%[a])
Gagner, Pomp 1997[71]	10	4 PDAC, 3 AMP, 2 pancreatitis, 1 CC	40	33	510	NR	22.3	17	50	0	7 (3–14)	0
Staudacher 2005[72]	7	2 PNET, 1 PDAC, 1 MM, 3 NR	43	100	416	325	12	0	0	0	26 (16–47)	0
Lu et al 2006[73]	5	4 DA, 1 PNET	NR	100	528	770	NR	20	60	20	NR	NR
Dulucq et al 2006[74]	25	11 PDAC, 4 AMP, 2 DA, 1 PNET, 2 pancreatitis, 1 RCC, 1 SCA	12	41	287	107	16.2	4.5	32	4.5	18 (NR)	0
Palanivelu et al 2007[75]	42	24 AMP, 9 PDAC, 4 MCA, 3 CC, 2 pancreatitis	0	0	370	65	10.2	7.1	NR	2.4	13 (8–21)	0
Pugliese et al 2008[14]	19	6 PDAC, 4 AMP, 2 CC, 1 mesenchymal tumor	32	54	461	180	18	23	37	0	12 (4–22)	0
Cho et al 2009[59]	15	6 mucinous adenoma, 3 MCA, 2 PNET, 1 AMP, 1 PDAC, 1 duodenal plasmacytoma, 1 pancreatic trauma	0	100	338	445	16.4	13	27	0	18.5 (NR)	0

Abbreviations: AMP, ampullary adenocarcinoma/ampullary dysplastic adenoma; CC, cholangiocarcinoma; DA, duodenal adenocarcinoma; MCA, mucinous cystadenocarcinoma; MM, metastatic melanoma; NR, not reported or not individually reported for laparoscopic enucleations; PDAC, pancreatic ductal adenocarcinoma; PNET, pancreatic neuroendocrine tumor; RCC, metastatic renal cell carcinoma; SCA, serous cystadenoma.

[a] For malignant pathology.

the most common causative factors.[14] The series by Palanivelu and colleagues,[15] however, boasts a remarkable 0% conversion rate in 45 procedures performed between 1998 and 2006.

Available evidence thus far does not indicate increased rate of pancreatic fistula development after laparoscopic PD, with reported frequencies ranging between 0% and 23% (see **Table 4**). Overall morbidity rates are described between 0% and 60%, although similarly high complication frequencies are described after open PD.[76] Although immediate perioperative complication data seem comparable to historical data associated with open PD, to our knowledge only 2 studies have attempted direct comparison between the open and laparoscopic approaches. Cho and colleagues[13] examined the outcomes of 15 laparoscopic and 15 open PD patients who were similar in age, sex, American Society of Anesthesia classification, and body mass index. Although statistically significant reductions in use of blood transfusion (0% laparoscopic vs 20% open, $P<.05$) and times of intravenous analgesic administration (1.1±1.0 laparoscopic vs 3.8±1.6 open, $P<.05$) were identified, operative time (338±48 minutes laparoscopic vs 287±117 minutes open), blood loss (445±384 mL laparoscopic vs 552±336 open), days to oral intake (7.7±2.5 days laparoscopic vs 6.7±2.6 days open), and length of stay (16.4±3.7 days laparoscopic vs 15.6±1.3 days open) were all similar. In another unmatched retrospective comparison by Pugliese and colleagues[14] between 13 laparoscopic and 41 open PD, complication rates, time to oral intake, time to ambulation, and length of stay did not differ significantly based on approach. Both studies lack stratification for tumor pathology; thus, oncologic implications of these reports are limited.

Other than cosmetic benefits, the key elements to improved outcome in any laparoscopically performed operation are effect on hospital length of stay and time to functional recovery. Neither metric is well established for patients undergoing laparoscopic PD as yet. Data concerning long-term oncologic outcomes of tumor recurrence and patient survival are not defined. Despite technical feasibility, in the absence of definitive improvements over the open approach, and in light of remaining uncertainties regarding long-term oncologic outcome, caution should be exercised in the assessment of the appropriateness of this operation for individual patients.

TUMOR BIOLOGY

Regardless of incision size or length of hospital stay, ultimate success of an oncologic operation rests on cancer-related long-term survival. This outcome is typically driven by disease biology rather than by treatment variables such as operative approach. More immediate surrogates for oncologic outcome include tumor margins and adequacy of node dissection. Because little data for even these outcomes exist, the targets for laparoscopic pancreatic resection have been mostly benign lesions and those of low malignant potential.

Cystic Pancreatic Neoplasms

Cystic pancreatic neoplasms represent a broad range of tumors that exhibit varying biologic behavior. These lesions present diagnostic and management dilemmas as they range in behavior from completely benign simple cysts, serous cystadenomas, and pseudocysts to potentially premalignant mucinous cystadenomas and intraductal papillary mucinous neoplasms (IPMN), to frankly malignant mucinous cystadenocarcinomas and malignant IPMN. In the absence of a tissue diagnosis, factors prompting resection of cystic pancreatic neoplasms include large tumor size, presence of mural nodules or symptoms, evidence of tumor growth over time, cyst fluid carcinoembryonic antigen level greater than 200 ng/mL, and general patient anxiety.[77–79]

Because cross sectional imaging does not distinguish well between mucin-containing lesions and those with serous fluid, definitive diagnosis usually comes after resection, unless CT-guided or endoscopic ultrasound-guided biopsy is available.[80] Most cystic neoplasms of the pancreas are benign.[81] Even the frankly malignant tumors can be indolent to some extent, and laparoscopic resections via left pancreatectomy, and, less frequently, enucleation, are performed with technical success and acceptable perioperative outcome.[35,38,82] In a multicenter analysis comparing 508 open and 159 laparoscopic left pancreatectomies, cystic lesions comprised 59% of the laparoscopically resected tumors and 46% of the laparotomy tumor group. Lesions involved with conversion were more likely to be solid (50%) than cystic (35%) versus laparoscopically resected cases (36% solid, 56% cystic), although this observation was not statistically significant ($P = .19$).[12]

An issue pertinent to MIS pancreatectomy for neoplasms is that of tumor manipulation and potential rupture, especially in the case of cystic tumors. Existing reports do not suggest that the incidence of tumor rupture is higher with the laparoscopic approach; however, this event may be under-reported. Nodal involvement is generally not a concern for cystic tumors; thus, these lesions represent ideal targets for pancreatic surgeons developing experience with laparoscopic resection.

Neuroendocrine Tumors

A large proportion of pancreatic neoplasms treated with curative intent using laparoscopic techniques are neuroendocrine tumors. In a European study by Mabrut and colleagues[35] evaluating 111 patients who underwent laparoscopic pancreatectomy between 1995 and 2002, 45% had neuroendocrine tumors. In the Spanish series by Fernandez-Cruz and colleagues[38] describing 96 successfully completed laparoscopic pancreatic resections from a single institution, 42% were performed for neuroendocrine tumors. In both studies, insulinomas were the most common subtype resected. Laparoscopic management (left pancreatectomy and enucleation) of insulinomas is a consistently successful application of laparoscopic pancreatic surgery for tumors.[83]

Neuroendocrine cancers often manifest a protracted course, even when metastatic, with patients surviving for years. Potential cure is achievable only with surgical resection. In the Mabrut[35] series, histologic analysis revealed a 16% malignancy rate within laparoscopically resected neuroendocrine tumors, including 2 insulinomas that were presumed preoperatively to be benign. In this series, negative margins were achieved in all malignant cases, with no evidence of recurrence at 7 to 47 months follow-up. However, the limited sample sizes preclude definitive conclusions with regard to survival.

To assess the adequacy of laparoscopic resection for pancreatic neuroendocrine tumors, Fernandez-Cruz and colleagues[66] examined 49 patients with these tumors from their considerable experience with laparoscopic pancreatic resections. After an 8% conversion rate, 23 (51%) laparoscopic left pancreatectomies and 21 (48%) laparoscopic enucleations were completed for neuroendocrine tumors. The perioperative outcomes were in accordance with other studies in the literature. Furthermore, the investigators describe negative surgical resection margins in all malignant lesions, which comprised 25% of nonfunctional, and at least 12% of functional, tumors. Despite some encouraging outcome data including biochemical complete response in nearly all patients with functional tumors, and up to 5-year survival despite distant recurrence in malignant cases, overall conclusions regarding oncologic outcome are still limited by small sample size with heterogeneity of diagnoses.

Pancreatic Ductal Adenocarcinoma

With data supporting the feasibility and safety of laparoscopic pancreatic resections, more surgeons are targeting these techniques toward aggressive malignancies such as pancreatic ductal adenocarcinoma (PDAC). PDAC remains a daunting malignancy with a dismal prognosis. With an estimated 42,470 cases diagnosed in 2009, it is expected that 35,240 deaths will occur.[84] It is unrealistic to assume that laparoscopic resection of pancreatic cancer will result in improved survival, but it may result in better quality of life, shorter hospital stay, and better cosmesis for selected patients. What must be shown is that the change in surgical approach (open to laparoscopic) does not compromise short-term oncologic outcomes such as node retrieval and tumor margin, and ultimately the long-term outcome of patient survival.

To date, 4 studies report cancer-specific survival in cohorts of patients with pure PDAC after laparoscopic resection (**Table 5**). Two of these are published reports and the others are abstracts presented at national surgical societies. The first is from is the study by Fernandez-Cruz and colleagues,[38] in which a subset of 13 patients with adenocarcinoma underwent MIS distal pancreatectomy. Negative margins were achieved in 90% of cases, and median survival was 14 months for these 13 patients.[38] The focus of this report was not to compare outcomes of MIS and open pancreatectomy, but to investigate outcomes among different approaches to MIS distal pancreatectomy and enucleation; thus, only preliminary conclusions regarding cancer outcome can be gleaned from this early report. The second is a feasibility study from Italy, in which MIS PD was attempted in 11 patients with ductal adenocarcinoma, of which 5 were converted to open procedure and overall survival was 18 months, in keeping with what is observed with open PD at many centers.[14] This report is encouraging, but realistic, in that conversion rate was high and the reconstruction was performed via minilaparotomy in almost half the cases.

To date 2 unpublished studies attempt to compare outcomes of MIS distal pancreatectomy for PDAC with those for the open approach. In an abstract presented at the 2009 American Hepato-Pancreat-Biliary Association, investigators from the Mayo Clinic in Rochester, MN, compared cancer results between 10 patients who had laparoscopic distal pancreatectomy with 35 patients who had open surgery.[85] Summary data for this study are provided in **Table 5**. Hospital stay was 1 day less (7 vs 8 days, $P = .05$) and median overall survival was similar between the groups (14.9 vs 14.6 months, $P = .64$). The investigators concluded that the laparoscopic approach seems to provide equivalent oncologic results.

At the 2009 Southern Surgical Society, the Central Pancreas Consortium presented their combined results of more than 200 distal pancreatectomies for PDAC.[86] Twenty-three patients had laparoscopic resections, and results from these cases were compared with those from 70 match controls who underwent open distal pancreatectomy. In this comparison, there were no differences in tumor margins, number of nodes retrieved, and overall survival between the groups (see **Table 5**). Mean hospital stay was shorter (7.4 vs 10.7, $P = .03$) among the laparoscopic group.

Although definitive survival benefits of extended lymphadenectomy during resection of PDAC have not been shown, adequate lymphadenectomy provides useful staging information that in turn influences decisions regarding adjuvant chemotherapy or chemoradiation therapy. In addition, the ratio of positive to procured lymph nodes has been shown to be of prognostic significance.[57,58] Adequacy of lymph node sampling

Table 5
Summary of reports describing at least 3 laparoscopic pancreatic resection for ductal adenocarcinoma, arranged by number of cases performed laparoscopically

Author, Year, References	Cases N (Percent of Total Lap Cases in Series)	Op Type	Conversion	Nodes Assessed	Margin Positive %	Survival (mo)
Kooby et al, 2010[86]	23 (100%)	DP	4 (17%)	14.0 ± 8.6	27%	16
Kooby et al, 2008[12]	16 (10%)	DP	2 (13%)	NA	13%	NA
Fernández-Cruz et al, 2008[38]	13 (16%)	DP	NA	NA	10%	14
Pugliese et al, 2008[14]	11 (58%)	PD	5 (45%)	13 ± 4	0%	18
Dulucq et al, 2006[74]	11 (24%)	PD	NA	18 ± 4	0%	NA
Fisher et al, 2009, abstract[85]	10 (100%)	DP	NA	14	0%	14.9
Palanivelu et al, 2007[15]	9 (36%)	PD	0 (0%)	NA	0%	NA
Taylor et al, 2008[39]	9 (20%)	DP	NA	NA	NA	NA
Melotti et al, 2007[36]	5 (9%)	DP	0 (0%)	NA	0%	NA
Mabrut et al, 2005[35]	4 (3%)	NA	NA	NA	NA	NA
Lebedyev et al, 2004[87]	4 (33%)	DP	NA	NA	NA	NA
Velanovich, 2006[55]	3 (20%)	DP	3 (100%)	NA	NA	NA
Laxa et al, 2008[40]	3 (9%)	DP	NA	NA	NA	NA

Abbreviations: DP, distal (left) pancreatectomy; PD, pancreaticoduodenectomy; NA, data not available.

during laparoscopic resection has been questioned. Mean number of harvested nodes was 14.5 (±3) in the Fernandez-Cruz and colleagues[38] left pancreatectomy series, 18 (±4) in the Dulucq and colleagues[74] laparoscopic PD series, and 14 (±9) in the CPC experience, all of which compare favorably with the large open series.

SUMMARY

There has been impressive growth in the number of reports concerning MIS of the pancreas during the past 5 years. Greater emphasis is being applied to patient outcomes (complications and hospital stay) and cost. Now, with the emergence of noninferior cancer-related data, the time is potentially right for a randomized trial to assess the true value of laparoscopic pancreatectomy for cancer. However, the greatest limitation to a meaningful, properly powered randomized trial assessing the effect of laparoscopic distal pancreatectomy for patients with body and tail adenocarcinoma will be the number of available cases.

If approximately 40,000 cases of pancreatic cancer are diagnosed each year in the United States, and only 25% will be operative candidates for potential cure (approximately 10,000), and only 10% to 15% will be those tumors arising in the body and tail (1000–1500 cases annually), the likelihood of accruing a sufficient number of cases that are amenable to laparoscopic resection is small. It is the author's belief that a trial of this design would be subject to failure from low accrual. Finally, the issue of patient survival is less likely to be related to resection technique than it is to tumor biology and potentially multimodal therapy. Perhaps, with the new retrospective data currently in press, there is enough information to proceed without a randomized trial.

In summary, current data are supportive of the use of laparoscopic distal pancreatectomy and enucleation for the management of indolent pancreatic tumors, and emerging data support the role of laparoscopic distal pancreatectomy for adenocarcinoma. The authors believe that, given the available data, cancer outcomes associated with laparoscopic PD are probably no different from those of the open procedure, but that perioperative improvement must be realized in a large comparative trial before this approach becomes routine.

REFERENCES

1. Clinical Outcomes of Surgical Therapy Study G. A comparison of laparoscopically assisted and open colectomy for colon cancer [comment]. N Engl J Med 2004;350(20):2050–9.
2. Cuschieri A. Laparoscopic surgery of the pancreas. J R Coll Surg Edinb 1994; 39(3):178–84.
3. Warshaw AL, Tepper JE, Shipley WU. Laparoscopy in the staging and planning of therapy for pancreatic cancer. Am J Surg 1986;151(1):76–80.
4. Warshaw AL, Gu ZY, Wittenberg J, et al. Preoperative staging and assessment of resectability of pancreatic cancer. Arch Surg 1990;125(2):230–3.
5. Conlon KC, Dougherty E, Klimstra DS, et al. The value of minimal access surgery in the staging of patients with potentially resectable peripancreatic malignancy. Ann Surg 1996;223(2):134–40.
6. Hochwald SN, Weiser MR, Colleoni R, et al. Laparoscopy predicts metastatic disease and spares laparotomy in selected patients with pancreatic nonfunctioning islet cell tumors. Ann Surg Oncol 2001;8(3):249–53.
7. Shoup M, Winston C, Brennan MF, et al. Is there a role for staging laparoscopy in patients with locally advanced, unresectable pancreatic adenocarcinoma? J Gastrointest Surg 2004;8(8):1068–71.

8. Guzman EA, Dagis A, Bening L, et al. Laparoscopic gastrojejunostomy in patients with obstruction of the gastric outlet secondary to advanced malignancies. Am Surg 2009;75(2):129–32.
9. Ghanem AM, Hamade AM, Sheen AJ, et al. Laparoscopic gastric and biliary bypass: a single-center cohort prospective study. J Laparoendosc Adv Surg Tech A 2006;16(1):21–6.
10. Khan AZ, Miles WF, Singh KK. Initial experience with laparoscopic bypass for upper gastrointestinal malignancy: a new option for palliation of patients with advanced upper gastrointestinal tumors. J Laparoendosc Adv Surg Tech A 2005;15(4):374–8.
11. Kooby DA. Laparoscopic pancreatic resection for cancer. Expert Rev Anticancer Ther 2008;8(10):1597–609.
12. Kooby D, Gillespie T, Bentrem DJ, et al. Left-sided pancreatectomy: a multicenter comparison of laparoscopic and open approaches. Ann Surg 2008;248(3):438–46.
13. Cho A, Yamamoto H, Nagata M, et al. Comparison of laparoscopy-assisted and open pylorus-preserving pancreaticoduodenectomy for periampullary disease. Am J Surg 2009;198(3):445–9.
14. Pugliese R, Scandroglio I, Sansonna F, et al. Laparoscopic pancreaticoduodenectomy: a retrospective review of 19 cases. Surg Laparosc Endosc Percutan Tech 2008;18(1):13–8.
15. Palanivelu C, Jani K, Senthilnathan P, et al. Laparoscopic pancreaticoduodenectomy: technique and outcomes. J Am Coll Surg 2007;205(2):222–30.
16. Luo Y, Liu R, Hu MG, et al. Laparoscopic surgery for pancreatic insulinomas: a single-institution experience of 29 cases. J Gastrointest Surg 2009;13(5):945–50.
17. Sweet MP, Izumisato Y, Way LW, et al. Laparoscopic enucleation of insulinomas. Arch Surg Dec 2007;142(12):1202–4 [discussion: 1205].
18. Schraibman V, Goldenberg A, de Matos Farah JF, et al. Laparoscopic enucleation of pancreatic insulinomas. J Laparoendosc Adv Surg Tech A 2007;17(4):399–401.
19. Crippa S, Bassi C, Salvia R, et al. Enucleation of pancreatic neoplasms. Br J Surg 2007;94(10):1254–9.
20. Sa Cunha A, Rault A, Beau C, et al. Laparoscopic central pancreatectomy: single institution experience of 6 patients. Surgery 2007;142(3):405–9.
21. Pisters PW, Lee JE, Vauthey JN, et al. Laparoscopy in the staging of pancreatic cancer. Br J Surg 2001;88(3):325–37.
22. Mayo SC, Austin DF, Sheppard BC, et al. Evolving preoperative evaluation of patients with pancreatic cancer: does laparoscopy have a role in the current era? J Am Coll Surg 2009;208(1):87–95.
23. Maithel SK, Maloney S, Winston C, et al. Preoperative CA 19-9 and the yield of staging laparoscopy in patients with radiographically resectable pancreatic adenocarcinoma. Ann Surg Oncol 2008;15(12):3512–20.
24. Vollmer CM, Drebin JA, Middleton WD, et al. Utility of staging laparoscopy in subsets of peripancreatic and biliary malignancies. Ann Surg 2002;235(1):1–7.
25. Hann LE, Conlon KC, Dougherty EC, et al. Laparoscopic sonography of peripancreatic tumors: preliminary experience. AJR Am J Roentgenol 1997;169(5):1257–62.
26. Pietrabissa A, Caramella D, Di Candio G, et al. Laparoscopy and laparoscopic ultrasonography for staging pancreatic cancer: critical appraisal. World J Surg 1999;23(10):998–1002 [discussion: 1003].
27. Zhao ZW, He JY, Tan G, et al. Laparoscopy and laparoscopic ultrasonography in judging the resectability of pancreatic head cancer. Hepatobiliary Pancreat Dis Int 2003;2(4):609–11.

28. Jhala NC, Jhala D, Eltoum I, et al. Endoscopic ultrasound-guided fine-needle aspiration biopsy: a powerful tool to obtain samples from small lesions. Cancer 2004;102(4):239–46 [see comment].

29. Chang KJ. State of the art lecture: endoscopic ultrasound (EUS) and FNA in pancreatico-biliary tumors. Endoscopy 2006;38(Suppl 1):S56–60.

30. Bergamaschi R, Marvik R, Thoresen JE, et al. Open versus laparoscopic gastro-jejunostomy for palliation in advanced pancreatic cancer. Surg Laparosc Endosc 1998;8(2):92–6.

31. Strong VE, Dalal KM, Malhotra VT, et al. Initial report of laparoscopic celiac plexus block for pain relief in patients with unresectable pancreatic cancer. J Am Coll Surg 2006;203(1):129–31.

32. Sussman LA, Christie R, Whittle DE. Laparoscopic excision of distal pancreas including insulinoma. Aust New Zeal J Surg 1996;66(6):414–6.

33. Gagner M, Pomp A, Herrera MF. Early experience with laparoscopic resections of islet cell tumors. Surgery 1996;120(6):1051–4.

34. Park AE, Heniford BT. Therapeutic laparoscopy of the pancreas. Ann Surg 2002;236(2):149–58.

35. Mabrut JY, Fernandez-Cruz L, Azagra JS, et al. Laparoscopic pancreatic resection: results of a multicenter European study of 127 patients. Surgery 2005;137(6):597–605.

36. Melotti G, Butturini G, Piccoli M, et al. Laparoscopic distal pancreatectomy: results on a consecutive series of 58 patients. Ann Surg 2007;246(1):77–82.

37. Eom BW, Jang JY, Lee SE, et al. Clinical outcomes compared between laparoscopic and open distal pancreatectomy. Surg Endosc 2007.

38. Fernandez-Cruz L, Cosa R, Blanco L, et al. Curative laparoscopic resection for pancreatic neoplasms: a critical analysis from a single institution. J Gastrointest Surg 2007;11(12):1607–21 [discussion: 1621–2].

39. Taylor C, O'Rourke N, Nathanson L, et al. Laparoscopic distal pancreatectomy: the Brisbane experience of forty-six cases. HPB(Oxford) 2008;10:38–42.

40. Laxa BU, Carbonell AM, Cobb WS, et al. Laparoscopic and hand-assisted distal pancreatectomy. Am Surg 2008;74(6):481–7.

41. Sa Cunha A, Rault A, Beau C, et al. A single-institution prospective study of laparoscopic pancreatic resection. Arch Surg 2008;143(3):289–95 [discussion: 295].

42. Strasberg SM, Drebin JA, Linehan D. Radical antegrade modular pancreatosplenectomy. Surgery 2003;133(5):521–7.

43. Shoup M, Brennan MF, McWhite K, et al. The value of splenic preservation with distal pancreatectomy. Arch Surg 2002;137(2):164–8.

44. Kim SC, Park KT, Hwang JW, et al. Comparative analysis of clinical outcomes for laparoscopic distal pancreatic resection and open distal pancreatic resection at a single institution. Surg Endosc 2008;22(10):2261–8.

45. Warshaw AL. Conservation of the spleen with distal pancreatectomy. Arch Surg 1988;123(5):550–3.

46. Bassi C, Dervenis C, Butturini G, et al. Postoperative pancreatic fistula: an international study group (ISGPF) definition. Surgery 2005;138(1):8–13.

47. Lillemoe KD, Kaushal S, Cameron JL, et al. Distal pancreatectomy: indications and outcomes in 235 patients. Ann Surg 1999;229(5):693–8 [discussion: 698–700].

48. Kleeff J, Diener MK, Z'Graggen K, et al. Distal pancreatectomy: risk factors for surgical failure in 302 consecutive cases. Ann Surg 2007;245(4):573–82.

49. Knaebel HP, Diener MK, Wente MN, et al. Systematic review and meta-analysis of technique for closure of the pancreatic remnant after distal pancreatectomy. Br J Surg 2005;92(5):539–46.

50. Sheehan MK, Beck K, Creech S, et al. Distal pancreatectomy: does the method of closure influence fistula formation? Am Surg 2002;68(3):264–7 [discussion: 267–8].
51. Diener MK, Knaebel HP, Witte ST, et al. DISPACT trial: a randomized controlled trial to compare two different surgical techniques of DIStal PAnCreaTectomy – study rationale and design. Clin Trials 2008;5(5):534–45.
52. Thaker RI, Matthews BD, Linehan DC, et al. Absorbable mesh reinforcement of a stapled pancreatic transection line reduces the leak rate with distal pancreatectomy. J Gastrointest Surg 2007;11(1):59–65.
53. Ferrone CR, Warshaw AL, Rattner DW, et al. Pancreatic fistula rates after 462 distal pancreatectomies: staplers do not decrease fistula rates. J Gastrointest Surg 2008;12(10):1691–7 [discussion: 1697–8].
54. Bilimoria KY, Bentrem DJ, Ko CY, et al. Multimodality therapy for pancreatic cancer in the U.S.: utilization, outcomes, and the effect of hospital volume. Cancer 2007;110(6):1227–34.
55. Velanovich V. Case-control comparison of laparoscopic versus open distal pancreatectomy. J Gastrointest Surg 2006;10(1):95–8.
56. Misawa T, Shiba H, Usuba T, et al. Systemic inflammatory response syndrome after hand-assisted laparoscopic distal pancreatectomy. Surg Endosc 2007; 21(8):1446–9.
57. Teh SH, Tseng D, Sheppard BC. Laparoscopic and open distal pancreatic resection for benign pancreatic disease. J Gastrointest Surg 2007;11(9):1120–5.
58. Matsumoto T, Shibata K, Ohta M, et al. Laparoscopic distal pancreatectomy and open distal pancreatectomy: a nonrandomized comparative study. Surg Laparosc Endosc Percutan Tech 2008;18(4):340–3.
59. Nakamura Y, Uchida E, Aimoto T, et al. Clinical outcome of laparoscopic distal pancreatectomy. J Hepatobiliary Pancreat Surg 2009;16(1):35–41.
60. Weber S, Cho C, Merchant N, et al. Laparoscopic left pancreatectomy: complication risk score correlates with morbidity and risk for pancreatic fistula. Ann Surg Oncol 2009;16(10):2825–33 2009 Jul 2816.
61. Amikura K, Alexander HR, Norton JA, et al. Role of surgery in management of adrenocorticotropic hormone-producing islet cell tumors of the pancreas. Surgery 1995;118(6):1125–30.
62. Patterson EJ, Gagner M, Salky B, et al. Laparoscopic pancreatic resection: single-institution experience of 19 patients. J Am Coll Surg 2001;193(3):281–7.
63. Ayav A, Bresler L, Brunaud L, et al. Laparoscopic approach for solitary insulinoma: a multicentre study. Langenbecks Arch Surg 2005;390(2):134–40.
64. Toniato A, Meduri F, Foletto M, et al. Laparoscopic treatment of benign insulinomas localized in the body and tail of the pancreas: a single-center experience. World J Surg 2006;30(10):1916–9 [discussion: 1920–1].
65. Liu H, Peng C, Zhang S, et al. Strategy for the surgical management of insulinomas: analysis of 52 cases. Dig Surg 2007;24(6):463–70.
66. Fernandez-Cruz L, Blanco L, Cosa R, et al. Is laparoscopic resection adequate in patients with neuroendocrine pancreatic tumors? World J Surg 2008;32(5): 904–17.
67. Roland CL, Lo CY, Miller BS, et al. Surgical approach and perioperative complications determine short-term outcomes in patients with insulinoma: results of a bi-institutional study. Ann Surg Oncol 2008;15(12):3532–7.
68. Martinez-Isla A, Griffith PS, Markogiannakis H, et al. A novel laparoscopic approach to lesions related to the posterior aspect of the pancreatic head. Am J Surg 2009;197(4):e51–3.

69. Isla A, Arbuckle JD, Kekis PB, et al. Laparoscopic management of insulinomas. Br J Surg 2009;96(2):185–90.
70. Falconi M, Mantovani W, Crippa S, et al. Pancreatic insufficiency after different resections for benign tumours. Br J Surg 2008;95(1):85–91.
71. Gagner M, Pomp A. Laparoscopic pancreatic resection: is it worthwhile? J Gastrointest Surg 1997;1(1):20–5 [discussion: 25–6].
72. Staudacher C, Orsenigo E, Baccari P, et al. Laparoscopic assisted duodenopancreatectomy. Surg Endosc 2005;19(3):352–6.
73. Lu B, Cai X, Lu W, et al. Laparoscopic pancreaticoduodenectomy to treat cancer of the ampulla of Vater. JSLS 2006;10(1):97–100.
74. Dulucq JL, Wintringer P, Mahajna A. Laparoscopic pancreaticoduodenectomy for benign and malignant diseases. Surg Endosc 2006;20(7):1045–50.
75. Palanivelu C, Shetty R, Jani K, et al. Laparoscopic distal pancreatectomy: results of a prospective non-randomized study from a tertiary center. Surg Endosc 2007; 21(3):373–7.
76. Diener MK, Knaebel H-P, Heukaufer C, et al. A systematic review and meta-analysis of pylorus-preserving versus classical pancreaticoduodenectomy for surgical treatment of periampullary and pancreatic carcinoma. Ann Surg 2007; 245(2):187–200.
77. Brugge WR, Lewandrowski K, Lee-Lewandrowski E, et al. Diagnosis of pancreatic cystic neoplasms: a report of the cooperative pancreatic cyst study [comment]. Gastroenterology 2004;126(5):1330–6.
78. Moesinger RC, Talamini MA, Hruban RH, et al. Large cystic pancreatic neoplasms: pathology, resectability, and outcome. Ann Surg Oncol 1999;6(7): 682–90.
79. Allen PJ, Jaques DP, D'Angelica M, et al. Cystic lesions of the pancreas: selection criteria for operative and nonoperative management in 209 patients. J Gastrointest Surg 2003;7(8):970–7.
80. Visser BC, Yeh BM, Qayyum A, et al. Characterization of cystic pancreatic masses: relative accuracy of CT and MRI [comment]. AJR Am J Roentgenol 2007;189(3):648–56.
81. Basturk O, Coban I, Adsay NV. Pancreatic cysts: pathologic classification, differential diagnosis, and clinical implications. Arch Pathol Lab Med 2009;133(3):423–38.
82. Talamini MA, Moesinger R, Yeo CJ, et al. Cystadenomas of the pancreas: is enucleation an adequate operation? Ann Surg 1998;227(6):896–903.
83. Fernandez-Cruz L, Cesar-Borges G. Laparoscopic strategies for resection of insulinomas. J Gastrointest Surg 2006;10(5):752–60.
84. Jemal A, Siegel R, Ward E, et al. Cancer statistics, 2009. CA Cancer J Clin 2009; 59(4):225–49.
85. Fisher JE, Donohue JH, Nagorney DM, et al. Laparoscopic vs. open distal pancreatectomy for pancreatic adenocarcinoma of the body and tail. HPB(Oxford) 2009;11(Suppl 1):1–104.
86. Kooby DA, Hawkins WG, Weber SH, et al. A multicenter analysis of distal pancreatectomy for adenocarcinoma: is laparoscopic resection appropriate? Proceedings of the Southern Surgical Association 2009, in press.
87. Lebedyev A, Zmora O, Kuriansky J, et al. Laparoscopic distal pancreatectomy. Surg Endosc 2004;18(10):1427–30.

Index

Note: Page numbers of article titles are in **boldface** type.

A

ACOSOG Z05031, for curable pancreatic cancer, 334–335
Adenocarcinoma
    pancreatic. See *Pancreatic adenocarcinoma.*
    pancreatic ductal, biology of, 440–442
AHPBA/SSO. See *American Hepato-Pancreatico-Biliary Association/Society of Surgical Oncology (AHPBA/SSO).*
Alimentary reconstruction, in pancreatic metastatic disease management, 279–280
American Hepato-Pancreatico-Biliary Association/Society of Surgical Oncology (AHPBA/SSO), 309
Anastomotic sealants, duct occlusion vs., for pancreatic metastatic disease, 278–279
Aspiration, fine-needle, in pancreatic malignancy diagnosis, 235
Autoimmune pancreatitis, 298–300

B

BD-IPMNs, management of, 389–392
Bevacizumab, for pancreatic malignancies, 370–371
Biliary drainage, stenting and, for pancreatic metastatic disease, 279
Biliary obstruction, palliation of, 356–357
    endoscopic palliation, 356
    radiologic palliation, 357
    surgical palliation, 356–357

C

Cancer(s)
    pancreatic. See *Pancreatic cancer.*
    pancreatico-biliary, evaluation of
        EUS in, **251–263.** See also *Endoscopic ultrasound (EUS), in pancreatico-biliary cancer evaluation.*
        IDUS in, 258
Capecitabine
    for pancreatic malignancies, 367
    gemcitabine with, for pancreatic malignancies, 368–369
CapRI trial, with chemoimmunotherapy, for curable pancreatic cancer, 335
Cetuximab, for pancreatic malignancies, 371–372
Chemoimmunotherapy, for curable pancreatic cancer, 333–335
Chemoradiation therapy (CRT), for pancreatic malignancies, **341–354**
Chemotherapy
    for curable pancreatic cancer, case against, 329–330
    palliative, for pancreatic malignancies, **365–375.** See also *Pancreatic malignancies, palliative chemotherapy for.*
    single-agent, for pancreatic malignancies, 366–367, 369–372. See also specific agents.

Surg Clin N Am 90 (2010) 447–456
doi:10.1016/S0039-6109(10)00026-5
0039-6109/10/$ – see front matter © 2010 Elsevier Inc. All rights reserved.